ETHICAL ISSUES
IN SEXUALITY AND
REPRODUCTION

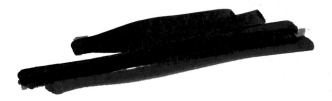

ETHICAL ISSUES IN SEXUALITY AND REPRODUCTION

MARGOT JOAN FROMER, R.N., M.A., M.Ed.

Private Consultant in Nursing Practice,
Washington, D.C.; Formerly Assistant Professor,
University of Delaware College of Nursing,
Newark, Delaware

The C. V. Mosby Company

ST. LOUIS · TORONTO · LONDON   1983

MOSBY

A TRADITION OF PUBLISHING EXCELLENCE

Manuscript editor: Carol Claverie
Book design: Kay M. Kramer
Cover design: Diane Beasley
Production: Barbara Merritt

Printed in the United States of America

The C.V. Mosby Company
11830 Westline Industrial Drive, St. Louis, Missouri 63141

Library of Congress Cataloging in Publication Data

Fromer, Margot Joan, 1939–
    Ethical issues in sexuality and reproduction.

    Bibliography: p.
    Includes index.
    1. Sexual ethics. 2. Bioethics. 3. Human
reproduction—Moral and ethical aspects. I. Title.
[DNLM: 1. Bioethics. 2. Sex behavior. 3. Repro-
duction. HQ 32 F931e]
HQ32.F76   1983   176   82-14460
ISBN 0-8016-1708-1

S/VH/VH 9 8 7 6 5 4 3 2 1   01/A/007

PREFACE

Everyone has a sex life of some type (heterosexual or homosexual, solitary or with a partner, in reality or in fantasy), and almost everyone has the capacity to reproduce, although action on that capacity is frequently a matter of conscious or unconscious choice. Sexuality and reproduction are human endeavors or behaviors, and all behavior is, or should be, guided by ethical principles. These activities are further characterized by the fact that they are almost never solitary (with the exception of masturbation and fantasizing about sex); other human beings are involved, which tends to increase individual vulnerability. Therefore, the potential for cruelty, exploitation, and other forms of harm exists in great measure. Human beings who relate to each other on any level or in any situation do so against a backdrop of a set of moral values and a code of ethical behavior; sexuality and reproduction involve activities and relationships where values and ethics are particularly crucial.

Topics discussed in this book will be based on principles of bioethics, which is defined as "the systematic study of human conduct in the area of the life sciences and health care, insofar as this conduct is examined in the light of moral values and principles" (*Encyclopedia of Bioethics* [Vol. 1], p. xix). Bioethics springs from the study of ethics (also known as moral philosophy) as it relates to human conduct in general; this book will apply principles of bioethics to specific areas of human conduct that involve sexuality and reproduction. For example, is homosexuality immoral, unnatural, or morally neutral? What should be done about an infant who is born with severe handicapping defects; should it be encouraged to live and develop, or should it be killed or let die? (Is there a moral difference between killing and letting die, especially in regard to infants?) What rights do the mentally retarded have as persons? Do various forms of reproductive technology (genetic manipulation, prenatal diagnosis, recombinant DNA, and the like) interfere with the natural reproductive process to too

v

great an extent, and should these practices be more stringently controlled, or even halted? These and other questions and issues will not be definitively answered, but they will be discussed in the rational light of moral examination methods, that is, applying universalizable rules and principles to the solution of ethical problems surrounding sexuality and reproduction.

The title of the book, and indeed the nature of moral philosophy itself, indicates that certain actions *ought* to be done or not done to and for others in the realm of sexuality and reproduction. Some will balk at this idea, particularly when it involves matters of sexuality. The live-and-let-live attitude that emerged in the 1960s and developed strength in the 1970s may continue well into the present decade. Although dogmatism is not a part of the style and content of the book, there *are* ethical issues in sexuality and reproduction. Study of ethics or moral philosophy is the study of what *ought* to be done to live a "good" moral life. Methods of ethical debate will be examined to provide closer and clearer views of problematic issues.

Because sexual activity almost always involves two people, and reproduction always involves at least two, plus a fetus, contractual arrangements can be said to exist, although perhaps not in the way we have been accustomed to think of a contract. Rights and obligations are inherent; there are actions that one or another person ought to take in relation to the contractual partner, and there are morally right and wrong (correct and incorrect) ways of behaving. Existence of a contractual agreement usually results in what is known as a "special relationship," that is, a relationship with another human being that creates duties and obligations not found in relationships with total strangers. Examples of special relationships are parent-child, sibling-sibling, friend-friend, and physician-client. A parent is obligated, by nature of the special relationship, to assume duties and obligations that would not exist in any other relationship, and a person behaves toward a friend in ways he is not necessarily obligated to behave in toward other people. Out of this relationship spring special obligations such as truth telling and promise keeping. Actions deriving from these special relationships involve the application of moral principles and will form a large part of the basis for discussion in this book.

Sexuality and reproduction cut across all social, cultural, political, and racial boundaries. One of the themes of the book will be comparisons of ethical absolutism and ethical relativism and how these two systems can be used in solving substantive problems. Ethical absolutism (sometimes referred to as basic moral rules) means that a particular ethical rule or principle should apply to all persons at all times, in all places. It should not be affected by cultural beliefs or social mores and institutions. Two examples of ethical absolutist principles are the Golden Rule, "Do to others as you would have others do to you," and Immanuel Kant's first formulation of the Categorical Imperative,

"Act only on that maxim whereby thou canst at the same time will that it should become a universal law" (*Fundamental Principles of the Metaphysics of Morals*, 1898). Ethical relativism (or derived moral rules) implies that ethical or moral principles are not universalizable and in fact affect and are affected by the vagaries of time, place, and culture. Ethical relativists maintain that different times and cultures *require* different moral standards; that is, behavior that may be morally correct in an industrialized society may be incorrect in a hunter-gatherer society. The most frequently used example is the Eskimo practice of placing old and infirm members of the community alone on an ice floe and permitting them to perish of the elements. Our society would regard such a practice as anathema. Ethical relativists maintain that what is morally right is what people *think* is morally right at a particular time, in a particular place.

Some areas of human endeavor make it easier to take a stand on ethical absolutism vs. ethical relativism. For example, in business ethics the maxim, "Do not cheat," would apply whether the transaction was conducted on a remote Pacific island with seashells as legal tender or the business arrangement involved ten supertankers loaded with crude oil and the legal tender was gold bullion.

In sexuality and reproduction there is more argument because of the nature and scope of the activity and because it affects people on their most basic emotional and ethical levels. Although physiologic elements are the same in all groups, social and cultural beliefs and the practices differ widely. Ethical relativism is powerfully tempting; it is so much easier to bend ethical rules or to create new ones in view of changing conditions. Rationalization is the tool of the relativist; absolutists are frequently seen as rigid and morally unprogressive.

Despite recent increases in depiction of sexual acts in the media and despite people's increased willingness to discuss sex, it remains a relatively private activity. Reproduction, however, hovers between the public and private domains and thus adds fuel to the fire of ethical controversies. What aspects of reproduction (and possibly sexuality) "belong" to the public, and what aspects do individuals have a right to keep private? And what exactly is privacy? For example, if I am in the "privacy of my own home" and am subjected to loud rock music from outside, has my privacy been invaded, or is it merely that my esthetic sensibility has been offended? For another, more serious, example, if a person is a carrier of a genetic disease that, if passed on to offspring, will have an impact on society, should the person's decision to bear children be private, or does society have a legitimate stake in the decision? If a woman has had an abortion or has given birth to a child she subsequently gave up for adoption, who has a right to that information? When, if ever, may a physician or other health professional violate the confidentiality of clients?

Technology has come to reproduction. Questions now exist that would have seemed like flights of fancy a decade ago: Shall we apply for in vitro fertilization?

Do I want a man to participate in the conception of my child? Shall we plan to conceive a girl or a boy? Because we are an infertile couple, will you be a surrogate mother?

To what extent can technology interfere in natural reproduction before the process or even the essence of human nature is changed? Do benefits to be gained from experimentation in reproductive technology outweigh risks? Do benefits exist? How is the balance to be assessed? Research will continue with or without the approval of the general public; in that case controls must be instituted, but debates rage about the existence and nature of those controls. Technology has a seductive power. We are constantly amazed at what it produces, and in our slack-jawed wonder, we sometimes forget to look *critically* at what we are marveling at, and we forget to ask how it will affect the quality of our lives.

An excellent example is the fetal monitor. When it was introduced in the mid 1960s, it was automatically assumed by the obstetric community to be a good thing, a piece of technology that would prevent much fetal distress and lower the intranatal death rate. Consequently physicians and hospitals rushed to purchase the most sophisticated fetal monitors available and used the machine on all parturients as a routine part of care during labor. As a result, cesarean sections increased dramatically. Subsequent research, however, showed that, although the fetal monitor was not a bad piece of technology and was indicated in certain circumstances, it should not be used in so universal a fashion. Reproductive technology should be analyzed in the same ways as other scientific advances: there must be a balance drawn between the risks and benefits to the individuals involved in its use; an assessment should be made of what qualities were sacrificed or spent so the technology could exist; and questions need to be asked about whether we need the technology and how it will affect our lives.

One of the problems in applying ethical rules and principles, some of them devised hundreds or thousands of years ago, is determining their adequacy in light of evolving scientific knowledge and modern technology. Would Socrates, sitting in the Stoa of Athens, or Aristotle, walking the paths of the Academy, be able to apply their incredibly brilliant and creative theories to today's ethical dilemmas? Would Descartes and Galileo, as they revolutionized the philosophy of science, be philosophically at home in a neonatal intensive care unit? Can "old" morality meet the challenge of new technology? I propose to show that it can by applying rules of moral behavior that do not change simply because the nature of the problems change. It is true that the *meaning* of many principles may have to be continually reexamined, but if we do not adhere to them and apply them, and if we constantly seek new rules to fit changing situations, we will be lost in moral chaos.

Discussions of values are important to contemporary lay and professional society. Societal values appear to be changing so rapidly that individuals are frequently uncertain of personal values; this tends to lend a certain shakiness to the moral underpinnings of one's life. A value refers to a belief or principle that is good or bad for a particular person or group (group may refer to a unit as small as a family or as large as a nation). The terms *good* and *bad* do *not* refer to personal preferences, as in "That was a bad restaurant," or "Ken is a good tennis player," but to assignment of moral qualification. Metaethics is the branch of philosophy that is concerned with the definition of "good," that is, what things are good in and of themselves (intrinsic values) and what things are good because they lead to other good (instrumental values), and with a description of the characteristics and boundaries of good. Chapter 1 contains a brief description of metaethics.

The subject of values will arise throughout the book; differentiations will necessarily be made between intrinsic and instrumental values and what the purpose of each is in relation to the issue under discussion. Some philosophers, for example, Jeremy Bentham and John Stuart Mill, believe that happiness (sometimes characterized as pleasure) is the only intrinsic value. Many thinkers believe there are others, such as health, power, justice, and life. From intrinsic values stem instrumental ones, such as knowledge, love, money, and beauty. It should be noted here that much disagreement exists over labeling values. For example, power can be seen as an intrinsic value to be enjoyed for its own sake, or it could be an instrumental value used to achieve happiness or pleasure. Values always have a moral meaning, even though the concept is frequently misunderstood and misused.

Life, its value and quality, is the central issue in any bioethical discussion. Nowhere is it more important than in the areas that deal with the beginning of life: sexuality and reproduction. Many, perhaps most, people maintain that sexuality involves the pursuit of pleasure, and it surely does, but its major physiologic function is procreative. That hundreds of millions of acts of sexual intercourse and other forms of sexual expression take place every day without resulting in the beginning of a new life, and without procreative intent, is irrelevant to the fact that intercourse must take place (with rare exceptions) to begin life. Therefore sexuality and reproduction are bound to each other and to life itself.

The value of human life is undoubtedly the single most perplexing philosophical question of all time. It is obvious that some value is placed on human life in all cultures and societies, or the culture would cease to exist. It is also obvious, by studying sociological and anthropological history, that the value of human life ranges from supremely important in most societies to considerably less so in others. It will be accepted as a given in this book that all human life is valuable to some degree and that all human beings have a right to life, up to a point. The phrases "to some degree" and "up to a point" are used advisedly because it will also be a given that not all human life is equally valuable and that not every person has the same right to life as every other person. For example, you have neither a moral nor a legal right to live if you are trying to kill me, and I have a right to kill you if I have concrete evidence that you will kill me. Other examples of the unequal right to life are the irreversibly comatose or the infant born with such tremendous brain damage that it will never develop the ability to think.

Use of the word *person* complicates ethical debate. How does one define personhood? Is a newborn infant a person at all, or in any way? If so, is it a person in the same sense as you and I in that we are fully developed self-conscious human beings conceiving of ourselves as distinct entities existing now and in the future? These questions are continually debated by philosophers; it is interesting to note how many refuse to grant the title "person" to a newborn and how much argument there still is about the question. If a newborn is a person, it surely differs from an adult in terms of self-awareness, consciousness, and even social worth. It differs, too, from a young child, who is in turn not the same as an adult. Adults also differ from each other in entitlement to the designation *person*. An individual may be fully grown physically but retain the mental and emotional capacities of a child or infant. Do these differences mean there should also be differences in the value placed on the life itself? Philosophical disagreement exists here also. Many of the arguments and moral bases for treating human life unequally will be examined in this book. For example, in what specific ways does human life differ from all other forms of life? The usual answer is that humans are "rational animals" or that they communicate by means of a formal language. But what do we mean by "rational," and how is rationality demonstrated? If a person loses his temper and is out of control for a short time, or if he is unconscious, does he lose his right to be treated as a rational animal for that period of time? If being a person involved dynamic change and growth, do rights change in relation to the person's capacity to deserve particular rights? Which rights are absolute and inalienable? Rights and personhood in relation to each other will be discussed in Chapter 1.

"Quality of life" is another phrase that has crept into our lexicon and seems to be based more on personal preference than on any concrete moral principles. We assume we know what is meant by the phrase, but most people, when questioned closely, can provide only a vague, subjective notion of the concept. Does quality apply only to the amount of happiness one can achieve? If so, what are the requirements for happiness? Does a person need to be fully functional mentally and physically to be happy? If not, what degree of handicap can be tolerated before the potential for happiness will be impaired? Perhaps quality refers to the amount of social utility one can provide for himself and others. If that is so, what characteristics of personhood are best suited to maximizing social utility?

In philosophical discussions, quality of life is used in one of three ways: descriptive, evaluative, and morally normative. A descriptive statement merely makes an observation about the presence or nature of a particular characteristic or property. Since all characteristics can be called qualities, everyone has a quality to his life. An example of a descriptive quality of life would be the fact that a person works at a particular job. In this sense, quality of life is morally neutral. An evaluative statement indicates that particular characteristics are assigned worth or value. When a characteristic is assigned a positive value, then the quality of life, with regard to that particular characteristic, is said to be positive. Value judgments can be made, but they generally have no basis in moral rules. An example of an evaluative statement is that a person is capable of performing his job better. A morally normative statement casts a moral judgment on particular qualities of life, which in effect says that a certain characteristic is good or bad. Ways of treating people are based on moral judgments; these modes of treatment can have grave consequences for the individual and may even spell the difference between life and death. A morally normative statement would point out that the poor quality of job performance resulted in someone's harm.

The purpose of this book on sexuality and reproduction is not to provide answers to what should or should not be done in particular instances but to demonstrate clear methods of examination and analysis of questions and issues. Simply accepting as morally correct what has always been done or what a majority of people think or believe to be correct does not necessarily make an action correct. Only when moral choices are submitted to the test of ethical rules and principles can a correct answer sometimes be obtained. This book will provide bases for examination, will suggest ways to ask questions, and will give examples of applications of moral rules. And it will try to demonstrate the truth of the Socratic maxim: "An unexamined life is not worth living."

Margot Joan Fromer

CONTENTS

ETHICAL ISSUES IN SEXUALITY AND REPRODUCTION

CHAPTER 1

ETHICAL THEORY

DEFINITIONS OF ETHICS AND MORAL PHILOSOPHY

Ethics or moral philosophy (the terms are frequently used interchangeably by philosophers) is a system or process by which decisions are made about which course of action is morally correct in a given situation. Decisions are made by using rational thought based on a set of rules or principles that exist because they have been demonstrated to be applicable and useful in solving moral dilemmas. Rational thought, and behavior based on that thought, is characterized by the fact that it is always open to consideration and evaluation; it is based on a set of values that has been incorporated into a person's life-style.

Descriptive ethics, as the name implies, delineates various ethical systems and describes different sets of values. A professional "hit man" who makes a rational decision to commit a murder for which he has been hired is operating from a set of values and ethical decisions that are based on given rules and principles. Determining whether these principles are morally correct falls into the realm of normative ethics, which will be discussed later in this chapter. A concise definition of ethics is provided by Taylor:

> Ethics may be defined as *philosophical inquiry into the nature and grounds of morality*. The term "morality" is here used as a general name for moral judgments, standards, and rules of conduct. These include not only the *actual* judgments, standards, and rules to be found in the moral codes of existing societies, but also what may be called *ideal* judgments, standards, and rules: those which can be justified on rational grounds. Indeed, one of the chief goals of ethics is to see if rational grounds can be given in support of many moral judgments, standards, or rules, and if so, to specify what those grounds are.[1]

It becomes obvious, then, that rationality, as opposed to personal preference or emotionality, is part of the foundation of ethics. This is an important observation to be noted throughout this book, which deals with issues that are subject to a great deal of emotionality. Sex is not usually thought of as the most rational area of human activity, and reproduction is almost as seriously mired in emotionality as is sexual behavior. This book does not intend to profess the view that we should all become unrealistically rational about sex; what it does intend is that thoughts and attitudes about sexual activity itself and sexual behaviors in general be examined in the cool light of rationality with a view toward evaluation of those thoughts, attitudes, and behaviors. Reproductive decisions can last a lifetime; therefore the reproductive process calls for even more rationality than does sexual behavior, parts of which can be quite fleeting (although admittedly the effects of sexual decisions can be long-lasting). Rationality will be heavily stressed throughout this book.

Moral theories, rules, and principles

Moral rules and principles are derived from moral theories, which can be defined as organized sets of beliefs that include not only sets of principles but also reasons why those principles exist and how they are applied to solve moral problems. The two aims of a moral theory are correctness and applicability. A theory is correct if it is true, if it conforms to known facts about the universe, and if it is consistent with empirical evidence as far as possible. A theory is applicable if it can be used to solve moral problems. Other branches of philosophy find varied uses for theories that exist only in the abstract. In moral philosophy a theory is not much use if it cannot be successfully applied to a dilemma.

A moral theory must also be universalizable by rational persons, that is, the rules and principles it contains must be applicable in all situations, even by people who hold different sets of values. For example, a theory called ethical egoism exists and is considered incorrect and nonapplicable by many modern philosophers. *Egoism* (a philosophic term that should not be confused with the psychologic term *egotism*) states that an action is morally correct if the consequences of that action bring happiness and pleasure *to the actor*, regardless of the effect the action has on others. It meets the conditions for a moral theory because egoism is an organized set of beliefs on which principles and rules can be based. However, it can be seen at a glance that it is a morally unworkable one. If *A*'s happiness would be increased if *B* did not exist, then *A* would be perfectly justified in killing *B*, regardless of the effect it would have on *B* or *B*'s family and friends. Moral chaos would reign if many people subscribed to and practiced egoism. The effect that an action has on others is irrelevant to the egoistic actor unless those consequences ultimately affect him.

To be universalizable, a moral theory must be sufficiently concrete to be understood by a vast majority of rational people. Those theories that are vague, too abstract, and about whose meaning philosophers cannot agree will not do. Differences in interpretation of theories are acceptable as long as there is acknowledgment about what those differences are.

Moral theories fall into two major categories: consequentialist and deontologic (sometimes referred to as nonconsequentialist). Consequentialist theories revolve around the consequences or results of an action, and deontological theories are concerned with the duties or obligations involved in the action, regardless of the consequences. These two theories will be discussed in detail in the section on normative ethics because they are most important in modern moral philosophy and because one or the other is practiced by the vast majority of people.

There are two other moral theories that should be mentioned briefly because of their historical interest and because they are also a part of the belief system of many people. The first, libertarianism, is characterized by noninterference with what belongs to other people in the actions they take. Contained in the concept of *belonging* is practically everything: body; mind; soul, if there is one; all physical possessions, whether purchased, bartered, or received as a gift; and anything else we take possession of that does not already belong to another. Each person may do exactly as he wishes with his own belongings, but he may do nothing with anyone else's, except with the express consent of the other person. Absolute respect for the liberty of others is the foundation of libertarianism.

Contractarianism is a modification of egoism that builds in some restraints on the absolute permissibility to do whatever will promote one's own self-interests. The constraints are those that are mutually beneficial, that is, a contractual moral theory that permits each individual to act so as to benefit himself as well as others. Agreements are made to help one another if the helpful act produces results that are better than if the individual had acted independently. Mutual advantage and adherence to agreements are the criteria on which moral praise and blame are based.

Moral theories, then, can be defined as sets of moral beliefs, on which rules and principles are based; that speak to certain acts or sets of acts. Moral theories are concerned with the rightness or wrongness of behavior. Nonmoral theories are different; they have nothing to do with morality and should not be confused with the word *immoral*. Examples of nonmoral theories are scientific ones such as the theory of relativity, psychological ones such as behaviorism, or social ones such as territoriality. Nonmoral theories are generally neither right nor wrong in and of themselves; however, the uses to which they are put can have strong moral overtones.

Moral rules and principles can be described as guidelines to action or yardsticks for the morality of behavior. They are tools to be used to determine whether an action is right or wrong. In the section of this chapter having to do with normative ethics, especially deontology and Kantianism, various moral principles will be defined, described, and applied to illustrative examples.

To introduce a discussion of principles, the Principle of the Value of Life will be discussed here. This principle, because it is so fundamental, is understood by many, if not most, philosophers to be the one on which all morality is based. It is certainly the most important to understand and analyze. It is also not as simple as one might automatically assume from its name. Generally the value of life is regarded as an inherent value, that is, one that is valuable for its own sake. (An instrumental value is one that is desired so that it can produce or obtain other values.) If life is an inherent value, then it is to be respected and protected. The value of life is also considered an inalienable right, that is, it cannot be sold, transferred, or given away. (It is interesting to note here that the three inalienable rights mentioned in the Declaration of Independence are life, liberty, and the pursuit of happiness.)

If the value of life is inherent, and the right to that value (life) is inalienable, there would seem to be no need to discuss the matter further. However, Blackstone[2] believes that three basic questions need to be posed about the Principle of the Value of Life. The first concerns the scope of the principle, that is, what forms of life have inherent value. The second question is about the degree of inherent value that different life forms possess: Do all living things have an inherent value, or do some have a greater value than others? If the value of life differs with different life forms, a hierarchy of morality could be established, not only from species to species, but also within the same species, for example, do some human lives have more value than others? The third question Blackstone asks relates to the stringency of the rule against killing. If life is inherently valuable, the rule against destroying it should be absolute, but it is well known that many instances exist where killing is morally permissible. Therefore what counts as a justifiable exception to the rule against killing?

A discussion of these three questions must center first on the scope of the principle. The value of life is held by many to refer only to human life, especially as it concerns the issues to be discussed in this book, or for that matter, any bioethical issue. Some would go so far as to not include all humans in the scope of the principle. This view is called moral inegalitarianism and might exclude some human life, such as infants born with severe handicapping defects, those individuals who are irreversibly comatose, or even people who are convicted mass murderers. Another view of the scope of the principle is to include other life forms. This view is usually confined to the higher forms of animals (most especially domestic pets and livestock), but a few people, notably Albert Schweitzer, include all life forms in the principle, even the lowest on the evolutionary scale. The latter, however, is not a widely held view and presents certain pragmatic difficulties.

In examining various justifications for overriding the moral rule against killing, we find an even wider variety of views. The most common is that killing is prima facie wrong, that is, we ought not to kill unless we can appeal to another more stringent or compelling rule that would justify breaking the rule not to kill. Self-defense is the justification that comes immediately to mind, although there are others, such as suicide in the face of extreme pain or misery, being ordered to kill for one's country in time of war (this is frequently seen as an extension of self-defense), and state execution of convicted murderers or traitors.

A discussion of the Principle of the Value of Life, no matter how brief or how complex, must lead one to wonder why it is important to discuss it at all. Taylor expresses this as the Ultimate Question as follows: "Is the commitment to live by moral principles a commitment grounded on reason or is it, in the final analysis, an arbitrary decision?"[3] The Ultimate Question is not in itself a moral question; it is a question about the justification of morality in general. Why live a moral life? Why worry about right and wrong? Why sacrifice happiness and pleasure for moral integrity? It is frequently easier to cast moral principles aside for the most expedient or hedonistic action, and many people who live that way seem to sleep well and to suffer no emotional ill effect. Why bother to confront ethical issues, especially those in the area of sexuality and reproduction where it is so easy to let nature and pleasure have their way?

Plato, in "The Myth of Gyges" (*Republic*, Book II), tries to show that moral virtue is its own reward and that only the morally upright person is truly happy:

> Then the actions of the just would be as the actions of the unjust; they would both come at last to the same point. And this we may truly affirm to be a great proof that a man is just, not willingly or because he thinks that justice is any good to him individually, but of necessity, for when ever any one thinks that he can safely be unjust, there he is unjust.[4]

Plato appears to be arguing that morality is an intrinsic value, one to be desired for its own sake, as is happiness. Since the ancient Greeks, philosophers have debated this view because morality often conflicts with happiness or self-interest; it is not always the same as happiness. Logical reasons exist both for following a moral course of action and for acting out of self-interest if morality and self-interest are not the same or do not result equally from the same action. Neither are pleasure and happiness always the same, although they are frequently used interchangeably. The Ultimate Question asks why a person should follow a moral path if an easier and more pleasurable one is as logical, even though it may produce different results.

Taylor believes the answer to the Ultimate Question lies in the logic of moral reasoning, that is, ethical decision making.

> Moral reasoning takes place whenever someone deliberates about whether he morally ought to do one thing rather than another in a situation of choice, and whenever someone tries to show that another's action, or a past action of his own, was the morally right (or wrong) thing to do, given the circumstances that held at that time.[5]

There are two basic parts to the process of moral reasoning: deliberation and justification. Deliberation involves the process by which one decides what *ought* to be done in a given situation; one thinks about reasons for prospective actions. It is the weighing of pros and cons of various alternatives open to the actor in the dilemma or conflict. The purpose is to arrive at a conclusion that can be translated into action. Justification involves a similar thought process, although it involves actions of others or of ourselves in the past. Reasons must be found to support the rightness or wrongness of an act already done. Deliberation involves prospective reasoning; justification is retrospective. In either case, the reasoning must be logical, that is, rules of inference or of specific forms of argument must be followed. Arguing from a set of rules and principles (note that we *always* return to rules and principles; moral philosophy cannot exist without them) is arguing logically.

> These principles are such that, if our reasoning is carried out in accordance with them, we can claim that we are rationally justified in making the moral judgments which we draw as our conclusions. We can claim to *know* that a certain act is the right or wrong thing to do in a given situation. Moral knowledge is possible only when there is a method for giving good reasons in justification of moral beliefs or, in other words, only when there is a logic of moral reasoning.[6]

Methods of moral reasoning must be universalizable, that is, the principles must be universally binding in that if they apply to situation A, they must also apply to situation B, *and* they must be able to be used by person X or person Y in situation A or B, assuming that all other considerations are equal. This may appear simplistic, and the reader may be wondering, if moral principles are universalizable, why dilemmas exist. Let us look at the following example: X wants to do R in situation A; Y disagrees and wants to do R_1 in the same situation. Each person thinks or believes he is making the correct moral decision. If X came to his decision to do R by means of logical moral reasoning, then the only *logical* answer is R; R_1 will be shown to be illogical and therefore incorrect. However, Y may strongly believe that R_1 is the correct thing to do, and he may very well take action on that belief. Even if no harm occurs as a result, it was the morally incorrect action because the decision was not based on universalizable moral principles. Therein lies the source of all moral dilemmas;

strongly held beliefs are not always logical or universalizable, but they are so much a part of the fabric of the individual's ethical operations that they cannot be discarded. Many of these illogical beliefs are theological in nature and are derived from divine revelation and will therefore never stand up to logical proof.

Belief is a difficult concept to analyze. People are notoriously reluctant to challenge the beliefs of others, but if we are to arrive at the truth of an ethical dilemma, beliefs *must* be challenged. To refuse to do so is to be mired in ignorance, prejudice, and superstition. Beliefs are grounded in hope, hypothesis, and sheer conjecture. If they had facts as their base they would not be beliefs. For example, when a person says he believes in God, what he is really saying is that he has no way to explain the inexplicable; thus he puts his hope in the belief that the unknowns of the universe are caused and controlled by God. He has taken what Kierkegaard has described as the leap of faith, that great leap over the chasm of truth and knowledge. When another person says he believes that a profoundly retarded neonate should not be allowed to survive because it will not have a satisfying quality of life, that person is expressing a guess about the infant's future *as* a belief.

It should be understood at the outset that a decision that cannot be proved correct by logical moral reasoning is not necessarily morally wrong or evil; it simply means that it is not universalizable and is always subject to argument. Even use of moral principles is not always the answer; there can be a variety of interpretations of almost any principle. For example, the Principle of the Value of Life can be interpreted at two extremes or at any number of positions between. One extreme, the position taken by Albert Schweitzer and a few others, is that *all* life forms, animal and vegetable, have intrinsic value and should be preserved and protected. The opposite extreme is that only life that is *fully human* (see sections in succeeding chapters on abortion and infanticide for a discussion of what constitutes a human being or person) has value and should be protected. There are many people in modern society who assume this position. Now, using the Principle of the Value of Life, let us come to a correct moral decision about whether to let severely deformed and retarded infants die. It will be impossible to use logical moral reasoning unless one comes to a decision about where on the continuum of the value of life one "stakes one's claim." Those who find themselves at or near the first extreme discussed would do everything in their power to save the infant's life. Those at or near the opposite extreme would let the infant die if they thought it was in the best interest of the infant or its parents to do so. Thus this and other dilemmas are not always solvable by logical moral reasoning, even if all persons were to agree that the Principle of the Value of Life is the fundamental philosophic principle on which all others should be based.

We still have not answered Taylor's Ultimate Question: Why make a commitment to lead a moral life grounded in reason when that commitment might be purely arbitrary? The question itself is seen by many as absurd. Those who would even ask the question already know, by the fact that they know enough to ask, that some actions are morally correct and some actions only perpetuate self-interest. The person who asks the Ultimate Question already has a fairly clear idea of what is right; he simply wants to know why he should do what he already knows to be correct. Therein lies the absurdity; he must do what is correct simply because it is his duty to do so *because* it is the correct thing to do. Therefore the question answers itself and probably needs to be asked only by those who would never think to do so.

Methods of ethical argument

The term *argument*, when applied to moral decision making, is a specific concept, sometimes called a function, based on the correspondence between sets of things, usually reasons or principles. The value or correctness of the argument depends on the logical relationship between things and has *nothing* to do with preference, numbers of people who hold a certain belief, or moral authority. The strength of a moral argument depends solely on its logic. If logical arguments can be given in favor of an action while at the same time logically refuting arguments against it, then the action is morally correct, no matter how the actors or agents *feel* about the action. Conversely, if one has a positive feeling about a particular action, it is not necessarily morally correct. One frequently hears the statement, "I just wouldn't feel right about doing thus-and-so, therefore I think it's wrong." Although their importance in our lives should not be negated, feelings play a small role in ethical argument. This transition from feelings to logic is most difficult to make and requires constant vigilance. Moreover, logic is often linguistic in nature and depends on a common understanding of the meaning of words. For example, the commonly used adage in logic, "Given A, then B follows," may have no meaning if the precise meaning of A is not clear to all concerned.

An ethical argument or moral judgment must be based on reasons; it may not be arbitrary, that is, equally fine if one agrees with it or not. There must be something substantive to argue about; one does not make ethical decisions about matters of taste or personal preference. The statement, "Sunny days are more pleasurable than dreary days," cannot be argued about, at least not by rational people (and rational people are the only ones who are concerned about ethics). However, the statement, "Homosexuality is wrong because it is contrary to natural law," is one about which we can make an ethical decision. The second statement is based on reason, not on personal preference. The statement,

"I dislike homosexuals," has the same lack of ethical substance as does the previous one about the weather and therefore cannot be said to be a correct or incorrect moral statement. A truth, then, about ethical argument is that

> when *moral* claims are being made, rational support is in order; the truth is simply the position that has the best reasons on its side. The attempt to determine what is true in morals, then, is always a matter of analyzing and weighing up reasons. Otherwise, morality degenerates into nothing more than prejudice, propaganda, and crass self-interest, without claim on any rational person.[7]

Brief mention was made about the necessity of refuting arguments against a logical moral argument. All criticisms are not easily dismissed, nor should they be if they are based on logic or principles. Scientists who find their hypothesis proved incorrect by empirical data do not discard the hypothesis; they use the new information to revise and improve the hypothesis. So too with moral arguments. The philosopher who discards his argument when faced with a rational refutation soon would be out of business. If a moral theory or argument can be easily refuted by logical criticism, it should be a clue that the argument was weak in the first place and must be reworked. If an ethical argument is based on a true judgment and a valid statement (one that is logically correct), it is most likely a correct argument.

METAETHICS

Metaethics (sometimes called analytic ethics) has as its aim understanding semantics, logic, and epistemology of the structure of moral philosophy. Metaethics is the effort to understand ethics. One wants to study the semantics of moral philosophy because without an understanding of the meaning of words and statements, they cannot be used to describe what ought to be done in a given instance. Logic is necessary to moral philosophy because one must grasp the relationship between concepts to arrive at moral conclusions from premises and supporting statements. Epistemology (the branch of philosophy having to do with the study of knowledge) is important because it is closely connected to logic and because in moral philosophy statements of knowledge are made frequently in support of moral arguments; epistemology helps us to know what we know.

Metaethics involves two major tasks: analysis of the meaning of terms and statements used in moral argument and examination of the rules of reasoning by which beliefs can be shown to be true or false. These tasks can be at least partially accomplished by the process of conceptual analysis and assessment of the positive and negative components of moral judgments, or the ways to answer moral questions.

Conceptual analysis

Conceptual analysis is the activity by which concepts or ideas are clarified; it strives to attain precision of meaning of words and phrases, particularly those used in moral discourse, about which there tends to be much debate.

Two components of conceptual analysis are necessary conditions and sufficient conditions. A necessary condition states the following: if X is a necessary condition of Y, then Y cannot be the case if X is not the case, that is, if not X, then not Y. For example, having a four-chambered heart is a necessary condition for being a mammal. It is given that X is a four-chambered heart, and Y is a mammal. If a creature does not have four-chambered heart (not X), then it cannot be a mammal (not Y).

A sufficient condition states that if A is a sufficient condition of B, then B will be the case if A is the case, or if A, then B. For example, being a flying machine with fixed-position wings is a sufficient condition for being an airplane. If A is a flying machine with fixed-position wings, then B, it is an airplane.

A necessary condition is not always a sufficient condition. For example, an animal with legs is a necessary condition for something to be a dog, but it is not a sufficient condition; there are many animals with legs that are not dogs. Something that is a house is a sufficient condition of being a dwelling place, but it is not a necessary condition; there are many dwelling places that are not houses, that is, it is not necessary for a dwelling place to be a house.

Necessary and sufficient conditions may seem a bit confusing at first, but one must understand them to clarify under what conditions certain concepts can be applied, that is, what conditions must be satisfied before a concept can be correctly used. Abortion is a dilemma in which understanding of necessary and sufficient conditions is crucial to the nature of the conflict. What conditions must be satisfied before the fetus has a right to be morally and legally protected? Is the state of being a fetus a necessary and/or sufficient condition to warrant noninterference with its growth and development?

Frequently, concepts defy philosophic or linguistic analysis, especially in bioethical issues, and this increases the intensity of debate. For example, a closed plane figure must have precisely four interior angles to be called a rectangle, although this is not a sufficient condition because a parallelogram also has four interior angles but is not a rectangle. What are the precise necessary and sufficient conditions to be considered a person, the value of whose life should be respected? Ethical debates about necessary and sufficient conditions sometimes are impossible to settle. However, it is important to strive to reach the highest degree of clarity possible; the more precise the understanding of a concept, the more likely dilemmas will be understood and possibly solved.

Moral judgments

Metaethics also has to do with the *process* of making moral judgments. A correct process, or one that works in all instances, may not exist, but there are pitfalls to be avoided, and some components of the judgment process can be agreed to by almost all philosophers. Regan[8] first lists the ways in which moral judgments should *not* be made.

1. Matters of personal preference are not open to moral judgment. This has been discussed previously and needs no amplification, except that it is important to note that personal preference does *not* require a reason (it is inappropriate to ask *why* one likes chocolate better than vanilla).

2. Although feelings are frequently related to moral judgments, they are not the same and do not necessarily have a causal relationship. One may feel personally squeamish about abortion or be saddened by having undergone one, but those feelings do not change the fact that one has made the moral judgment that abortion is morally permissible.

3. Thinking that something is morally correct does not necessarily mean that it *is* morally correct (or incorrect). The statement, "I think infanticide is all right in some cases," has as little value as *feeling* that infanticide is permissible. It is essentially a statement of personal preference unless it is qualified and explained by logical moral reasoning. The several hundred members of the Flat Earth Society think, feel, and believe that the earth is flat. They are wrong because they are unable to prove it by logical reasoning.

4. There may be strength in numbers, but not truth, either moral or scientific. No matter how many people believe something to be morally correct, it is not correct unless it can be logically shown to be so, by even only one person. All the polls in the world do not give credence to moral judgments. One has only to take a cursory glance at history to see that this is true. Hundreds of thousands of Christian crusaders believed they were doing the right thing by slaughtering millions of nonbelievers (nonChristians) in the Middle Ages on their marches to Jerusalem. They thus perpetrated one of the greatest mass slaughters in history. The United States government believed it was doing the morally correct thing when it imprisoned thousands of Japanese-Americans during World War II. Denying liberty to innocent American citizens was politically expedient but morally wrong. Moral truth does not depend for its existence on numbers of people; it exists for its own sake.

5. There is no such thing as a moral authority to whom one can appeal for final decisions about ethical judgments. Those who have studied philosophy are more familiar with modes of inquiry and the nature of dilemmas

than are nonphilosophers, but they are no closer to real answers than is anyone else. This immediately raises the question of God, or a god, as a moral authority. Theological theories of moral philosophy will be discussed later in the chapter, but for now, suffice it to say that there is no such thing as a *human* moral authority. Clergymen and judges are frequently called on to settle moral disputes, but the best they can do is to *interpret* scriptural, constitutional, and statutory law *as they see it*. Judgments they make may have elements of morality, but they are not to be considered definitive or the final word on the dilemma.

Then how should moral judgments be made? Regan lists several criteria that are essential to logical moral reasoning.

1. Conceptual clarity. One cannot debate an issue unless its meaning is known. If the dilemma centers on euthanasia, for example, we must have more than a vague general notion of "mercy killing"; we need to know as precisely as possible what does and does not constitute euthanasia and which of its four major types are under discussion.

2. Factual information. An issue cannot be logically argued if one or both parties in the argument do not know the facts and will be unable to predict consequences of actions. For example, in an argument about the morality of homosexuality, the cause of logical reasoning will not be furthered if the many myths surrounding homosexuality continue to be believed. If one knows little or nothing about the variety of homosexual behavior or life-styles, then there is little to debate about.

3. Rationality. The ability to understand relationships between ideas and concepts, to understand why some statements are true and what makes them true, and to be able to conceptualize abstract thoughts is the hallmark of the rational person. A rational person is sometimes said to be logical, although the terms are not precisely synonymous. What is likely meant is that a rational person does not deliberately contradict himself, that is, he cannot possibly be committed to sets of beliefs that are not all true at the same time. Each one of a person's set of beliefs must be true in and of themselves. For example, a person cannot be a pacifist and in favor of capital punishment at the same time. By definition a pacifist is opposed to using violence (against persons) under all circumstances with no permitted justifications, not even self-defense. Capital punishment involves extreme violence; therefore a pacifist would contradict himself if he were to favor capital punishment. By the same token, a person who is a vegetarian because he believes it is wrong to kill animals for human consumption would contradict himself if he wore leather shoes. A person who habitually contradicts himself is not rational.

4. Impartiality. One who holds a particular set of beliefs is naturally partial to those beliefs, but in forming moral judgments, impartiality refers to an unquestioning, extreme sort of bias that has no real basis in reason. Judgments that are clouded by bigotry, bias, or prejudice cannot be moral or logical.

5. Coolness. This is a term Regan uses to refer to a state that is the opposite of extreme emotionality such as passion, anger, fear, or grief. Everyone has had the experience of making statements or decisions in the heat of excitement that were later regretted. That is the state in which it is best *not* to make moral judgments or even to engage in ethical debate. This is often easier said than done. We start a discussion with the intention of remaining cool, and the very nature of the issue being debated inflames us; we lose our heads and consequently our rationality—at least temporarily. The less cool we are, the more likely we are to make errors of judgment that have potential for disastrous consequences.

6. Free will. For a person to make a moral judgment he must have free will. "Beings who lack free will cannot control how they behave; the only way they *can* behave is the way they *do* behave, which makes it pointless to say how they *ought* to behave."[9] Free will is a human characteristic that exists on a continuum and might be defined as autonomy; that state in which a person has the liberty to act on freely chosen plans. An autonomous person is self-determined, self-contained, and free. It is obvious that a severely mentally retarded person has diminished free will. It is also true, but perhaps less obvious, that a person bound by the shackles of bigotry, ignorance, and blind adherence to cultural prejudice also suffers from diminished free will.

NORMATIVE ETHICS

Normative ethics (sometimes called prescriptive ethics) is concerned with determining correct moral principles and theories by which *all* rational people ought to be guided. At the heart of normative ethics is the proof that a particular moral theory is indeed correct and should be used as a life guide by everyone. It is obvious to any aware reader that no ethicist or moral philosopher from Socrates to the present has presented conclusive proof, to the satisfaction of all thinkers, that one moral theory is superior to all others. But the search continues, and it is with this search that we will be concerned here.

The reader may be a bit thrown by use of the word *proof* in relation to moral principles and theories, as if proofs were no more complicated than chemical formulae with which one can prove an equation if it "comes out right." Of course a moral theory is more difficult to prove than a scientific one, but it can be done, and the remainder of this chapter will be concerned with that process.

A normative ethical theory is developed when a philosopher determines that a set of rational obligations can be established that results in a set of moral criteria by which actions can be judged correct or incorrect. The purpose of normative ethics is not merely to inquire about people's belief systems but to determine their *truth* or *falsity* when judged against moral criteria. If an action cannot be judged by a particular set of criteria derived from a moral theory, then the theory is not universalizable and is therefore incorrect or incomplete. To the casual reader of moral philosophy or to the believer in the "live-and-let-live" school of moral thought, this description of normative ethics sounds harsh or even self-righteous. It is not. If no system of normative ethics existed, we would be quickly thrown into a state of moral chaos, and life would be truly unlivable.

Consequentialist theories

Normative ethics is divided into two major types of theories: consequentialist and nonconsequentialist. It is with the former that we will be concerned first. Consequentialist theories are frequently referred to as *teleological* (from the Greek *telos*, meaning end) because they refer not so much to the actions themselves but to the rightness or wrongness of the end results of those actions. A consequentialist theory holds that the moral correctness of an action is a function of its end result or consequence. The purpose, and thus the moral correctness, of an action is to increase the balance of good over evil. There are three major types of consequentialist theories: ethical egoism, which was defined earlier in the chapter; ethical altruism; and utilitarianism.

Ethical altruism holds that an action is morally correct if the consequences of the action produce good for everyone *except* the actor. Consequences for the actor are irrelevant unless those consequences in turn affect everyone else. Altruism is almost the precise opposite of egoism and may seem at face value to be unrealistic. "Pure" altruism, that is, doing acts that are totally "other-regarding," is not a commonly held philosophy, but forms of altruism have been the source of a great deal of beneficence throughout history.

UTILITARIANISM. Utilitarianism is the consequentialist theory that makes the strongest claim for moral correctness and has the greatest number of adherents. However, it has serious flaws and has been used to justify clearly immoral acts. Because of both its popularity and shortcomings, it deserves serious consideration.

Utilitarianism holds that an action is morally correct if the consequences of that action produce the greatest amount of happiness for the greatest number of people, including the actor.

The Principle of Utility, which is the basis of utilitarianism, was first proposed by Jeremy Bentham (1748–1832), a British economist and moral philosopher who was also trained in the law. He was somewhat of a radical, but it must be remembered that the eighteenth century was a time of political and social enlightenment, characterized by industrialization, political revolution, and entirely new ways of looking at people's lives. The eighteenth century saw the greatest advances in political, social, and moral thought since the golden age of Greece. It was a time of great philosophical excitement, and it was therefore appropriate that Bentham should put forth his "radical" ideas. One of Bentham's leading followers was John Stuart Mill (1806–1873), who wrote prodigiously on utilitarianism and did much to promote the welfare of all citizens and to counteract the prevalence of the divine right of kings and natural moral law. Both Bentham and Mill could be classified as skeptics and were therefore not much beloved by the Catholic Church, whose philosophers and theologians had greatly influenced philosophic thought up until that time, which was the beginning of the Age of Reason. It should be noted that Thomas Jefferson was a contemporary of Mill and was greatly influenced by the writings of both Bentham and Mill.

Classical utilitarianism, as defined earlier, is characterized by three main features, all of which must be present in judging an act to be morally correct or incorrect, according to the Principle of Utility: (1) No action is right or wrong in and of itself; actions are right or wrong *only* as a function of their consequences. For example, lying or promise breaking are wrong only if their use results in bad consequences. (2) Goodness or badness of consequences is measured or determined by *happiness* or *unhappiness*. Therefore the more happiness that results from an action, the more morally correct the action. (3) Each individual's happiness is *equally as important* as another's happiness. All persons count equally in determining total amounts of happiness, no matter what the social or political status.

At first glance it seems impossible to believe that utilitarianism is anything less than the perfect moral theory, especially in view of its emphasis on happiness, consequences, and equality. However, some of the most grossly immoral acts have been condoned and justified by the Principle of Utility. Slavery is the most frequently cited example. Slavery by definition is the withdrawal of all human liberty and freedom from a small segment of society. Slaves are nonpersons who have no rights whatsoever and who customarily belong to a racial or ethnic minority. It is easy to use utilitarianism to justify slavery. Whatever unhappiness a small minority of people experience as a result of being enslaved is more than compensated for by the increased happiness of the majority of slave owners or nonslaves. Thus slavery will result in a greater amount of happiness for a greater number of people than will a society in which slavery is not permitted *if* the existence of slavery is the only criterion for happiness in relation to this particular societal dilemma. The fact that the system of slavery is unfair and unjust and totally disregards the liberty and autonomy of a segment of that social system is completely irrelevant to utilitarianism. It should be noted that neither Bentham nor Mill, nor any modern utilitarian, endorses slavery, but they do not seem bothered by the fact that utilitarianism ignores certain fundamental principles and rights.

Utilitarianism can be subdivided into act- and rule-utilitarianism. Act-utilitarianism holds that the rightness or wrongness of each particular action is determined by its own specific set of consequences. Rule-utilitarianism holds that individuals should adopt rules or principles of conduct by which happiness of consequences tends to be maximized. Following general rules will thus prevent the necessity of determining the balance of happiness for each individual action. Rule-utilitarianism is seen by many philosophers as less rigid than act-utilitarianism, but it does not conform as specifically to the tenets of classical utilitarianism as does act-utilitarianism.

Problems of application exist for both forms of utilitarianism. In act-utilitarianism the end result of maximized happiness frequently permits acts that are clearly immoral. For example, a woman who is past menopause has some abdominal symptoms for which she seeks medical advice. After a series of tests, exploratory abdominal surgery is performed, and a small benign tumor is removed from her bowel. The surgeon also removed her uterus because he found it to be slightly fibrous and believes it could become a site for future problems. When the woman recovers from anesthesia, he tells her about the benign tumor but deliberately neglects to tell her about removing the uterus. He reasons that she will experience depression and other emotional trauma if she knows she has had a hysterectomy. The surgeon predicts future unhappiness for both the woman and himself if he tells her about the hysterectomy. Indeed, the woman makes a rapid and uneventful recovery and continues her life happy in the fact that nothing serious was wrong. The surgeon is happy because he does not have to confront the possibly traumatizing aftereffects of hysterectomy. Total happiness has been increased, and the act-utilitarian would applaud the surgeon's action. However, it is clear that the surgeon acted immorally. He not only lied to the woman, he performed a surgical procedure without her consent, thereby ignoring respect for her autonomy. This is a clear example of why many modern philosophers not only cannot adopt act-utilitarianism but feel compelled to condemn it on the grounds of justice, fairness, and human rights.

The rule-utilitarian would view this situation differently. If an action can be subsumed under a rule that is justified by the Principle of Utility, then that rule can be universalizable and actions can be judged on the basis of the rule. For example, lying and all that it implies (lack of freedom and autonomy for the dupe) generally tends to minimize happiness for both the liar and the dupe. Therefore truth telling is a rule or principle that can be subsumed under the Principle of Utility as generally maximizing happiness. The rule-utilitarian would thus judge the surgeon's action as morally wrong because he lied to the woman.

One major problem with rule-utilitarianism is that it frequently ignores principles of justice. For example, according to the FBI's Uniform Crime Report, black males between the ages of 18 and 30 commit more rapes than any other group of men; those rapes occur most frequently at night. The rule-utilitarian could, therefore, justify requiring that all men of that group somehow not be permitted to come into contact with women during certain hours. The general populace would likely feel safer, and rapes might decrease. If people feel safer, they are happier, as they surely are if women are raped less frequently; therefore the restriction would be consistent with the Principle of Utility. It would not, however, be consistent with the principles of justice and fairness.

Utilitarianism was founded and promoted by two eminently decent men, if one can make this kind of judgment based on their writing. Mill, in particular, in his essay, "On Liberty," gives the reader the impression that he views individual freedom, autonomy, and liberty to be absolutely sacrosanct. His battle against the state's interference with personal privacy of action (unless that action resulted in harm to another) is evident to even the most casual reader of his work. It is puzzling, then, that utilitarianism as a moral theory so frequently ignores some of the very principles that Mill espoused. Most modern utilitarians (Beauchamp, Brandt, Singer, and others) write from the rule-utilitarian view; many of their philosophies and beliefs are almost indistinguishable from nonconsequentialist theories because of their emphasis on rules and principles. Act-utilitarianism seems to have lost favor with most contemporary philosophers.

Deontologic (nonconsequentialist) theories

Deontology (from the Greek *deon*, meaning duty or obligation) holds that an act is morally correct because of the rightness or wrongness of features or characteristics of the act *regardless* of the consequences. We immediately run into the problem of determining *what* features of an act make it right or wrong and *why* this is so. There are several ways of vindicating moral judgments. Some philosophers appeal to divine revelation such as interpretation of the Ten Commandments. Others prefer to justify rightness or wrongness by comparing it with natural law, which can be defined as prescriptive statements of morality based on the laws of nature (e.g., the Thomist prohibition against suicide because "everything naturally loves itself"). Some philosophers find common sense and intuition sufficient to determine rightness or wrongness (the philosophy of intuitionism is based on this school of thought). Others use a social theory or a social contract base for making judgments, taking into account justice, fairness, and rights. Whatever basis is used for justification of deontological theories, they all have one thing in common—the consequences of an act, although not completely discounted, are far less important than the moral characteristics of the act itself.

Deontology, like utilitarianism, can be divided into two major types, monistic and pluralistic deontology. Monistic deontology holds that there is only one single rule or principle from which can be derived other rules by which to judge moral actions. The classic example is Immanuel Kant's Categorical Imperative, against which he tested all maxims of action. If a maxim of action could not be universalizable, that is, if it could not fit the Categorical Imperative, then it could not be a maxim for morally correct action. Kant devised more than one formulation of the Categorical Imperative, and it is clear that they are not equivalent. Therefore it may be that even Kant was not a purely monistic deontologist (more about Kantianism in the next section).

Pluralistic deontology is more widely accepted than monistic deontology. It allows for a choice of moral rules and principles to be applied to judgments. Modern philosophers believe that there are several basic and irreducible principles, such as fidelity, truth telling, beneficence, and justice, that can be applied to any moral dilemma to determine moral rightness or wrongness. At first glance pluralism seems to be a more practical and human alternative than does monistic deontology; however, basic principles come into conflict with each other. For example, if a client tells a physician something in confidence that he knows will be seriously harmful to another person, the physician faces the conflict between nonmaleficence and maintaining the confidential relationship. He cannot adhere to both principles, although they are both basic and irreducible. Several philosophers have attempted to arrange principles in a hierarchy, but aside from a general agreement on nonmaleficence (doing no harm) being assigned highest priority, there is little other concordance about the remaining principles.

Deontology in general is founded on sets of rules and principles that identify classes of action as right or wrong. For example, the principle of truth telling would make all mendacious actions wrong; the principle of fidelity would obligate one to keep all promises and would make actions such as adultery, treason, and betrayal of friendship wrong. Deontology is also based on duties or obligations. Therefore the principle of nonmaleficence obligates us never to hurt another person, and the principle of beneficence creates the duty to do good. Frequently one must face the problem of when, if ever, a basic moral rule can be overridden. Obviously circumstances will occur in which it is permissible to override a rule, but it is equally obvious that those circumstances should be few and far between and should not occur if the moral rule is an absolute. As previously mentioned, the deontologist does not totally ignore the role of consequences in determining moral rightness and wrongness; at times the consequences of adherence to rules would clearly be worse than breaking them. An example that is frequently used is the matter of European Christians hiding Jews in their homes during the Holocaust. When the Nazis pounded on the doors of these Gentiles demanding to know if Jews were there, the truth would surely result in concentration camps and torture for *both* Jews and Gentiles. Therefore the obligation to tell the truth is overridden. There are, however, some rules that are absolute; for example, murder (unjustified killing) is always prohibited, as is doing harm without the ultimate goal of doing good. Knowing which rules are absolute and which can be overridden, when, and for what reason creates ethical dilemmas for the deontologist.

KANTIANISM. The German philosopher Immanuel Kant (1724–1804) had a profound influence on modern philosophy and ethical theory. He believed that a good person followed certain moral rules simply because it was *right* to do so. He was less interested in the consequences of an action than in the universalizability of the maxim or rule that directed the action. He was precise and positive about which rules were to be obeyed, and he formulated reasons for obeying particular rules.

Kant believed that when a person contemplates a particular action, he should first ask himself what rule he would be following if he did the action. The person should then ask himself if he would be willing for *everyone* to follow the same rule in similar situations. If so, the rule may be obeyed, and the action is therefore permissible. If the person must answer in the negative, the rule must not be followed, and the action is not permissible. This, Kant believed, is the supreme basis of morality, which he termed the Categorical Imperative: "Act only on that maxim whereby thou canst at the same time will that it should become a universal law." A maxim is defined as a rule governing human actions, and Kant gives several examples: "Do not make a lying promise" (a promise that one does not intend to keep); "Do not commit suicide"; "Assist others in distress." The Categorical Imperative derives its name from the fact that the maxims it covers are indeed imperative; and because there are no exceptions to the rule, it is binding on all humans regardless of feelings of personal preference.

Kant distinguished the Categorical Imperative from a hypothetical imperative. The latter is based on a precondition of desire: *if* you want X, then you *ought* to do Y. *If* you want to buy a house, then you *ought* to save money. The admonition to save money rests on the precondition that the desire to buy a house is present. A hypothetical imperative is optional; the Categorical Imperative is not.

> We should follow such rules, Kant says, not merely because we have desires that would otherwise be frustrated, but because it would not be rational to reject them. Compliance with the Categorical Imperative is required by reason itself; it is the supreme principle of rationality in conduct. We can begin to see why Kant says this if we consider that it would be *inconsistent* of us not to act on the principles that we would want others to accept, or to act on principles that we would want others to reject. For example, suppose I refuse to help others in distress, but when I am in distress I want others to help me. The "maxim" in question is "assist others in distress", and consistency requires that, if I think that others ought to follow this rule, then I ought to follow it myself.[10]

Treating persons not merely as means, but as ends in themselves is a strong concept in Kantian ethics. Kant, in fact, believed so strongly that we should not use persons as mere means that he devised an alternative formulation of the Categorical Imperative: "Act so as to treat humanity, whether in thine own person or in that of any other, in every case as an end withal, never as a means only." Many Kantian philosophers see these two formulations of the Categorical Imperative as clearly different from each other, although by no means mutually exclusive, and therefore as two separate imperatives. For the purpose of this book, they will be labeled the first and second formulation of the Categorical Imperative and will be considered to carry equal moral weight.

The second formulation has to do with respect for persons, which Kant believed to be a moral obligation. He held that respect for persons derives from respect for law, although one can easily see how a person could meticulously obey all laws and yet have utter contempt for his fellow beings as persons. If one does not kill another or abridge any of his rights, it does not necessarily follow that respect exists. Respect for persons also implies a clear understanding of the nature of persons, both in terms of one's own consciousness and of that of others. This is not easily accomplished; in addition to defining individuals as persons, there is the problem of defining the term in a societal context. Much has been written about the concept of personhood, on both physical and metaphysical levels. On a moral level, that is, a person being an individual to whom one owes moral duties and obligations, the concept is even more elusive and complex. R. S. Peters believes that the moral components of personhood reach their zenith when one enters and sustains a personal relationship in which the bonds that tie the people together derive from their own choice and their own appraisal of each other as persons, not from societal status or position. They create their own voluntary obligations that sustain the relationship and are felt to be far more binding than those that are externally imposed.[11]

This is essentially what Kant meant by respect for persons and is the basis of the second formulation of the Categorical Imperative. If respect for persons exists, it should follow that one will not use another person as a means only; respect implies using the person as an end also.

What did Kant mean when he prohibited using a person as a mere means? For example, if I were to cultivate your friendship for the sole purpose of meeting your uncle who is in a position to offer me a job I want very much, I am using you *only* as a means to get to your uncle. Kantian ethics would prohibit that action. If, however, I genuinely like you and enjoy your company and continue to see you *whether or not* your uncle offers me a job, I am using you as an end also, the end being friendship, and am thus engaging in a morally correct action. In the first instance I have contempt for you as a person; in the second there is respect for your personhood.

The principle of autonomy and the principle of human worth spring directly from respect for persons as expressed by Kant in his imperative concerning duties toward others:

> The natural end which all men have is their own happiness. Now humanity might indeed subsist although no one should contribute anything to the happiness of others, provided he did not intentionally withdraw anything from it; but after all, this would only harmonize negatively, not positively, with *humanity as an end in itself*, if everyone does not also endeavor, as far as in him lies, to forward the ends of others. For the ends of any subject which is an end in himself ought as far as possible to be *my* ends also, if that conception is to have its *full* effect with me.[12]

Here Kant is discussing the universalizability of morally correct actions, that is, one *ought* to do that which a person would will to be done for him. This maxim is implicit in the principle of autonomy: we ought to treat other people as total persons who control the direction and actions of their own lives, as we want others to allow us in similar situations to direct our own lives.

A common example of disregard for autonomy is a woman who is *told* by an obstetrician how she will deliver her child. If the obstetrician chooses the position she will assume, controls the persons who will accompany her in the labor and delivery rooms, and informs her when and under what circumstances she is permitted to have physical contact with her newborn baby, the physician demonstrates lack of regard for her autonomy because he has disregarded respect for her as a person and ignored the principle of human worth. The physician owes both a professional and a moral obligation to the woman to direct the circumstances of her own delivery insofar as her health and safety permit. Both formulations of the Categorical Imperative lead directly to the principle of autonomy and respect for persons.

JUSTICE. One of the major criticisms of utilitarianism is that justice is not taken into account in determination of morally correct action. In the previous example of justifying slavery, we saw how the utilitarian came to a moral decision based on total amount of happiness. The fact that the system is grossly unfair to slaves is ignored. Deontology seeks to solve that problem by employing justice as a basis for deciding whether the characteristics of an act are morally correct. John Rawls and other philosophers have built entire moral theories around the existence of justice and its role in social contracts.

Justice is most frequently defined in terms of fairness or *desert*; justice has been served when an individual or group receives from another individual or group what is due or owed. Determination of societal goods or benefits (as well as societal burdens) that are owed to individuals or groups creates judicial moral dilemmas. We are familiar with the term *special interest group*, particularly as the term is used in the political sphere. Lobbies for special interest groups attempt to convince politicians that the groups have been treated somehow unfairly in the past and now "deserve" a particular societal benefit. Or the special interest group may make an effort to convince society that if a particular burden is imposed (or benefit denied), injustice will occur. The dilemma then caused is sorting out which burdens and benefits do indeed accrue to special interest groups or to any other group or individual. Different types of dilemmas require different concepts of justice.

Comparative justice means that competing claims of individuals or groups are balanced against each other, and the merits of each claim are compared. The person trying to solve the dilemma decides how much each person is due. Comparative justice is frequently used in civil lawsuits, such as settling child support payments after a divorce or determining financial reward in a malpractice suit. In each of these two examples both parties claim competing benefits; the court must decide which party has all or some rights to the claim.

Distributive justice applies only when conditions of scarcity exist, as in certain types of health resources. If everyone in society were sympathetic to the needs of everyone else, conditions of scarcity would occur much less frequently and fewer dilemmas involving distribution would arise. For example, if more people signed the Uniform Anatomical Gift Act (a document stating the intent to donate all or some body organs after death), more kidneys would be available for transplant. As a result, fewer people would die of kidney failure or would be forced to undergo dialysis for protracted periods of time. People are not, however, as fairminded as they ought to be; therefore scarcity and deprivation exist for certain portions of the populace, and distributive justice must be used in an effort to equalize societal benefits and burdens.

> The rules of justice serve to strike a balance between those conflicting interests and also between claims that repeatedly occur in society. Since law and morality are our explicit tools for balancing conflicting claims, there is a close link between the lawful society and the just society. Nonetheless, the law may be unjust; and not all rules of justice are connected to the law or to legal enforcement. Accordingly, parties with conflicting claims must often justify their claims by appeal to basic moral rules.[13]

This is essentially a description of and reason for civil disobedience—the belief that certain laws can be disobeyed because the laws themselves are unjust.

Formal justice states that equals ought to be treated equally and unequals unequally as long as the respects under consideration are equal. Stated negatively, formal justice holds that no person should be treated unequally from all other persons unless it can be shown that the person is unequal *with regard to* the matter under consideration. For example, two bank robberies occur under almost identical conditions, and both robbers are caught in the act and brought to trial. One robber is a white business executive who has been unemployed for 2 years and is unable to feed his family. He thus resorts to bank robbery out of desperation. The other robber is a black adolescent who is on a lark and decides to rob a bank just to see if he can get away with it. Neither person has ever done this before. Formal justice requires that each robber be treated equally because the only matter under consideration is bank robbery. Conditions of social class, race, or motive are not relevant.

The only problem with formal justice is that the theory often does not work well in practice. One is not likely to argue with the theory that persons ought to be treated equally, but relevant differences between individuals always exist, even if they are difficult to detect or to specify. In the example given, although the crime was "equal," the circumstances that led to its commission were different, thus unequal. Although bank robbery is always wrong and should always be punished, a judge might believe himself justified in inflicting unequal punishment for an equal crime because of circumstances surrounding its motive. A man in a desperate attempt to feed his family may be viewed as slightly less guilty than the adolescent who robs a bank for sport. On the other hand, the unemployed executive may be viewed by the court as mature enough to have known better than to rob a bank, and the adolescent may be excused for his youthful prankishness. Judgment of the equality of the crime may depend on community standards, the values of the judge, or even less rationally based variables.

What, then, are some material principles that are relevant to the distribution of justice if formal justice is not applicable in practice? Rescher[14] has delineated five principles that are accepted by many philosophers: (1) to each person an equal share; (2) to each person according to individual need; (3) to each person according to individual effort; (4) to each person according to societal contribution; and (5) to each person according to merit. Any combination of these five principles can be applied to any dilemma involving justice, although they are most frequently used in distributive justice where conditions of scarcity exist and resources must be allocated on a just basis. For example, in a country in which all physicians and other health professionals work for the government and are assigned by the government to work in particular places for specified periods of time, communities will be assigned health professionals on the basis of need. Merit, societal contribution, or any of the other principles would not apply. But a large private foundation, awarding 100 fellowships from among 1000 applicants, would use the principles of individual effort, societal contribution, and merit.

Beauchamp and Childress demonstrate how, in the distribution of justice, the principle of need is based on relevant properties and public policies.

> The principle of need declares that distribution is just when it is based on need. But how are we to understand the notion of a need? The term is subject to different interpretations, and a meaning must be fixed before meaningful distribution would be possible. In general, to say that a person needs something is to say that *without it he will be harmed* (or at least detrimentally affected).[15]

Therefore people of equal needs should be treated equally with regard to satisfaction of those needs. Common sense must be applied to determination of needs. A basic need (without which one would be harmed) is sufficient food to maintain health. Therefore resources should be divided equally on this basis. If, however, certain individuals experience a need to have their protein requirement met in part by caviar and their carbohydrate requirement by champagne, these "needs" must be met by ability to pay because it cannot be reasonably shown that a person will be harmed without caviar and champagne.

John Rawls, more than any other modern philosopher, has written about the integration of justice in the fabric of society. He maintains that justice is inherent in the social contract but is only one of the virtues that contribute to a good society. Justice is not to be confused with equality, nor, according to Rawls, is it the *same as* fairness, although fairness is fundamental to justice. That is, justice cannot exist without fairness, although the two are not identical. Justice implies equality in some form, as in equal pay for equal work, whereas fairness implies that while equality might not necessarily exist, the participants are content with decisions made. The two concepts, however, are interdependent. Rawls' working definition of justice in the usual sense "is essentially the elimination of arbitrary distinctions and the establishment, within the structure of a practice, of a proper balance between competing claims."[16]

Rawls further refines his concept of justice by formulating two principles:

first, each person who participates in a practice has an equal right to the most extensive liberty compatible with a similar liberty for all other persons. Second, inequalities of practice are arbitrary unless it is reasonable to expect that the inequalities will work out to everyone's advantage and that the positions and offices to which the inequalities are attached are open to all. In the first principle, if all liberty were compatible with everyone else's liberty, injustice would not exist; in the second principle, inequalities would not be considered inequalities if they were to conform to the necessary constraints. Rawls, then, envisions justice as a complex of three ideas: liberty, equality, and reward for services contributing to the common good.[17]

RIGHTS. Rights are difficult to pin down to a precise definition; they are usually seen as justified claims that individuals or groups make against other individuals or groups in society. The key word is "justified" because, although anyone can claim anything from anyone else, not all such claims are justified. We might receive a clearer idea of which claims are justified and which are not by further defining the nature of rights.

A moral right is different from a legal right. A moral right is universal, that is, it transcends political, jurisdictional, or cultural boundaries; any person may claim a moral right. A legal right is restricted to and depends on jurisdictional boundaries, which may be a country, a state or province, a municipality, or some other politically defined jurisdiction. A legal right in one country may not exist in another and may change from state to neighboring state. One may claim a legal right only if it exists in the jurisdiction in which the person makes the claim. Moral rights are always equal rights; legal rights are not necessarily equal. For example, if the pursuit of happiness is a moral right, then every individual has the same and equal right to pursue happiness. The right to purchase and consume liquor in a public place is a legal right that is not necessarily equal. State A may permit only those persons over age 21 to do so, while state B may allow all those who have reached the age of 18 to drink in public. State C may not grant the right at all.

Moral rights are inalienable, that is, they cannot be transferred (lent or sold) to another person; legal rights are not inalienable unless they are also moral rights. A moral right can sometimes be forfeited. For example, a person who has murdered another can forfeit his own *right* to life, according to some philosophers, even though he is not necessarily expected to forfeit the life itself. Moral and legal rights are sometimes the same; frequently they differ. For example, one has a moral right to the truth, although such a right does not exist in law except in the case of telling the truth under oath in court.

Another important distinction in the matter of rights is the difference between positive and negative rights. A positive right is the right to other people's positive actions; a negative right is the right to other people's forbearances. If X has a positive right to something, then Y must take positive action to fulfill that right. If *X* has a negative right to something, then *Y* must refrain from doing something. The distinction can be clarified by examining the abortion controversy and the Supreme Court decision *Roe v. Wade* (1973). The case was fought mainly around a woman's right to privacy; she is permitted to abort the fetus during the first two trimesters, within certain limits. The court granted women negative rights in that the state is not permitted to interfere with her privacy, nor is it permitted to prevent her from seeking an abortion within the limits specified. The Supreme Court did *not* grant a woman a positive right to an abortion; that is, the ruling in *Roe v. Wade* did not specify that the state or a private physician *must* provide a woman with an abortion, only that they may not prevent her from obtaining one.

A natural right is one that accrues to a person by simply being born a human being. No other requirements are necessary. The one natural right that all philosophers agree exists is the right to life. Although some maintain that it can and should be forfeited under certain conditions, we will ignore that stipulation for the moment and state that all human beings have a natural, universal, and inalienable right to life. Liberty or freedom is another right generally believed to be natural, universal, and inalienable; some also believe that a natural right to happiness, or at least the search for happiness, exists. The last of these three rights is the most controversial, probably depending on one's definition of happiness and what is involved in its attainment.

Any discussion of rights is incomplete without a corresponding discussion of duties and obligations (the terms *duty* and *obligation*, although they are not precisely synonymous, will be used interchangeably here). There is a logical correlation between rights and obligations; existence of a right *implies* a corresponding obligation, either on the part of the person himself, or more usually, on the part of someone else. Moral rights incur moral obligations, and legal rights incur legal obligations. For example, if *X* has a moral right to be treated with autonomy and respect for his person, then *Y* has a duty to do those things that promote and maintain respect, such as respecting X's autonomy, not harming him, and doing good when the situation requires it. If *X* has a legal right granted by a particular jurisdiction, then *Y* is obligated to secure that right or to do nothing to interfere with it.

Fulfilling duties and obligations arising from rights does not depend on feelings or personal preference; one is obligated to do certain things whether one wants to or not. Much of today's social ferment and dissatisfaction with social and political life stems from misunderstandings about the nature of rights and obligations. Homosexuality can be used as an illustrative example. It is a matter of indifference to the discussion of rights whether homosexuality is morally correct or incorrect behavior, nor is it important that people like or dislike the fact of homosexuality or choose to participate in homosexual acts.

Let us look only at the rights of homosexuals and the obligations owed them by virtue of those rights. One must first separate the homosexual as a human being from the homosexual as a person who is a member of a minority group. As a human being, a homosexual has all the rights and obligations, both moral and legal, that pertain to all other human beings. Does, however, the fact of his homosexuality change any of those rights, and if so, in what way? Can a political jurisdiction remove or abridge any legal right a homosexual has accrued by virtue of being a person, and can individuals be released from their moral obligations to persons who are homosexual? Based on what we know about justice and rights, the answer must be no. It is as unfair to imprison a homosexual for his activities with a person of the same sex as it is to enslave another person because his skin is a different color from that of the majority in a particular society. One is not obligated to *like* homosexuality any more than one is obligated to like persons of a different race or religion; one is obligated only to uphold their positive, negative, moral, and legal rights *as persons*.

There is a difference between a moral requirement and a logically derived obligation arising from a right, although that difference is often obscure. For example, charity is a moral requirement rather than an obligation because no one has a *right* to charity. We may feel obligated to contribute time or money to charity, but the perceived obligation springs from our own set of values; it does not arise extrinsically from the right of others. Another example is love. No one has a right to be loved, although we all may desire it. Parents are obligated to provide certain conditions and actions for their children, but the obligation springs from the nature of the parent-child relationship and from the legal and moral rights arising from the "contractual" agreement that exists between parent and child. (Use of the word *contract* in regard to this relationship may appear a bit callous, but the action of bearing a child and agreeing to raise it by not giving it up for adoption implies a contract, recognized by law, to do certain things for the child.) The parent is not, however, obligated to love the child because the right to be loved does not exist.

Mill characterized this distinction as the difference between duties of perfect obligation and duties of imperfect obligation. The former are those that are based in a correlative right and usually are duties of justice. The latter do not involve a right and belong to other spheres of morality such as generosity or beneficence.

One further distinction in the matter of rights is the difference between option rights and welfare rights. An option right involves freedom of choice and the exercise of autonomy. An example of an option right is the right to pursue any career one wishes as long as it does not infringe on the rights of others. A "career" as a bank robber is not an option right! Within a certain sphere of action an individual is sovereign and may do as he pleases; the boundaries of that sphere are usually set at the point where other individuals are in danger of being harmed in that there is a possibility that their rights will be abridged. Golding[18] provides an interesting example of sovereignity in regard to option rights. Persons generally have the right to do whatever they choose with their own bodies (certain kinds of self-mutilation are illegal in some states, but we shall ignore that exception for the moment); in that respect their option rights are sovereign. However, they may not infect themselves with the bacteria or virus of a contagious disease because in so doing they would be causing harm or potential harm to other persons and would thus step outside the boundary of an option right.

A welfare right is the entitlement to some societal good or benefit such as sufficient food or decent housing. Welfare rights are the subject of heated controversy, and many people believe that, except in certain specific instances, they do not exist. Welfare rights arise from constitutional or statutory law, which in turn springs from societal values at the time the law was enacted. For example, there is no guaranteed legal right to health care in the United States, although it is a common belief in the latter part of the twentieth century that such a right *should* exist.

Some welfare rights have become a historic tradition as well as a legal right (the right to a free public education), some are subject to fluctuating public opinion (the right not to be discriminated against for reasons over which a person has no control, e.g., skin color), and some are more important than others (sufficient food is more important than paved roads). If welfare rights are seen as mandatory, that is, rights that involve duties of perfect obligation or rights that cannot be renounced, then they are separate and distinct from option rights. However, if welfare rights are not mandatory and involve choice in some way, then they could be viewed to some degree *as* option rights and thus result in moral dilemmas. The question of welfare rights as mandatory tends to fall under the rubric of ethical relativism; that is, societies view rights in different ways from time to time depending on the social and political mood of the group. The best example is the right to a certain minimum level of education that varies with the group in question (usually a minority one) and what its position is vis-à-vis other social and political groups in the society.

The language of rights tends to be both overused and misused in today's society. Individuals tend to demand rights from others when they have no moral or legal claim to those rights, and rights that do and should exist tend to be ignored or abrogated because of personal preference or bias. When we speak of rights, we must be careful to do so in a logically correct manner and to understand the legal and moral bases on which they rest.

INTUITIONISM. Intuitionism is a part of deontologic theory that tends to be obscure and murky, mainly because not all people tend to intuit the same things. Intuitionism claims that determination of moral rightness or wrongness depends on the intrinsic nature of a particular act. This intrinsic nature is composed of "right-making" *and* "wrong-making" properties (and some that are neutral as well); intuitionism involves a two-stage process of determining which properties will "win," thus making an act morally right or wrong. It tends to be a fairly arbitrary process.

The first stage consists of identifying all the right-making and all the wrong-making properties of any given act; the second stage involves determining the relative importance or moral "weight" of each property, and then calculating the total. If an intuitionist is asked how he knows, not only what are right-making and wrong-making properties, but also how important each of the properties are, he is likely to reply that he knows this by intuition. This would seem to be no help whatsoever, but perhaps an example involving abortion can clarify the process. The right-making properties of an abortion (depending on the situation) may involve saving the life of a pregnant woman or alleviating the mental anguish of being pregnant. A wrong-making property might be killing the fetus. Depending on what moral weight is ascribed to these properties, the intuitionist can make a moral judgment.

Intuitionism is probably not of much practical use to the layperson who is trying to solve a moral dilemma because of its lack of rules and principles to apply to the situation at hand.

> The distinguishing mark of intuitionist theories ... is their irrationalism; that is to say, at certain crucial points in the process which is supposed to end with an answer to a moral question, they appeal, not to argument, but to our alleged ability to know, without argument, the truth of certain moral facts.[19]

In the minds of many who have a more empiric or pragmatic bent, this knowledge without argument sounds suspiciously like the leap of faith required by theologic theories. Without rational argument, it is difficult to prove a philosophic theory.

Theologic theories

Many philosophers, particularly those modern thinkers who are influenced by the writings of British empiricists, such as Hume, Locke, and Berkeley, and the Logical Positivists, such as Ayer, Wittgenstein, and Carnap, believe that reason and theology are contradictory. Twentieth century philosophy has been notable for a dependence on the scientific method and the almost total repudiation of God as a moral force. Bertrand Russell believed that knowledge did not exist unless it could be scientifically proved. The positivist A. J. Ayer declared, "All utterances about the nature of God are nonsensical."

Proof of the existence of God has occupied theologians and philosophers since the beginning of rational thought. Atheists maintain that the convoluted efforts and mental acrobatics that theologists go through to prove the existence of God proves the opposite: that God does not exist, and all the intellectual machinations in the world will not create a God or gods.

Atheists seem to have logic and reason on their side, but it is interesting to look at some of the ways in which theologists "prove" the existence of God.

1. Moral proof. There are universal signs of conscience in all human beings that cannot be explained simply in terms of self-interest or social conditioning. The source of this conscience is God. Kant believed that each person engaged in a quest for the highest good, which implies existence of a moral being and an end to the quest, which must necessarily be God.

2. Mental proof. The only possible explanation for the power of reason and humanity that is unique to our species is God. Reason exists separate from and outside the human mind and is responsible for whatever valid and logical thoughts occur in humans. Therefore reason must exist in God as the next highest being. Knowledge that God exists comes from inferring God's existence from the known existence of other beings; that is, if A exists, then there is no reason why B cannot exist also.

3. Experiential proof. If so many people have religious experiences, there must indeed be something to them. The commonality among the experiences proves that they are not merely mental aberrations or the result of wishful thinking.

4. Teleologic proof. The complex structure and function of the universe is proof that it was designed by a being with powers far superior to those of humans. Skeptics argue that nature operates in so capricious a manner that proof exists that the universe merely evolved haphazardly rather than having been specifically designed.

5. Ontologic proof. This somewhat convoluted reasoning states that if it is even *possible* that God exists, then by reason of logic, God must exist in actuality.

6. Cosmologic proof. Thomas Aquinas argued that all effects that exist in the world have a cause and that cause and effect relationships are an endless chain beginning with the first cause, the Prime Mover, which is God. Cosmologic proof also states that because atheists cannot prove absolutely that God does not exist, then God must indeed exist beyond a reasonable doubt.

Theologic ethics, which is predicated on belief in God, means that one takes into consideration reflections on belief in God when one is thinking about morality and making decisions about moral dilemmas. Theologic ethics also examines the moral beliefs of religions or even secular humanistic philosophies.

Carney[20] maintains that three kinds of normative judgments are basic to theologic ethics: judgments of obligation, virtue, and value. Judgments of obligation ask what morally *ought* to be done in a given situation, that is, which actions are right and which are wrong. Judgments of virtue ask what qualities about a person, provided the person is responsible or accountable for the qualities, are commendable or reprehensible. Thus a person may be considered praiseworthy or blameworthy for particular characteristics. Judgments of value ask what objects or states of affairs are good or bad. This largely determines rightness or wrongness of behaviors, actions, or outcomes. These three types of ethical judgments are frequently described together simply as values or as value judgments, thus creating confusion about what a value is. The description of theologic ethics may appear indistinguishable from secular moral philosophy; the difference between the two schools of thought is the orientation brought to their study.

THEISTIC ORIENTATION. The major distinguishing characteristic of theologic ethics, as opposed to secular moral philosophy, is a theistic orientation. In addition to belief in God (or gods), a theistic orientation calls on human beings to make some response to God. The response depends on how God is perceived and on the tenets or requirements of a particular religion. A wide variety of human responses exists, some of which are justice, compassion, humility, sorrow, mercy, commitment, obedience, and acceptance. Again, theistic orientations fall into the following three basic categories:

1. God is the author of a universal ordering of appropriate human response; humans must perceive this ordering to abide by it. For example, Catholics use the doctrine of natural law, and Hindus developed a conception of karma (a person is and receives today what he deserves from his past).
2. God has intervened in the history of the world to establish a relationship with humankind; therefore every event in history is illustrative and interpretive of all other events. The believer in God makes certain events central to the understanding of human existence that should give meaning to the event and to one's own existence.
3. Emphasis is placed on the characteristics of God rather than on the order established by God in the world. The believer then tries to imitate the positive characteristics of God and to be awed by the negative ones.

These orientations are not necessarily mutually exclusive because they all rest on a foundation of belief in God and are different ways of viewing and worshipping God.

A theistic orientation must relate to moral ideas or there would be no point to theologic theories of morality. There are several ways in which the relationship can be viewed. A historic relation points to the origins of a particular moral idea, such as agape from early Christianity. However, the original moral idea could have begun elsewhere (as perhaps it did), and the historic relation does not ignore subsequent moral and religious development and interpretation. A logical relation implies that a practice derives from a belief and that a particular belief implies a practice. Theistic orientations justify moral judgments. A psychologic relation denotes that a theistic orientation motivates obligations or duties, that is, reasons for developing one's character in certain ways or for doing certain actions arise from a theistic orientation. An epistemologic relation implies that one *can* know that a theistic orientation contributes to morality. This relation holds that certain truths are known *only* through a theistic orientation. The ontologic relation holds that the existence of moral obligations is vitally connected with the existence and activity of God. If everything in existence depends on the existence of God, then morality also depends on the existence of God.

The idea of morality runs as a strong thread through theologic theories, particularly in Judaism and Christianity. Obligation or duty is a large part of both moral philosophy and theology; the major difference lies in origins of obligations. The obligation to do good, for example, can be justified because it is commanded by God or because good exists and therefore ought to be done. Obligations to love thy neighbor can spring from respect for persons or from an interpretation of the Ten Commandments. Those who hold a theistic orientation do so out of a belief in, and obedience to, God.

Double effect

The principle of double effect, which is used almost exclusively by Roman Catholic philosophers and theologians, holds that one may rightfully cause evil if the following four conditions are present and verified: (1) the act itself, for which the evil is caused, is good, or at least morally neutral; (2) the good effect of the act is what the agent (actor) primarily intends, and the evil is only secondary; (3) the good effect may not come about *by means of* the evil effect; and (4) there must be some proportionately grave reason for permitting the evil effect to occur.

Permissibility of double effect rests on the premise that there is a morally significant difference between *intending* evil and *permitting* evil and on the premise that it is wrong to use an evil means to obtain a good end. The purpose of the principle is to determine to what extent, if any, evil can be caused in pursuit of good. It is used today in bioethical theory to solve problems where death or serious harm will occur as a result of an action intended to do good. The example of abortion is the one most frequently used in explaining the principle of double effect. Catholic doctrine insists that abortion is always morally wrong, and therefore impermissible, except where the principle of double effect can be applied. For example, if a woman is suffering from an ectopic pregnancy of the fallopian tube and it is known (as it always is) that continuation of the pregnancy will result in rupture of the fallopian tube, peritonitis, and subsequent death, an abortion may be performed because the intent is to save the life of the pregnant woman, not to kill the fetus. Although death of the fetus is an unavoidable and foreseen evil effect, it was not the effect that was intended. All four conditions described earlier are present and verified: (1) the act of saving the woman's life is good; (2) the physician, in performing the surgery, intends to save the woman's life, and the evil of killing the fetus is only permitted, not intended; (3) the good effect (saving a life) comes about through no evil ends, that is, the woman's life is not saved *by means of* killing the fetus; and (4) the proportionately grave reason for permitting death of the fetus is the certain death of the pregnant woman if the surgery is not performed.

The principle is also used to justify removal of a cancerous uterus of a pregnant woman, although direct abortion (without the simultaneous removal of diseased maternal tissue) cannot be justified, even if there is grave physical danger to the woman, because the third condition has not been satisfied; that is, the good effect of decreasing danger (even saving life) *will* be brought about by evil means.

Considerable debate exists about the principle. Some philosophers believe that the second distinction is an example of moral quibbling and a specious argument. Whether evil was intended or merely permitted is irrelevant; the end result is the same—evil occurs. Whether the death of the fetus was a direct or indirect action means nothing; the fetus is still dead. Defenders of the principle claim that the difference in consequences is great because of the intent of the agent. True, evil still occurs, but the intention places a different moral significance on the act. For an analogy, it is granted that it is evil to kill dogs with one's car. However, there is a significant moral difference between deliberately aiming for and hitting a dog that was crossing the road and swerving one's car to avoid a person in the road and being forced to hit the dog who was in the path of the swerving car. The dog is hit in both instances, and in both instances the driver knows he will injure or kill the dog; the difference is in intent.

May[21] believes that the argument over the principle is waged over some critical issues in ethics. If one accepts the principle, then there are very few evil actions that may be taken on the way to good actions. For example, the many forms of medical research or perhaps even mass reductions in the work force in an effort to improve the economy. Those who reject the principle are more "liberal" in allowing certain evil actions.

Situation ethics

Situation ethics has often been described as "morality without rules." It is, however, more accurately defined as a type of act-utilitarianism. The situation ethicist would not absolutely discard moral rules and principles but would use them only as rules of thumb to be applied as a general guideline *if* the situation at hand warrants their use. Moral rules can be used or discarded at will. What, then, keeps the proponent of situation ethics from doing all sorts of harm if he is not beholden to any moral rules? He must make all moral decisions on the basis of act-utilitarian theory, that is, determining the net gain in happiness, now and in the future, if a particular action is taken or not taken. Human happiness is the criterion, not moral rectitude. If duty or obligation is involved at all, it is the obligation of the actor to achieve the best possible results in terms of happiness. "Thus duty means to do what is best in the situation, which may mean either obeying or flouting any given rule."[22]

It is this phrase that sometimes causes persons who prefer to use moral rules or principles to accuse act ethics of "the end justifies the means." Fletcher believes the accusation is warranted because "nothing we do (no means) is morally justifiable except by the good end it seeks." Given this premise, the situation ethicist can break even the most commonly accepted rules with impunity. He would not believe himself compelled to tell the truth, keep promises, fulfill a contract, and so on. The proponent of situation ethics is motivated by human well-being as characterized by human happiness and will make all ethical decisions accordingly. The situation ethicist might or might not permit a person to exercise autonomy, depending on the situation. If he decides that a paternalistic withholding of autonomy would result in greater happiness, he would not hesitate to do so, although in another situation he might respect absolutely the person's autonomy. For example, a woman needs advice from a surgeon for a lump in her breast she has recently discovered. The surgeon has a wide variety of choices in establishing a relationship with the woman and in treating her. On one extreme he can do a biopsy, report the findings to her (assume for the moment that the lump is malignant), explain all the treatment options available, and then let her decide what she chooses to do. On the other extreme, he can adopt the "stick-with-me-kid" attitude, do the biopsy, and then amputate her breast even before she comes out of anesthesia. If the surgeon is a situation ethicist he will adopt the course of action he believes will result in the greatest present and future happiness for the woman and her family. If he would *prefer* to behave paternalistically but *knows* that disrespect for her autonomy will cause greater unhappiness than will the results of the breast cancer (no matter what treatment modality is chosen), he will respect her autonomy. If, however, he knows that breast amputation will ultimately be the best course of action, he will amputate her breast.

Situation ethicists are accused of breaking all fundamental moral rules and are frequently viewed in a most unfavorable light. Although few philosophers espouse act-utilitarianism or situation ethics as a stated belief, it is not uncommon to find situation ethics practiced routinely in business, commerce, and particularly in health care.

SUMMARY

Ethics is a system of thought by which decisions are logically made about what course of action, in a choice of two or more, is morally correct. Moral judgments, rules, codes, standards, and values are used in the decision-making process. Rational logical thought is the process by which ethical decisions are made, and moral theories, rules, and principles are the bases of decisions.

Ethical argument is based on correspondence or relationship between two sets of things, usually moral rules or principles, and depends *only* on logical relationships, not on personal preference, feelings, or moral authority. The strength of a moral argument depends solely on its logic.

Ethics is divided into two branches: metaethics and normative ethics. Metaethics is concerned with the structure of moral philosophy: its language, argument forms, conceptual analysis, logic, and epistemology. It is the effort to understand ethics. Normative ethics is concerned with determining correct moral principles and theories by which *all* rational people should be guided. It is prescriptive in nature and is generally composed of two types of theories: consequentialist and nonconsequentialist (deontologic).

A consequentialist (teleologic) theory holds that an action is morally correct as a result of the function (moral correctness) of its consequences. The most common consequentialist theory is utilitarianism, which holds that an action is morally correct if the consequences of the action produce the greatest amount of happiness for the greatest number of people, including the actor. Deontology holds that an action is morally correct because of the rightness or wrongness of features or characteristics of the act, regardless of the consequences. Conflict occurs in determining what features of an act make it right or wrong and why this is so. Deontology is also based on duties or obligations; their presence contributes to the rightness or wrongness of the act. Some of these duties include respect for persons, justice, beneficence, autonomy, adherence to rights, and knowledge about right-making and wrong-making properties of acts, sometimes called intuition.

Theologic theories of morality rest on belief in the existence of God, although many philosophers believe that reason and theology are contradictory. Much philosophic effort has gone into proving God's existence, although skepticism is still strong. A theistic orientation to morality calls for an individual to make one of a variety of responses to God when making moral decisions, which usually involves obedience to God's commandments. Duties and obligations to persons exist in theologic morality, and origin of duties is believed to arise from God rather than from rationality and a more secular sense of why individuals are required to do or forbear certain actions. The moral correctness of actions is frequently the same whether the path to the decision did or did not lead through belief in God.

Notes

1. Taylor, P. W. *Principles of ethics*. Encino, Calif.: Dickinson Publishing Company, 1975. p. 1.
2. Blackstone, W. T. The search for an environmental ethic. In T. Regan (Ed.). *Matters of life and death: new introductory essays in moral philosophy*. New York: Random House, Inc., 1980. pp. 301–304.
3. Taylor, p. 208.
4. Plato. *Republic* (Bk. 2.). In P. Shorey. *What Plato said*. Chicago: University of Chicago Press, 1933.
5. Taylor, p. 211.
6. Taylor, p. 213.
7. Rachels, J. Euthanasia. In Regan, p. 40.
8. Regan, T. (Ed.). *Matters of life and death: new introductory essays in moral philosophy*. New York: Random House, Inc., 1980. pp. 7–14.
9. Regan, p. 13.
10. Rachels, J. *Understanding moral philosophy*. Encino, Calif.: Dickinson Publishing Company, 1976. pp. 183–184.
11. Peters, R. S. Respect for persons. In Rachels, pp. 207–208.
12. Kant, I. Foundations of the metaphysics of morals. In Rachels, pp. 207–208.
13. Beauchamp, T. L., & Childress, J. F. *Principles of biomedical ethics*. New York: Oxford University Press, Inc., 1979. p. 170.
14. Rescher, N. *Distributive justice*. Indianapolis: The Bobbs-Merrill Co., Inc., 1966. (chap. 4.)
15. Beauchamp & Childress, pp. 173–174.
16. Rawls, J. Justice as fairness. *The Philosophical Review*. 1958, *67*, 165.
17. Rawls, p. 165.
18. Golding, M. P. The concept of rights: a historical sketch. In E. L. Bandman & B. Bandman (Eds.), *Bioethics and human rights*. Boston: Little, Brown & Co., 1978. p. 44.
19. Hare, R. M. Non-descriptivism. In W. T. Reich (Ed.), *Encyclopedia of bioethics*. (Vol. 1.) New York: The Free Press, 1978. pp. 447–448.
20. Carney, F. S. Theological ethics. In *Encyclopedia of bioethics*. (Vol. 1.), pp. 447–448.
21. May, W. E. Double effect. In *Encyclopedia of bioethics* (Vol. 1.), pp. 319.
22. Fletcher, J. Situation ethics. In *Encyclopedia of Bioethics* (Vol. 1.), pp. 422–423.

Bibliography

Baier, K. Deontological theories. In W. Reich (Ed.), *Encyclopedia of bioethics*. New York: The Free Press, 1978.

Bandman, E. L., & Bandman, B. *Bioethics and human rights*. Boston: Little, Brown & Co., 1978.

Beauchamp, T. L., & Childress, J. F. *Principles of biomedical ethics*. New York: Oxford University Press, Inc., 1979.

Bentham, J. *An introduction to the principles of morals and legislation* (1789). London: Oxford University Press, 1948.

Carney, F. S. Theological ethics. In *Encyclopedia of bioethics*.

Fletcher, J. Situation ethics. In *Encyclopedia of bioethics*.

Golding, M. P. The concept of rights: a historical sketch. In Bandman & Bandman.

Hare, R. M. Non-descriptivism. In *Encyclopedia of bioethics*.

Kant, I. *Foundations of the metaphysics of morals* (1898). (L. W. Beck, trans.) Indianapolis: The Bobbs-Merrill Co., Inc., 1959.

Kant, I. *Lectures on ethics*. (L. Infield, trans.). New York: Harper & Row, Publishers, Inc., 1963.

May, W. E. Double effect. In *Encyclopedia of bioethics*.

Mill, J. S. *Utilitarianism* (1861). New York: The New American Library, Inc. 1974.

Modernizing the case for God. *Time*, April 7, 1980, pp. 65–68.

Peters, R. S. Respect for persons. In Rachels.

Rachels, J. *Understanding moral philosophy*. Encino, Calif.: Dickinson Publishing Company, 1976.

Rawls, J. Justice as fairness. *The Philosophical Review*, 1958, *67*, 164–94.

Regan, T. (Ed.). *Matters of life and death: new introductory essays in moral philosophy*. New York: Random House, Inc., 1980.

Ross, W. D. Difficulties for utilitarianism. In Rachels.

Taylor, P. W. *Principles of ethics*. Encino, Calif.: Dickinson Publishing Company, 1975.

CHAPTER 2

SEXUALITY AND SEXUAL ETHICS

PSYCHOSEXUAL DEVELOPMENT

Sexuality is one of the most complex forms of human behavior, sometimes the most exquisitely pleasurable, sometimes emotionally and physically painful and degrading, but most times somewhere in between. The subject of sexuality is endlessly interesting to most people, although many find it difficult to discuss for a variety of personal and sociocultural reasons. This chapter will place sexuality in a perspective in which it is not usually related, that is, it will be treated as a series of ethical dilemmas in terms of both interpersonal activities and activities about sex, for example, sex research and therapy.

To better understand sexuality and sexual ethics, we need to know how we became the way we are. Psychosexual development is a crucially important part of human development and begins at conception with determination of gender: XX chromosomes for the female and XY for the male. Also during fetal life sexual differentiation takes place. Anatomic and physiologic structures separate, and by the beginning of the second trimester the fetus takes on the physical appearance of either a male or a female. As systems develop and mature, sex hormones begin to appear. Some researchers, such as Money and Erhardt,[1] believe that hormones play a significant role in the sexual behavior of persons after birth, although little human experimentation has been done in this area.

After birth, psychosexual development begins in earnest, and the infant is almost immediately aware of pleasurable, even erotic, sensations. Freud was the first to write extensively about psychosexual development, and his views are still believed by many to be the fundamental work in the area. However, Freud is currently not popular in all quarters (particularly with feminists who disagree with his "anatomy is destiny" theory); moreover psychologists since Freud, notably Erikson and Piaget, have devised developmental theories of their own. But as Freud's writings are still the most pervasive, we will concentrate on his theories of psychosexual development. He labeled the first stage of psychosexual development the oral stage, during which the infant uses his mouth as the major channel through which to receive sexual pleasure. However, even very young infants have been found to be capable of sexual arousal, even orgasm, and do a great deal of touching and stroking their genitals. Because infants' cognition is not sufficiently developed, they probably derive a similar sense of pleasure (although the physical sensations themselves might differ) from both the mouth and the genitals. During the first year of life, infants require much stroking, cuddling, and all types of affectionate touching to be able to function as a fully sensual human being in later life.

By about 2 years of age children progress into what Freud called the anal stage. They are in the midst of toilet training and begin to experience conflict with the pleasure received from urination and defecation and the negative social signals they receive from their mothers about both the acts and the results produced. Masturbation is also becoming a more conscious act, as is the negative reinforcement that usually results.

By 3 years old children know the difference between boys and girls, and more attention is directed toward the genitals (Freud's genital or phallic phase), both one's own and those of one's playmates. Childhood games involving sexuality are played ("I'll show you if you'll show me"), and toddlers often imitate adult sexual behavior by much hugging, kissing, and touching. There is also enormous fascination with the differences in the way boys and girls urinate. Many parents have found a wet bathroom floor after experimentation with the opposite sex's way of urinating! This exploration and experimentation are as essential to children's psychosexual development as creative play is to their intellectual and emotional development.

Freud described the period between 5 and 12 years of age as the latency period, in which sexual feeling is less intense and emphasis is placed on social and intellectual development. Sexuality does not disappear from the child's life, however, as evidenced by games such as "house" and "doctor," which can include some very specific sexual play. Boys of this age frequently engage in group masturbation, which seems to serve as many social purposes as sexual ones. Children of both sexes engage in homosexual play, almost all of which is discarded in adult life. There has been no demonstrated correlation between homosexual play in children and adult homosexuality as a chosen preference or natural orientation. During this phase about 10% of all children have their first "real" sexual encounter, that is, sexual activity that involves another person and that is not primarily masturbatory in nature[2]; it sometimes involves an adult who is known to the child, frequently a family member. Sexual exploitation of children is more common than most people believe and has long-lasting negative influences on psychosexual development. It is probably safe to say that all sexual activity between children and adults is exploitive since children are not in a position to give truly informed consent about their desire to engage in sex. This is particularly true when a child is in some way dependent on the adult in question.

Adolescence is the psychosexual transition between childhood and adulthood, characterized physically by fertility and emotionally by reawakened feelings of sexuality. Masturbation increases, and adolescents begin sexual activity with other persons, although the age at which loss of virginity occurs and patterns of subsequent sexual activity vary greatly with sociocultural factors. Sexual conflicts rage; desires and feelings and the natural inclination to give vent to them conflict with parental pressure to repress them. Sex fantasies increase in variety and intensity and are often accompanied by guilt and the loneliness of thinking that one is alone in having "dirty" thoughts.

The male-female double standard of sexual permissiveness becomes more apparent and is a source of guilt and frustration. Both boys and girls masturbate to orgasm, although girls are less likely to recognize the orgasm for what it is, both because there is no physical discharge to "prove" orgasm has taken place, as occurs with boys, and because girls are subject to more social and cultural repression than boys. Girls are frequently led to believe that they do not need sex as much as boys and that they should be passive recipients of sex and take little or no active pleasure in feelings of sexuality or sexual activity. This double standard, although it has been diluted somewhat in the past decade, is still extremely powerful and contributes to many of the sexual and social stereotypes that interfere with healthy psychosexual development.

Sexual activity among adolescents is often characterized by experimentation, exploration, guilt, excitement, shame, and a sense of adventuring into forbidden territory. Sometimes the sex is joyless and resentful, engaged in more out of peer pressure than from a real desire to make love. Boys feel they must "prove" their manhood and frequently believe the locker room stories told by other boys and thus feel a need to "keep up with" the crowd. Girls feel pressure to acquiesce to boys' advances to "keep" a boyfriend, to maintain popularity, or because they need to bolster the constantly fluctuating self-esteem of adolescence. Often real love and feelings of intimacy accompany the sexual activity, but it is almost always developmentally immature. These feelings of love are intense and should not be denigrated by adults, especially parents. The sexual activity of adolescence, whether autoerotic or with a partner, always involves learning, and most adolescents emerge from the experience relatively unscathed emotionally.

Psychosexual development continues throughout life, but basic patterns are established by the end of adolescence. Adult development essentially consists of expanding one's sexual horizons, for example, engaging in a wider variety of sexual practices and experiencing deeper sensual feelings, perhaps making a foray, temporary or permanent, into bisexuality or homosexuality or establishing an increasingly intimate relationship with one person. Adulthood implies independence and establishment of careers and social lives; it also implies making sexual choices from a wide variety of sexual life-styles, including celibacy. All choices can be temporary or permanent; more likely they are the former because needs and desires change, and social, emotional, and intellectual development continue.

Adulthood is also the time to begin to resolve psychosexual conflicts. In doing so, one must perceive oneself as a separate moral entity to be able to separate one's needs and desires from those of one's parents, friends, or even a segment of society. A set of sexual values must be established that is congruent with the moral values of the rest of one's life. If this sense of congruency between one's sexual and nonsexual life is not established, conflict will ensue that will cause emotional problems for the individual and possibly harm sex partners. For example, a man who behaves with sensitive courtesy to his business and social associates but acts in a violently aggressive manner with his sex partners has not established congruency and is not applying the same moral theory to his sexual and nonsexual lives. He is not only in emotional trouble but is behaving unethically toward others.

Psychosexual development is intrinsically tied to moral development in that, except for masturbation, sexual activity always involves another person, who is usually physically and emotionally vulnerable. Sexuality, almost more than any other area of human endeavor, requires respect for persons. Any form of sexuality that involves depersonalization, that is, treating the sex partner as anything less than a freely autonomous person, signifies a failure of both sexual and moral development. Instances of depersonalization can range from the quietly insidious ("Come on, baby, you *know* you want it.") to the overtly blatant ("Women are only good for one thing.") and the physical violence of rape and other forms of sexual assault. Seduction, a widely popular sexual "sport," involves depersonalization that uses coercion as its method. Enticements to depersonalize sex are increasing in Western culture as a result of media depictions of sexuality in nonsexual contexts (a scantily clad woman advertising an automobile) and the advent of both "soft" and "hard" pornography. The culmination of this increase in depersonalization is the tremendous annual increase in the number of rapes, 49% in the period 1969 to 1974, even when the FBI estimates that over 50% of rapes are unreported.[3] This is not meant to imply that all sexual depersonalization is as violent as rape, but the person who treats a sex partner with anything less than full autonomy is operating on the same continuum that has rape at the end point. The difference is in degree, not in kind.

Kaplan[4] believes that errors or failures in psychosexual development cause sexual dysfunction in adulthood; her view is based on Freudian theory. It is not the purpose of this book to discuss various sexual dysfunctions (except where the dysfunction results in a moral dilemma), but it is important to understand that much "abnormal" sexual behavior is thought to be caused by unconscious repression and resistance of sexual thoughts and fantasies. These dysfunctions have always been thought to be a private matter between sex partners and the therapist, but many forms of sexual dysfunction involve violence, depersonalization, and coercion. When this occurs, sexuality becomes criminality, and the behavior no longer falls completely into the realm of private consentual acts. The moral dilemmas of sex research and therapy will be discussed later in this chapter.

Sexual identity

If one used the phrase *sexual identity* at the beginning of this century, the speaker would be thought to have a problem with language. After all, boys were boys and girls were girls, and the fact was as noncontroversial as the fact that the sun rises and sets each day. Now we read accounts of people with identity crises, hear that an Olympic athlete was subjected to chromosomal examination to determine gender, and are aware of the phenomenon known as transsexualism (the belief by a person that he has been assigned the "wrong" body, that is, a person of one gender feeling mentally and physically opposite in terms of gender identity). Sexual identity is not as clear-cut as previously thought. What has been previously thought of as natural sexual behaviors that were closely tied to gender and social roles and patterns are now being questioned. Sexual desires and proclivities are currently acknowledged as more androgenous than had been believed; this creates confusion about what is "right," what is "natural," and even what is morally acceptable. If a man behaved in a warm, gentle, and tender manner, he was believed to be less masculine than he should be, and if he preferred to take a passive role sexually, either sometimes or always, he frequently thought there was something seriously wrong with his ability to function. The conflict arose from differences between his own needs and desires and societal expectations.

Sexual identity is more accurately seen as a continuum, affected by variables such as personal preference, sociocultural factors, self-perception, parental attitudes, needs, and desires. Solomon and Sanders[5] group sexual identity into four categories: biologic sex, gender identity, sexual orientation, and sexual ethics. Biologic sex refers to anatomic structures and physiologic functions. It depends on chromosomal configuration, presence of sex gonads, presence and levels of sex hormones, internal reproductive structure, and external genitalia. Most of the time the combination of these five factors result in a biologic male or female. But increasing numbers of cases are being identified in which one or more of these characteristics are absent or in incorrect proportion to the others. Structural or functional anomalies can create components of both sexes in the same person.

Gender identity has always been thought to be a direct outgrowth of biologic sex and can be identified as the cultural and social role one plays as a result of one's biologic sex. Boys and girls have traditionally been socialized differently, and it is only within the last decade or so that this sharp distinction is becoming somewhat blurred. Sex role behavior has usually been learned on an imitative basis, but since traditional roles are no longer seen as absolute, imitation becomes confused with cross-imitation (men imitating certain female behaviors and vice versa). Past patterns and practices and stereotypical behaviors frequently no longer apply to modern social and emotional life.

Several patterns of atypical gender identity have been observed: homosexuality, in which biologic sex is consistent with gender identity, but sexual orientation is inconsistent with the usual way of "using" one's sexual identity, that is, in an attraction to the opposite sex; transvestism, in which a person takes pleasure from, and is usually sexually aroused by, wearing the traditional clothing of the opposite sex (transvestism is almost exclusively a male phenomenon); and transsexualism, described earlier, in which a person (90% of the time a man) wishes to anatomically and physiologically change gender.

Sexual orientation has to do with one's choice of sex partner and with preferred sexual activity. Researchers such as Money and Ehrhardt[6] and others have tentatively indicated that there may be a correlation between fetal hormones and sexual behavior. Most studies, however, have been done with rats and other animals; therefore conclusions about humans cannot be drawn. Sexual orientation results from many variables, such as social standards, parental influence, biologic factors, and personal preference. People choose sex partners and activities because they feel the choice will provide pleasure; the line between normal and abnormal, perverse and idiosyncratic, is difficult to draw and frequently involves matters of sexual ethics, which will be discussed in more detail later in this chapter.

SEXUAL BEHAVIOR
Forces of culture and tradition

Attitudes about sexuality and sexual behavior involve linkages of thoughts and feelings and result from socialization, which in turn results from the attitudes of the people one associates with. Attitudes change with age and with stages of moral development; what was believed to be particularly positive or negative about sex in adolescence may change by the time the person enters the middle years. Cultural norms are one of the most prevalent factors affecting attitudes about sexuality because they are usually incorporated into the life-style of the family and thus influence patterns of childhood behavior. Cultural norms can be rejected in adulthood, but it is usually difficult and accomplished only after much trepidation and guilt. Socioeconomic class and education are related to sexual attitudes. Kinsey[7] found that the more education a person had, the more he engaged in premarital sex, masturbation, and sexual activity not directly related to intercourse (fellatio and cunnilingus). Kinsey also found that the higher the social class, the more sexuality was connected to morality, that is, he found a strong sense of right and wrong in certain sexual behaviors and attitudes. The lower classes thought less about what was moral and more about what was natural. This represents the classic metaethical distinction between what *is* and what *ought* to be.

Sociocultural factors also affect the quality of sexual activity. A lower class couple, living in cramped quarters with thin walls and the threat of a baby about to burst into tears at any time, may find themselves rushed during sex and being forced to make love silently or with less freedom than they would wish. Sex is then unlikely to be consistently satisfying, surely of far different quality than the experiences of a single woman with her own apartment, a constant supply of candlelight, and a stereo for musical accompaniment.

A task orientation to sex will create a far different bedroom atmosphere than will a sensual orientation. A person who believes the only purpose for sex is orgasmic will bring a different attitude to bed than will the person who believes that sensuality is the most important ingredient in sex. Upper class women tend to have a higher rate of orgasm than do lower class women because they expect their partners to satisfy them and perhaps because they have a greater degree of sexual freedom, that is, an upper class woman will look for a satisfying partner, whereas a lower class woman will be more reluctant to experiment and has less opportunity to do so. Reasons for this phenomenon are mainly sociocultural. The more education and money a woman has, the higher are her expectations of life satisfaction, including sexual satisfaction. Education and money also tend to create a more sophisticated way of looking at life's options and the realization that there are many life-style choices.

Although it is not universally true, money and education mean greater freedom of social movement and therefore a wider circle of persons from whom to choose as friends, associates, and sex partners.

Sociocultural factors also have a strong influence on the psychosexual development of children. Cultures that have a strongly moralistic attitude about sex generally imbue children with a false sense of purity if they are able to repress all sexual thoughts and actions before marriage. Since it is impossible for children and adolescents not to think about sex and almost impossible not to experiment with masturbation and sex play with peers, the child grows up guilty and in conflict about adult sexuality. This sense of moralism and punitive behavior occurs mainly in highly religious cultures and among fundamentalist religious sects (all religions have branches or sects that are highly conservative or fundamentalist). Those cultures that do not encourage social interaction among children seem to produce adults who have trouble establishing mature and healthy sexual relationships. This is also true of people who were raised in families where parents did not display physical and emotional affection to each other.

Childhood socialization is more important than any other sociocultural factor in establishing adult sexual behavior patterns. American and many other Western children have been socialized along traditional gender-associated roles, that is, boys are taught to be aggressive, assertive human beings and therefore aggressive, assertive lovers. Women are expected to be passive and to wait for and wait on men. This socialization has frequently resulted in both men and women believing that men's sexual needs are more important than women's. Children receive constant reinforcement about conforming to sexual stereotypical behaviors in the toys they are given, the adult roles they are expected to fill, and the way they are treated and handled by their parents. Although there are some changes in these traditional patterns, mostly as a result of the women's movement, they are not as pervasive as feminists and nontraditionalists would prefer. Changes in traditional sociocultural sexual attitudes also follow class lines. The higher the class, the less resistance to change is observed.

Parental enculturation is frequently reinforced by the psychiatric establishment. For example, Hélène Deutsch[8] describes the typical feminine woman as leaving initiative to men, experiencing herself through others, possessing the quality of "feminine intuition," collaborating with and inspiring men, and being easily influenced by and adaptable to their companions. They may be gifted and original but do not enter into competitive struggles; they are willing to sacrifice their own achievements and then do not view it as a sacrifice. Deutsch wrote this description in 1944, but many psychiatrists still use it as an accurate view of women. Women who do not or will not conform to this stereotype are seen as masculine, and no matter how much professional or business success they achieve, they are seen as failures as women. A woman who wishes to compete with men in a traditional male world is frequently seen as maladjusted and outside the pale of womanhood.

Men too are irrevocably harmed by these sexual stereotypes in that if they choose a life-style not characterized by aggression, assertiveness, and competition, they are viewed as something less than masculine. If a woman is encouraged to be a dependent recipient of a man's social, economic, and sexual largesse, men are forced to assume all the responsibility for the dyadic relationship, that is, a man is enculturated to assume economic responsibility for several other human beings, his wife and children. If he is somehow unable to do this, or to do it less well than he or his family expects, his status in society is seriously diminished, and even worse, his self-esteem is threatened. Although conventional sex stereotyping obviously works against women in a harsher way, men are not immune from its detrimental effects.

In discussing the contemporary sociocultural aspects of sexuality, London believes that an increasingly permissive society has created conflicts. "People's sexual expectations have been turned up, as it were, but their anxiety and guilt continue to operate from more conservative platforms than their behavioral expectations. The moral anxiety produced by this ambivalence has behavioral consequences in symptoms that have been classical since Victorian times."[9] London lists these classic anxiety symptoms as a variety of physical sexual dysfunctions; adolescent behavioral problems resulting from performance anxiety rather than moral anxiety; increased numbers of people seeking sex therapy, which may or may not be appropriate or competent (sex therapy will be discussed in more detail later in this chapter); and lack of certainty about the limits of sexual permissibility. London also questions whether sexuality and sexual mores will or should remain a topic of ethical concern. He uses the analogy of moral injunctions about certain kinds of food; some Jews now eat anything without regard to traditional dietary laws, and many Catholics can barely remember that eating meat on Fridays was forbidden. A person who adopts the "anything goes as long as it feels good" attitude about sex might be analogous to the Jew who eats a ham sandwich with butter. Nontraditionalists will find this analogy imprecise, but "If sexual norms were to follow a similar course, then common attitudes and behavior connected with it, like those that predominate today with food, might become matters of preference, of health and manners, not of religion and morals."[10] Many believe that sexual attitudes *should* be a matter of personal preference, and equating religion and morality as opposed to preference is erroneous and confusing. Religious views about sexuality may or may not be similar to secular ethical views, and persons with similar attitudes may have arrived at them through different routes.

Masturbation is a sexual activity that has run the gamut of permissibility and is an excellent example of changing sociocultural norms. In the eighteenth and nineteenth centuries it was regarded as a serious physical and social disease that resulted in bodily deterioration because of loss of seminal fluid and mental deterioration because of the clandestine and subversive nature of the act. It was considered much worse than sexual intercourse (also not regarded with great favor) because it was unnatural and therefore debilitating. A long list of horrifying consequences was believed to result from masturbation, the worst of which was permanent insanity. In the latter part of the nineteenth century, although masturbation was still regarded as evil, it was also considered a disease in much the same pattern as the phenomenon of alcoholism. Masturbation was "cured" by all manner of ghastly procedures, most commonly clitoridectomy and castration, although there were some more lenient approaches such as "prescribing" prostitutes, cold baths before bedtime, and a variety of tonics.

The concept of masturbation changed from a moral evil to a disease, then to a condition that was thought to be second best to sex with another person but not quite as evil or harmful as had been previously believed. In the past decade or so, masturbation has been thought by many psychiatrists and sex therapists to be actively healthy, and it is recommended as a tension reliever, as a means to learn one's own sexual responses, and as a practice exercise, even when one is sexually active with a partner. Thus masturbation has come a full 180 degrees from a practice that was considered reprehensible and sick to one considered socially and medically approved. It is safe to say that attitudes about all forms of sexuality follow a similar pattern, determined by time, culture, socioeconomic conditions, and other circumstances.

THE SEXUAL REVOLUTION. The sexual revolution, which dates its beginning anywhere from the end of World War I to the counterculture movement of the 1960s, depending on who is defining and describing it, is a result of technology and publicity. Technology implies the means to sexual freedom or liberation: automobiles to make love in or to get to places where one can have sex, increased housing and affluence to ensure privacy, improvement in safety and availability of contraception, and the greater economic independence of women. The publicity of sex includes a wide variety of media—professional, popular, and pornographic. Although Freud, Kinsey, and a few others engaged in scholarly sex research, it has been only in the last decade or so that this research has been done on a widescale basis and has received government and private foundation funding. Medical, psychologic, and sociologic journals publish the results of the research, which is in turn picked up by the popular press. It is rare for a week to go by without a "serious" discussion of sex on television, and the theme of many situation programs has a sexual base.

Comedians' sex jokes have come out of private nightclubs and onto the public airways, and subscription cable television in some areas shows the most pornographic of films.

Pornography, both the soft and hard variety (the difference is the presence or absence of penile penetration), is a multibillion dollar business. A visit to an adult bookstore will boggle the mind with the variety of sex practices depicted in books, magazines, and films. Sex practices and beliefs that were once considered to be unspeakable perversions (homosexuality, transvestism, incest) are now casually discussed in public and private. This, then, is the sexual revolution: increased thinking and talking about sex and more sexual activity of a wider variety.

Is the sexual revolution good, bad, or morally indifferent? A utilitarian would make a moral assessment by calculating the total amount of happiness produced in the past two generations as a result of increased sexual awareness. If one compares Morton Hunt's 1972 survey and Kinsey's two studies of sexual behavior published in 1948 and 1953, it would seem that sexual happiness is indeed increased, at least among respondents to the survey who belong mainly to the educated upper-middle class. In every age group people reported more positive than negative feelings about sex and reported that they were having sex more frequently and were engaging in a greater variety of sex acts in 1972 than 20 years before. If we can assume that positive attitudes and practices about sex lead to increased happiness, then the utilitarian would view the sexual revolution as good and something to be encouraged and continued.

A deontologist, in determining goodness or badness of the sexual revolution, would look at individual characteristics and practices of various aspects of the phenomenon to see what is inherently good or bad about them. Pornography is a case in point. Can the portrayal of sex acts, and the selling of those pictures and films, be considered morally permissible? A Kantian would apply both formulations of the Categorical Imperative and would arrive at a negative answer each time. In the Kantian view pornography is immoral in all instances; that is, it is not universalizably permissible to portray and sell pictures of sex acts because pornography frequently involves the exploitation of those involved in its manufacture and distribution. The industry also uses persons as means only; for example, the models in the photographs and films are paid fees that are far from commensurate with the profits reaped. Moreover they are used as mere sex objects for the ultimate purpose of securing considerable profit for the manufacturers and distributors.

The deontologist would assess right- and wrong-making characteristics. Right-making ones would be exercise of First Amendment rights (free speech), whatever sexual pleasure is brought to the viewers of the material, and perhaps even profits in the free enterprise system. Wrong-making characteristics would include the illegal maneuverings involved in the industry, sexual exploitation of the models, financial exploitation of the purchasers (the profit margin on pornography is excessively high), and the incitement to sexual violence (studies conflict about whether this does indeed occur). The fact that certain types of pornography may be in poor taste, or esthetically displeasing is irrelevant to its morality.

Those people who argue about the sexual revolution on an ethical basis usually do so in relation to other areas of contemporary morality that seem to be eroding. In other words, sex is used as a barometer of morals in general, which may or may not be accurate or fair. If church attendance is down and violent crime is up, one wonders what this may have to do with the sexual revolution. Are the people who used to be in church out robbing banks or at home making love, or are the bank robbers and love makers not the same people who used to be in church? Is increased incidence of oral and anal sex, masturbation, and premarital intercourse necessarily a symptom of society's moral decay, or can it be part of the increase in leisure activities in general? Many sociologists and psychologists point to the increase in licentious sexual behavior just before the fall of the Roman Empire and make similar dire predictions for American civilization. It seems unlikely, though, that an increased variety of sexual behavior will win out over rampant inflation, irresponsible government, personal and corporate crime, bureaucratic inefficiency at all levels, a corrupt judicial system, massive pollution, and the energy crisis as causes of an eventual crumbling of American society.

Male-female social relationships

Sexual behavior is most frequently a function of societally induced and expected roles and relationships. If social training requires that a man be generally aggressive and a woman generally passive, then these behavioral expectations will spill over into the bedroom. If the sex partners wish it to be otherwise, a conscious effort must be made to evaluate and redirect the nature of the sexual relationship.

Changes in sex roles and behaviors generally conform to changes in other aspects of socioeconomic life. In the years during and following World War I through the mid-1920s women's roles changed radically. The women's movement began to form; women's suffrage came into existence; and women began to experiment with their new-found freedom. In the period following World War II and for about two decades afterward, as the country basked in peace and experienced tremendous economic growth, social roles solidified into the traditional male dominant–female passive pattern. In the late 1960s through the 1970s (and probably the remainder of the 1980s) an upsurge in social freedom for previously subjugated groups (blacks, women, and homosexuals) occurred, as did the beginning of economic independence for women as a result of increased career opportunities. Both men and women began to view their sexual relationships with new freedom.

Sexual stereotyping and social relationships have a strong effect on each other. The Freudian belief, ascribed to by many psychologists and psychiatrists even if they do not see themselves as strict Freudian practitioners, that men are superior to women because of the presence of a penis led to the erroneous belief that men *should* feel socially and sexually superior because they are biologically different from women. Thus the common practice of giving social and economic advantage to men was reinforced. Freud's "anatomy is destiny" proclamation that women will be forever relegated to inferior social and economic positions because of their childbearing capacity kept them economically dependent. Other psychologists have followed this Freudian model by "proving" in a variety of ways that a woman's major function was motherhood simply because she has the biologic capacity for such a role. All Western religions place women in an inferior position and generally respect only their roles of homemaker and mother. Women have rarely been permitted to play a role in religions' administrative or ecclesiastical functions, and as these are the primary reason for the existence of any religion, women were again viewed as less important than men.

The inequality of socioeconomic positions shows a partially causal relationship with sexual roles and functions. Adolescent girls wait for the telephone to ring, wait for the boy to make the first "pass," and then frequently make a decision to engage in sex more on the basis of what the boy wants (or says he needs) than out of mutual choice. Advancing age changes little. A married woman who is economically dependent on her husband has little choice in the matter of sex. If she consistently refuses to meet his sexual needs, she can be faced with the threat of further economic deprivation if he leaves her and if she has no other means of economic support. Although this situation is slowly changing in the United States, many women still feel obligated to meet their husbands' sexual needs.

By far the greatest impetus to change traditional stereotypes of belief and practice has been the women's liberation movement. The movement began in the midnineteenth century in the United States and has waxed and waned ever since. Early feminists such as Lucretia Mott, Elizabeth Cady Stanton, and Susan B. Anthony were most concerned with suffrage, domestic enslavement, and economic exploitation. After women received the right to vote, the movement moved into a quieter, less public phase that was mainly concerned with bettering women's "female" roles, that is, improved maternal and child health services, better working conditions, and more equitable domestic laws. The

World War II experience raised the consciousness of American women, and after two decades of quietude (and mounting anger), the modern women's movement burst into the open. It is not the purpose of this chapter to delineate the history of the movement but to show how it affected relationships between men and women and how that in turn affects sexual ethics.

The primary goal of the movement is achievement of economic and social equality for women. When this equality is achieved, women will be on the way to full independence. Socioeconomic independence will pave the way for love relationships based on mutual respect for persons, not on the need for one or the other partner to perform certain societally expected roles in return for other expected behaviors. Although it is too simplistic to draw a direct causal relationship between socioeconomic inequality and physically violent or psychologically coercive sexual relationships, it can be said that a woman or man who has achieved a measure of personal or financial independence is in a better position to make sexual choices and can behave in a way that is desired rather than one that is expected or even demanded. If a woman can earn her own living, she need not view men as "meal tickets" (if a single woman pays for her half of the evening's entertainment, she need not feel obligated to sleep with her dinner partner, and this lack of obligation can heighten her sense of freely choosing what she is doing and thus increase sexual pleasure). At the same time, a man who is not totally financially responsible for a woman and children will experience a decrease in anxiety with a resultant increase in the ability to relax and enjoy sex. A woman who is not economically dependent on a man need not be exploited by him.

Another goal of the women's movement is the fulfillment of women's talents and potentials outside the traditional female role, that is, the ability to exercise choice about life-styles. Freedom of choice in terms of education and career could lead to freedom of choice in sexual activity. A woman who knows what she wants in the nonsexual aspects of her life is likely to be a woman who knows what she wants sexually and will take steps to find a satisfying sex partner. Freedom not to be a mother, or to be one only in certain circumstances, leads to greater freedom of choice in sexual life-styles. Those women who wish not to marry, or to marry and remain childless, will be free to pursue the sexual life-styles they wish without the unwanted burdens of motherhood. In the event that a completely safe and reliable method of contraception becomes available, this freedom will be complete, as long as it is accompanied by economic independence and the kind of society that practices equality of the sexes.

The women's movement has resulted in conflict as well as independence. Centuries of traditional functioning cannot be changed without emotional trauma and serious attempts at thwarting that change. Women may not feel prepared for a larger social and economic role and may be comfortable with a false sense of security in a dependent role. Many men feel threatened by women's increasing independence, particularly as the latter begin to climb the career ladder as equals. Men have traditionally held all the domestic, occupational, and political power, and many are not willing to relinquish it easily. This conflict is likely to lead to anger and resentment, which can manifest itself in increased sexual exploitation and decreased sexual pleasure.

Kaplan[11] cites several areas in which poor social relationships result in less than satisfactory sexual relationships. Striving to attain some kind of mythical sexual perfection such as mutual orgasm or perfect bliss during each sexual encounter will undoubtedly lead to frustration. This is usually a result of either ignorance or "too much" information. What one sex manual or another describes as the height of sexual ecstasy may be unsuitable for particular individuals or couples. Social conflict between partners almost always results in sexual conflict. A man who resents his wife's increasing involvement with her job may "punish" her by refusing to perform her favorite sexual activities; by the same token, a woman who must always ask her husband for spending money will feel less inclined to do his favorite sexual things. Fear of failure in sexual performance can frequently cause failure. "Our experience suggests that generally insecure men and men whose behavior is excessively governed by a need to excel and to compete are particularly vulnerable to the fear of sexual failure."[12]

There is no reason to believe that this cycle of anxiety and sexual dysfunction does not apply equally to women, especially as they move out of the home and into the world of business and professional competition. Many couples are troubled by one or the other partner having an excessive need to please the other, although this phenomenon is much more common in women than in men because of traditional socialization: pleasing men by having perfect bodies, by always making certain the man has an orgasm, and by having one themselves so the man will think himself an adequate lover. A woman's expected need to please her partner can result in sex under less than pleasing circumstances, lovemaking that is too rushed, and worst of all, the need to fake an orgasm. Kaplan reports many instances of women who are highly orgasmic during masturbation but who cannot achieve orgasm during lovemaking with a male partner because they are trying too hard to please him.

Many couples continue to function in a relationship that has long since lost all emotional and sexual pleasure for both partners. This is sometimes the result of inertia, but more often there are practical reasons for not parting: economic dependence, lack of insight into the cause of the problems, the belief that children will be negatively affected, fear of being alone, and many others. It is almost impossible to have a gratifying sexual relationship when the social relationship has deteriorated.

"NORMAL" AND "ABNORMAL" SEXUAL ACTIVITY. The words *normal* and *abnormal* have been placed in quotations because there is no clear-cut definition of what is normal in the realm of sexuality. A sexual practice that makes one person cringe in horror at its very thought is practiced routinely and with great pleasure by another person. We might use the term *normal* to describe sexual activities practiced by significant numbers of people but that would be more indicative of changes in sexual "fashion" than in identifying the morality or health of the practice. For example, far more people in the 1972 Hunt survey admitted to practicing oral and anal sex than was acknowledged in the 1948 and 1953 Kinsey studies. Did oral and anal sex become more normal or more popular in two decades? The comparison of these two studies showed a great increase in the amount of both premarital sex and adultery. We can assume that the ethical correctness or incorrectness of these two activities has not changed in 20 years; has it become more or less normal? If normal means increased incidence, then adultery is more normal, but common sense tells us that this indicator is absurd. Intercourse with animals is more common among farmers than among nonfarmers; it would be ridiculous to assume that city folk are more sexually normal than rural folk. We need a better definition of normalcy, particularly in an age when almost any sexual activity is considered normal as long as it provides pleasure to those participating. Is there anything that is so bizarre or out of the ordinary that it is considered abnormal, and if so, is it also unethical? Solomon and Sanders[13] answer the question by discussing the philosophic and psychologic purposes of sex. They have isolated four different conceptions or models of sexuality: the reproduction, the pleasure, the metaphysical, and the communication models.

The reproduction model is what its name implies—any sexual activity that leads to reproduction is natural and therefore normal; all excessive sexuality should be avoided. Men and women, actually husbands and wives, have a God-given duty to reproduce, but pleasure during this reproductive function is unnecessary. Male orgasm is, of course, essential for reproduction, while female orgasm is not. A woman's orgasm is thought to be permissible if it happens to occur during intercourse, but to take specific action to bring about female orgasm is a perversion. Mutual pleasure, if it is prolonged beyond the point necessary to achieve intercourse, is seen as superfluous and therefore impermissible. The reproduction model is viewed as the correct one by people who practice a traditional and fundamental religion; Darwinists see it as essential for preservation of the species. The latter are not specifically opposed to pleasure as long as intercourse always takes place.

The pleasure model might be interpreted as a liberal reaction to the conservative reproduction model. It can also be called the Freudian model because it was Freud who was first responsible for the theory that sex is enjoyable for its own sake and has purposes other than reproduction. The pleasure model, at least as postulated by Freud, is male oriented because in addition to being a vehicle for pleasure, sex is also used to relieve physical and psychic tension, culminating in a physical discharge. The real foundation of the pleasure model is that sex *ought* to be pleasurable, that is, "good" sex provides a maximum of pleasure; "bad" sex fails to satisfy either or both partners. Using this model, nothing that provides pleasure is a perversion or is impermissible.

The metaphysical model is based on the classical platonic expression of love (despite current usage, Plato never conceived of the model as sexless) as the fusion of two half souls to form a unity. Neither reproduction nor pleasure is the purpose of sex in the metaphysical model; the meaning of the love relation-ship becomes the primary goal. This meaning can be enhanced by sexual pleasure, even by reproduction, but these aspects are secondary to the fusion of souls.

The communication model addresses itself to the many varieties of sexual experience that are not based on reproduction or everlasting love but that exist for a deeper purpose than mere pleasure. This model views sex as a form of physical expression of feelings: domination or submission, tenderness, concern, passion, anger, and an almost endless variety of others. The communication model shifts the emphasis from the purely physical or metaphysical to aspects of interpersonal communication in the form of body language. Sexual activities and positions often symbolize certain feelings and expressions, for example, holding a partner's body in such a way that freedom of movement is curtailed can symbolize anger or the need to dominate. Sex in a side-lying position or standing up can indicate equality in the relationship or perhaps just the mood of the moment. "What marks the communication model from the three more traditional models is its emphasis on expression of interpersonal emotions and attitudes. These expressions are recognized by the other models, but not as essential and primary."[14]

It now becomes evident that the question of normalcy in sex remains an unclear issue. It depends primarily on how one views the purpose of sex, although it is unlikely that one's view will fit neatly into only one of the four categories, except perhaps for the most conservative traditionalists. Normalcy in sexual matters also depends to some extent on the biologic and chromo-somal makeup of the individual, as well as his social conditioning. A homo-sexual orientation, for example, may be considered one of several variations on sexual orientation and may thus be viewed as perfectly normal, just as pre-ferring intercourse using the rear-entry position may be viewed as a normal choice of many positions for intercourse. "If sexual normalcy includes sub-jective preference and psychological as well as biological considerations, then any definition of sexual normalcy will necessarily give priority to certain preferences and models over others. But which ones?"[15] What ought to be considered normal remains an ethical dilemma. An ethical absolutist becomes hopelessly lost in a sea of cultural differences and personal preferences, none of which are right or wrong if they do not harm. There are no objective standards for defining sexual normalcy, but the study of ethics in sexuality should not be abandoned; it merely must take into consideration the great diversity of sociocultural values.

SEX RESEARCH

Sex research is carried out in several important ways. One is a survey of reported sexual attitudes and practices. Alfred Kinsey and his associates produced the first major survey of American sexual habits; its purpose was to dispel myths and correct misinformation about sex. The Kinsey associates conducted two major surveys, one in 1948 and the other in 1953, while the nation was experiencing a period of socioeconomic calm and prosperity that some might describe as somnolence. Neither survey represented an accurate cross section of Americans; respondents were mainly Protestant upper-middle class, well educated, urban and suburban, and lived east of the Mississippi. Although the sampling methods were less than desirable, the interview techniques were excellent and the information obtained was valid and reliable. The Kinsey reports constituted a major revelation about American sexual attitudes and habits.

Morton Hunt's 1972 survey for the Playboy Foundation was a more accurate representation of the diversity of Americans, although only 20% of those who received questionnaires participated in the survey. The questionnaire contained over 1000 questions; therefore one might assume that those who responded had a particularly great interest in thinking about and discussing sex, as well as the time and verbal skills necessary to communicate those attitudes.

Another type of sex research is ethnographic, or the participant-observer method. A researcher joins a group of people, usually a subculture, and participates in the sociosexual activities of the group. This method is frequently used in studying homosexual activities and life-styles. If the researcher is well trained and experienced, ethnographic studies can be accurate, interesting, and useful.

Masters and Johnson were the first to publish results of sex research using direct observation methods in a laboratory. Their research was directed primarily toward understanding the physiology of sex, that is, exactly what happens in and to various genital and nongenital organs during sexual activity. Cameras, microphones, and other recording and measuring devices were used to assure accuracy. The research required volunteers who were not bothered by the fact that their sexual activity was observed by humans and machines, who were capable of sexual response in such situations, and who had normal genitals. They also had to be capable of accurately communicating their experiences and reactions to them. These requirements guaranteed that Masters and Johnson would have a relatively small, nonrepresentative sample of volunteers from which to choose. The first sample consisted of 11 members of an academic community with prostitutes as partners (coyly referred to as "surrogate sex partners"). As Masters and Johnson continued their research, however, the number of volunteers grew, and the sample became slightly more representative.

Ethical issues

Is sex research different in form, content, and function from other types of physical and social research, and if so, how is it different, and how can general ethical principles of research be applied? Kolodny[16] believes that sex research is significantly different from other research, mainly because of both positive and negative public attitudes toward sex research. However, the public also has extremely strong emotional responses to other biomedical research, for example, the tremendous hue and cry over recombinant DNA and other types of genetic engineering studies and the public reaction (at least the members of the public who care about such things) to fetal research.

There are, however, areas of sex research that contain particularly hazardous pitfalls. The first is the research design: determining the appropriateness of the study itself (*why* is the information necessary, and *how* will it benefit human life?), choosing a population to be studied, and deciding how the information will be gathered. Some sex research studies use subjects who are already clients of sex therapists, and some use volunteers. Both groups present problems. Should the clinician therapist also be the researcher? If so, objectivity of the study may suffer, but subjects will not be placed in the position of having to reveal the most intimate physical and emotional parts of themselves to two groups of clinicians. In addition, the more people involved with any one subject or couple, the more chances for absolute confidentiality are decreased. Some studies use two groups of subjects, an intervention group (therapeutic) and a nonintervention control group (nontherapeutic). This poses problems also. Random selection is impossible because subjects already know they are engaging in sex therapy, and those people in individual sex therapy (as opposed to couple therapy) cannot be assigned to a random partner except under certain limited conditions. Comparing results of the two groups is almost impossible because of the unlimited number of human variables involved in sexuality.

Recruitment of subjects is also fraught with ethical dangers. The advertisement or announcement must be worded in such a way that the potential subject knows the nature of the research, but if it is too detailed, potential subjects may be repelled. The interview that precedes the subject's decision to volunteer must contain all the elements of informed consent, and this necessarily involves a discussion of the potential subject's sexual attitudes and behaviors *before* the subject and researcher agree to work together. If no agreement is reached, the subject has still participated in the research to some degree by revealing private aspects of himself. Although he is not officially a subject, he has subjected himself to the researcher's questioning. To protect potential subjects' privacy, the selection interview must be considered confidential.

Protection of subjects and scrupulous regard for their rights are particularly important in sex research because there is a strong tendency among researchers to take a slightly more cavalier attitude toward sex research subjects than toward those of biomedical research that deals with physical or mental disease. There are many scientists and laypersons who think:

> research in sexual functioning or sexuality violates an implicit moral code that precludes sex from the realm of investigation. There are, unfortunately, scientists, politicians, theologians, and educators who regard sex research as a bastardization of science and an unwarranted intrusion into the private lives of our citizenry.[17]

For the very reason that sex is surrounded by so many myths and taboos, sex researchers must be particularly careful about protecting subjects' rights.

In many states particular sexual acts are forbidden by law, the most common of which are sodomy, fellatio, and cunnilingus. Because a study would lose its validity if some sex practices were excluded, what is the ethical position of the researcher who asks subjects to knowingly break the law? Research findings must be used with great caution, and there may even be data that should be suppressed. This latter possibility is a serious ethical dilemma. Does the research subject have the right to all information that pertains to him? What if, for example, during the course of research a man, who was quite contentedly functioning as a heterosexual, were found to have strong latent homosexual desires, but they had not surfaced in his conscious mind. This is information about him, but how can the researcher know that he (1) wants the information and (2) would not be irrevocably harmed by it? This is a classic bioethical dilemma because it causes ethical principles to come into conflict. The principle of truth telling requires that the researcher tell all he knows about the subject, but the principle of nonmaleficence requires that he carefully consider all the ramifications before doing so.

The reader is referred to the vast amount of literature on the principles of informed consent in general, but some considerations specific to sex research should be mentioned here. The first is inadvertant violations of confidentiality if persons known to the subject are on the research team (confidentiality will be discussed in more detail later in this chapter), if records are carelessly kept, or if communication with the subject is carried out in a less than confidential manner. The second area of risk is possible long-term effects arising from having agreed to participate in the study: guilt, changed sexual patterns as a result of having been so closely observed, and social ostracism as a result of having participated. This is an interesting issue because scholarly sex research is so new an endeavor that researchers are not aware of the variety of long-term effects and thus cannot be expected to warn subjects about them. Some risks cannot be foreseen and some cannot be avoided. A researcher may know that some subjects will experience guilt or regret, but he cannot accurately predict when and where it will occur. There are human limitations on the amount and kind of information a potential subject can reasonably expect, and the subject must realize that he is participating in *research*, which by its nature contains unknown outcomes. The subject must be willing to take a certain amount of risk, and the researcher is obligated to keep that risk to a minimum.

The topic of deception in social and behavioral research must be addressed. Many researchers believe that psychosocial research (sex research cuts across the boundaries of social, psychologic, and physical research) is almost useless unless it has some elements of deception built into the design. How, they ask, will they be able to determine how people will behave in a variety of circumstances if subjects are told beforehand the exact circumstances of the research situation and have time to rehearse behaviors? Researchers can be tempted to use deception, not in the interest of doing conscious wrong, but because "good" science is likely to result. Few researchers intend to harm subjects, but during the course of justifying and rationalizing the deception, ethical standards tend to slip. The Department of Health and Human Services (DHHS), in a 1979 amendment to the guidelines established by the National Commission for the Protection of Human Subjects of Biomedical and Behavioral Research, established the following about deception in research[18]:

1. Deception will not materially affect the ability of the subject to assess the harm or discomfort of the research.
2. Sufficient information must be disclosed to give the subject fair opportunity to decide whether or not to participate.
3. The research must be of the nature that it could not be reasonably carried out without deception.
4. Deception must not be for the purpose of eliciting participation.
5. Whenever possible, the subject will be debriefed after participation.

Aside from these rather sketchy guidelines, DHHS appears to ignore the matter of deception in research. This is in sharp contrast (and seemingly contradictory) to the guidelines pertaining to informed consent that rest on the principle of truth-telling.

Another major area of concern in sex research is using surrogate partners, usually prostitutes who receive a consultation fee. For those who believe that sex with anyone other than a spouse is morally wrong, using surrogate partners would be impermissible, no matter how important the results of the research or how ultimately beneficial to either the subject or to the general populace. It is interesting to note, however, that female surrogates are found less objectionable than males. This is most likely a function of the double standard, or perhaps because we are more used to thinking of women than men as prostitutes. There would seem to be one major advantage for the surrogates themselves; a prostitute who participates in sex research risks fewer of the well-known hazards of her profession than if she were having sex with her usual customers. Her job safety increases significantly in the sex researcher's laboratory.

Sex research has been the target of enormous amounts of publicity, especially since Masters and Johnson first published their research results. Subsequently, the number of quacks, charlatans, and outright imposters has proliferated. There is little, if any, protection for the public when they fall into the hands of nonscientific sex researchers. Many states do not require a license for marriage counseling or other types of psychotherapeutic help. Any group of individuals can band together to form an "institute" for sex research, and as long as they receive no federal funds, they are not bound by the DHHS guidelines for the protection of human subjects. This leaves the door wide open for all kinds of mischief done under the guise of sex research.

CONFIDENTIALITY AND SUBJECTS' PRIVACY. The terms *confidentiality* and *privacy* are not precisely synonymous, but for the purpose here they will be treated as such. A relationship, as that between subject and researcher, that is confidential is also necessarily private. The goal of confidentiality in professional relationships in general and in sex research in particular is that as few people as possible know that a particular subject is participating in the research and that *no one* will have the information unless the subject gives consent in writing.

Maintaining confidentiality serves the researcher's interests as well as the subject's. If the subject does not feel as though he has been given as much privacy as possible during the course of the research, either in discussing sex or in participating in it, he is unlikely to be candid, and the study will be less valid and less reliable.

The United States Constitution does not specifically guarantee rights to privacy, but several amendments of the Bill of Rights can be interpreted with an eye toward protecting citizens' privacy. Supreme Court cases have upheld individuals' rights to privacy in sexual matters. *Griswold v. Connecticut* (1965) struck down the state's mandate to prevent individuals from using contraception, and *Eisenstadt v. Baird* (1972) guaranteed that persons are protected from unwarranted governmental intrusion in childbearing decisions.[19] From these and other decisions one can infer the right to privacy in the matter of sex research, especially if the researcher has guaranteed it in writing. In addition, early in 1976 the Code of Federal Regulations (Chapter 1, Title 42 CFR) was amended to establish a procedure in which a person conducting mental health research could apply for authorization to protect the privacy of subjects, that is, the researcher could not be required to reveal the identity of subjects without consent of the subject, unless the subject's health or safety were threatened. The amendment is not all-encompassing because it is project-specific. The researcher must reapply for authorization with each new study, but it is not automatically granted.

Because much sex research is done with the aid of federal funds, subjects' privacy was in serious jeopardy before the Privacy Act was passed in 1974, which required federal agencies to protect the privacy of citizens in the following ways:

1. An individual may determine what records are collected, used, and disseminated by all federal agencies.
2. Dissemination of records may not be done without consent of the individual.
3. The agency is liable for civil suit for violation of regulations.
4. Individuals may have a copy of all records and may correct or amend them.
5. The federal agency must determine that all information is accurate and current and that safeguards are exercised during use of the records.

Although the Privacy Act appears to protect individuals, in reality it is far less effective than it should be. Most people do not know the act exists, and it is only theoretically possible to contact every single federal agency to find out what records exist for each individual. Exceptions to the Privacy Act are so numerous and so loosely worded that information can flow freely from one agency to another (or to persons or groups not a federal agency) with almost total impunity. Because a sex researcher who receives federal funds becomes a federal agency, the subject is protected by the Privacy Act, but this privacy may be jeopardized by the 1966 Freedom of Information Act, which requires the government to publish in the *Federal Register* information pertaining to research activities. Names of individual subjects may be omitted, but other federal agencies can obtain names under certain circumstances and for certain needs: national security, welfare or personnel files, investigation by law enforcement agencies, and a variety of others. Thus it appears that the federal government provides confidentiality to subjects with one hand and removes that right with the other.

The concern about privacy and confidentiality in the conduct of research and surrounding data storage and retrieval reflects our society's conflict of values. A policy that protects confidentiality of researchers and of human research participants conflicts with our national policy of freedom of information. This conflict may be particularly germaine for the scientific community as research and, increasingly, therapy are publicly financed. Some accommodation between the competing values of confidentiality and freedom of information is necessary.[20]

In other words, if government pays for sex research (or therapy), does it then have the right to information about people's sex lives and attitudes? Release of information may be self-defeating in the long run because of the decreased accuracy of research mentioned previously. One must, however, also weigh the value of the sex research projects that are being increasingly criticized by professionals and the laity.

Sex research is a relatively new area of endeavor and has taken on some bandwagon characteristics; there is little actual empirical work available, and it does have a somewhat titillating nature (a sex researcher can guarantee that his study will be read with avid interest!). However, enthusiasm must be tempered with questions: What is the purpose of the research? How much new knowledge will it provide? How will the knowledge improve the quality of people's (sex) lives? What is the potential for exploitation of the knowledge in relation to its social usefulness?

SEX THERAPY

Sex therapy focuses on relief of sexual symptoms or dysfunctions that are bothersome to the client. Treatment techniques usually consist of a combination of traditional, although perhaps abbreviated, psychotherapy and prescribed sexual experiences. A sexual dysfunction is defined as an impairment of the physical components of the sex response. This seemingly simple definition springs from a host of sociocultural and emotional factors that combine to interfere with an individual's erotic experience. Kaplan[21] believes that for an individual to be able to function well sexually, he must be able to abandon control to some degree, to give up some present contact with his environment, and to give himself over to the erotic experience. Any conscious or unconscious monitoring of sexual activity can cause interference with the autonomic reflexes resulting in physical symptoms, for example, inability to achieve or maintain an erection, loss of function of Bartholin's glands, premature ejaculation, and an almost infinite variety of others. Much sexual dysfunction is temporary, and although it causes the individual concern, it usually disappears spontaneously. Everyone is subject to sexual dysfunction from time to time. It is usually the result of physical or emotional disturbances.

Sexual dysfunction that is permanent or long-lasting frequently responds to therapy. The purpose of this section is to discuss the *implications* of therapy, not its technique, but a brief overview of the most common methods of sex therapy is essential to understand resulting ethical dilemmas.

Some forms of sex therapy concentrate almost solely on exercises designed to either increase or decrease conscious control over sexual function, for example, exerting manual pressure just below the glans penis when a man feels he is ready to ejaculate to control premature ejaculation or bringing a woman to orgasm by manual stimulation of her clitoris with no responsibility on her part to do anything but be the recipient of sexual pleasure. This is called the "here and now" technique because it concentrates almost entirely on physical function. Another form of sex therapy involves marriage or couple counseling if it is thought that the dysfunction arises from the couple's faulty interpersonal relationship. This method may or may not involve physical exercises along with counseling.

Some sexual dysfunction is so severe and deep-rooted that it requires intensive psychotherapy or psychoanalysis, which can continue for years and is not always ultimately successful. Sexual dysfunction that responds to long-term treatment usually is a result of failures of or interruptions in normal psychosexual development during childhood. These may arise from excessively rigid or negative parental attitudes and behaviors or a childhood trauma such as rape or incest.

There is as wide a variety of causes of sexual dysfunction as there are dysfunctions themselves; sex therapy has frequently been successful in treating the dysfunctions, but it has just as often done no good at all. Success depends on many factors, such as recognition that a problem exists in the first place, the relationship with both the partner and the sex therapist, the cause of the problem, and the individual's attitude toward the problem. For example, if a man is impotent whenever he tries to engage in sex with another person, he must acknowledge that the problem is his, not his partner's. He should be ready to examine his sexual and nonsexual human relationships and his attitude toward alleviating the problem.

There are different varieties of sex therapy, depending on the theoretic orientation of the therapist. The Freudian therapist generally concentrates on failures of psychosexual development and attempts to resolve conflict originating in childhood. It is generally male oriented with a goal of full sexual satisfaction from penile penetration of the vagina. Other forms of sexual expression are acceptable as "normal" as long as the ultimate goal is intercourse. Freudian therapy views the height of sexual satisfaction as orgasmic response to intercourse for both the man and woman. Few people would deny that pleasurable intercourse, including orgasm, is a worthwhile goal, but it need not be the *only* goal, and in this respect Freudian therapy is traditional and tends to place a limit on choice in sexual therapy. A Freudian therapist would tend to brand a woman as less feminine, and therefore less adequate as a human being, if she prefers to reach orgasm by having her clitoris stimulated by her partner's tongue rather than by engaging in sexual intercourse. Freudian therapy is viewed with great justifiable skepticism by feminists and others who do not accept the "anatomy is destiny" philosophy for either men or women.

Jungian therapy is as traditional as is Freudian, although in a different way. Jung saw women as spiritual Earth Mothers who were destined to be mystical, fertile, and fulfilled by a man. Therefore Jungian sex therapy concentrates on achieving total satisfaction through a man's vaginal penetration of the passive woman recipient. Women who are socially or sexually aggressive or assertive are viewed by Jungian therapists as masculine and thus unable to come to terms with their feminine nature. Both Freudian and Jungian therapy rely heavily on verbal analysis of factors leading to sexual dysfunction; there is little discussion of the sexual process itself. The primary goal for the therapist is not treatment of the sexual dysfunction per se but the underlying factors that cause it to exist. The client who seeks help only for sexual dysfunction may find himself embarked on a long course of analysis before he realizes that his goals and those of the therapist differ. Extricating oneself from therapy is difficult.

Behavior modification is a form of therapy that is increasing in popularity and consists of reinforcing positive, pleasurable sexual activity and avoiding negative or nonpleasurable activity. Many references exist about behavior modification techniques; in sex therapy concentration is placed on increasing pleasurable sensations of any kind by giving the partner verbal or physical rewards. B. F. Skinner is the psychologist most closely associated with behaviorism; he believes that sexual behavior, as all behavior, is simply a measurable psychologic and physical response to a stimulus. Errors in response can be corrected by redirecting either the stimulus or the response to it. Aversive therapy (application of intensely unpleasant, usually painful, sensations to negatively reinforce certain kinds of behavior) is used to treat the extremes of socially unacceptable behavior such as pederasty, incest, and rape.*

General ethical issues

Whatever mode of sex therapy is chosen, the most important ingredient is the relationship between the therapist and the client; this relationship depends to a great degree on the ethical sensitivity of the therapist. Several areas exist in

---

*Although rape is not considered a sexual activity, sex organs are used in the commission of the crime, and it is therefore thought by some to be a sex crime.

which it is common to find violations of ethical principles. The most common occurs when the therapist engages in sexual activities with clients, the "let me show you how it should be done" approach. In almost all instances the therapist is a man and the client a woman who is in a particularly vulnerable state of mind, as is common among clients of psychologic counseling. There is no possible justification, from either a utilitarian or a deontologic point of view, for a therapist having sex with a client, no matter how therapeutic the rationale might appear. Therapists who have problems with their own sexual adequacy or functioning have no business counseling others with similar difficulties. It is safe to say that sex between therapist and client is always unethical.

Another common area of ethical violation is the attempt to project a new set of sexual values on the client or to undermine the client's sense of sexual morality. The purpose of sex therapy is to improve function, not to change values or beliefs.

Sex therapists (if they are indeed therapists) sometimes misrepresent their credentials or qualifications. Sex therapy is a field that is ripe for exploitation, particularly as most states have no licensing requirements, and almost anyone with a reasonably good business sense and persuasive manner can practice sex therapy with almost complete impunity.

Under what circumstances should a person seek sex therapy, that is, is sex therapy ever morally obligatory and not merely a matter of personal preference to increase happiness or pleasure? A bit further down the continuum of obligation is the question of whether the state can ever morally require an individual to undergo sex therapy. A case in point is nonviolent sex offenders, for example, exhibitionists (those who receive sexual pleasure from exposing their genitals) and voyeurs (those who are sexually stimulated by watching sexual activity). These two variants of sexual behavior, which are usually accompanied by masturbation to orgasm, are not considered a problem, except perhaps to the exhibitionists and voyeurs themselves, until the behavior takes place in public, and the individual is arrested, usually many times. Although "flashers" and "peeping Toms" are breaking the law, and people are shocked and offended, the crime is not serious in itself, and almost never is anyone physically harmed. No one benefits from jailing the offender, and a fine serves only to fatten the community's coffers; it does not solve the sexual or social problem. However, the public fears these nonviolent sex offenders because it is commonly believed that these activities are a forerunner to sexual violence, that harmless peeping will turn to violent action. There are no statistics to prove that such a causal relationship exists, but because the public believes it to be so, punishments remain as they are.

The public's right not to be subjected to exhibitionists and voyeurs must be protected; thus it would seem that enforced sex therapy is a reasonable, helpful, just, and humane course of action. But is it?

> Being arrested or in jail is a trauma that allows the sex offender to seek treatment. Ordinarily, sex offenders do not feel any more hurt or disabled because of their sex lives than do nonoffenders. They know their behavior is socially stigmatized and punishable, but the threat of punishment is not traumatic enough to induce them to seek treatment. Thus, to fail to provide treatment at the time of arrest or imprisonment is, in most instances, to fail forever.[22]

In his belief in the benefit of treatment, Money fails to take into account several considerations—if the offender does not feel disabled, he is a poor candidate for therapy because he is not convinced of its necessity. This lack of conviction will inhibit him from voluntarily giving informed consent for treatment. If he does submit to treatment to get out of jail or to lighten his sentence, one must immediately suspect coercion. The nonviolent sex offender, after his second or third arrest, usually has two choices: serve out the current prison sentence, and be almost certain of rearrest for repetition of the behavior, or enter sex therapy. In the first choice the individual must regard himself (and be regarded by society) as a criminal; in the second choice the label is mental illness. Both carry great social stigmata. Is either designation morally correct?

Society, by legally forcing its citizens to cover certain parts of their bodies (except in specific places such as private homes and nudist colonies), is exercising a collective personal preference in matters of taste, which should have no bearing on what is or is not morally correct. It is a matter of preference, with strong Puritanical overtones, that penises should be covered in public while feet may be exposed—or knees or earlobes. The human tongue is used as an instrument of sexual pleasure almost as frequently as the penis, yet we are not required to go about in public with adhesive tape over our mouths! Therefore why is it morally wrong for a man to want others to admire his penis while it is morally neutral to want others to admire his face? Exhibitionism, then, can be seen as a matter of collective public preference, not a matter of morality.

With regard to the criminality of exhibitionism or voyeurism, this again reflects the standards and values of what individuals deem appropriate for public view. The crime is considered by many to be victimless because no one has been physically harmed (surprised and outraged, perhaps, but not harmed), and one wonders why the already strained resources of the criminal justice system are wasted on this crime. Some believe exhibitionism to be far from harmless because of the psychologic shock that is created, especially if the "victim" is a child. As the situation stands now, however, the exhibitionist or voyeur is regarded as both mentally ill and as a criminal, and the issue is whether he is obligated to undergo sex therapy or can be coerced to do so.

Although treatment is likely to be less effective if it is not voluntary, the utilitarian would undoubtedly agree that a greater amount of happiness will exist if the person enters treatment than if he does not. In fact, the only person whose happiness might decrease is the offender, and then only because he is being denied a form of sexual pleasure. If treatment is successful, he too will be happy (assuming that persons are happier out of jail than in). John Money's position, quoted earlier, is a strongly utilitarian one.

A Kantian will immediately reject the idea of obligatory treatment by applying both formulations of the Categorical Imperative. A person cannot be coerced into undergoing treatment in this instance because the action is not universalizable; if it were, any form of physical or psychologic treatment could be made mandatory. This is clearly an untenable moral position. It is not even universalizable that the exhibitionist or voyeur should feel an internal moral obligation to submit to treatment if he chooses not to. Moreover, requiring treatment is a clear example of using the nonviolent sex offender as a mere means toward an end of which he is not willingly a part. The goal, or end, is to protect society from having to play an unwitting role in an individual's variant sexual activity. Aside from the observations on personal preference cited earlier, the goal is more or less morally neutral. However, using the exhibitionist or voyeur as a means to that end without his willing consent and without his ultimately being a part of that end is a morally incorrect action.

Another ethical consideration in sex therapy is the making of societal decisions about which variant sex practices will be tolerated and which will not, or in other words, who is normal, who is "a little weird," and who is bizarre enough to be labeled sick—and why. And who makes the decisions about what will and will not be tolerated.

Let us use the example of a man who, in addition to experiencing sexual gratification, including orgasm, from all the usual forms of sexual activity, derives exquisite pleasure from having steel clothespins attached to his nipples. The pressure of the metal biting into his flesh causes intense pain that results in an orgasm; no stimulation other than the painful sensation on his nipples is required to bring him to orgasm. It is his personal form of masturbation. His wife found out about his practice (she had been convinced that the marks on his nipples were caused by another person; he reluctantly admitted to his masturbatory activities to dispel her unfounded fears of infidelity) and is repelled by it. Their sex life, which had been quite satisfying to them both, has deteriorated because the wife believes that she is less satisfying to her husband than a steel clothespin. He insists (and knows it to be true) that his unusual form of masturbation is only a variety or diversion and does not detract from the pleasure he finds in making love with her. She is, however, so disturbed by his variant sex practice that their sex life worsens, and they enter therapy.

Answers to ethical questions in this situation will determine what *should* be done in the course of therapy, even though it is highly likely that the man *could* be conditioned or persuaded to stop this form of masturbation. Ethical questions can be divided into two categories: is either the husband or wife doing anything morally wrong, and what is the ethically correct course of action now that they have entered therapy? Of all people in a given population who masturbate, probably a miniscule number do it in the way that this man does, but as we have seen in Chapter 1, the moral correctness of an action has no bearing whatsoever on the number of people who engage in that action. Masturbating with steel clothespins is as much a matter of personal preference as wearing green clothes or liking one's steak exceptionally well done; it is not a function of morality. Masturbation is, by definition, something one does to oneself; therefore it is impossible to hurt another person in so doing. It seems clear, then, that this form of masturbation is morally neutral.

But what of the wife? She appears hurt by her husband's revelation, and their sex life has deteriorated as a result. Her husband has not deliberately hurt her (he even took care to prevent her from finding out about the clothespins); it then seems that the emotional pain she is experiencing comes from her own psyche and is not caused by another person. This is indeed troublesome, but it is morally neutral also.

If no morally incorrect action is taking place, what is the function of sex therapy and the role of the therapist? The goal of therapy is to reestablish a satisfying sex life between husband and wife, but the stumbling block is the wife's perception of and reaction to her husband's masturbation, not the masturbation itself (their sex life was satisfactory until she found out about his solitary activity). There appear to be four available courses of action: (1) the husband will stop masturbating with steel clothespins, and their sex life will continue as before; (2) the husband will continue to masturbate but will use appliances that will not leave marks on his nipples so he can tell his wife he has given up the practice, thus providing her with peace of mind and him with continued sexual gratification; (3) the husband will refuse to give up his clothespins, and he and his wife will deal with the problem as best they can with the help of the therapist; or (4) the wife could enter therapy alone to discover why she is so distressed by her husband's practice and why she is unable to see it simply as a choice of masturbatory technique.

The ethically correct solution, of course, depends on whether utilitarian or deontologic theory is applied, but even more important than the answer to this dilemma is examination of its components to determine which have a moral value and which are morally neutral. When this example in particular and sexuality in general are closely examined, it is almost always true that various forms of sexual behavior are, in and of themselves, morally neutral; it is only the intent (and actions surrounding the behavior, such as lying) of the agent that creates a moral value. Masturbating with clothespins is morally neutral; using that behavior to somehow hurt another person is another ethical matter.

> Among those variant forms of human sexuality that constitute the paraphilias, some are harmless and others are harmful to the partner or to the self. Harmless forms are often defined as crimes in today's law. Even so, they do not pose as great an ethical challenge to the therapist or the researcher as do the harmful paraphilias that constitute crimes with victims. . . . I draw an ethical dividing line between harmless and harmful paraphilias on the basis not simply of the criterion of partner consent—for one can encounter cases such as that of a masochist who consents to, and indeed stage-manages, his own murder. Harmful sexual practices are those that invade the personal inviolacy of one or both partners and bring about severe and injurious personal abuse, up to and including death. Like child abuse, these are intolerable practices that demand some degree of obligative, nonelective intervention and help with a view to bringing about change.[23]

There are two major areas in which one could disagree with Money. The first is the persons involved. There are those who feel it is unethical to harm others, but harming oneself is a matter of personal choice in much the same manner in which suicide is considered by some to be morally neutral because one's life belongs to oneself. The second area of disagreement is the obligation to nonelective therapeutic intervention. Many people believe that when harmful sex practices result in injury to another, the offender should be considered a criminal in the same way that a mugger is considered a criminal in the course of a street robbery, that is, sexual assault should be treated in the same way as any other assault—as a violent crime punishable by law. If the offender wishes to enter therapy, he should surely be allowed to do so, as should any other violent person, but he should not be obligated to do so, nor should the fact of therapy negate or dilute the fact that he has harmed another.

Therapy implies the presence of sickness; sex therapy implies that the sexual practice or dysfunction for which the client seeks counsel is sick. Is it, and if so, when? It is not the purpose of this chapter to engage in a psychoanalytic discussion of which sexual practices are sick and which are not, but it is appropriate to discuss the ethical aspects of a person who has assumed a sick role, or who has been cast into that role by societal values. The sick person is generally not blamed for his condition. In sexual sickness this view is sometimes manifested by excusing sexual violence because the person "couldn't help it" or because his violence is somehow caused by socioeconomic conditions. The sick person is also excused from some or all social obligations if he seeks help and makes an effort to recover from the sickness. The sick role can usually be tolerated for a finite, if variable, amount of time. There are exceptions to this description, but the person who is sexually sick can fit the model *if* sexual variance is considered a sickness instead of a personal preference and if no criminal harm is involved. If physical violence occurs, the person takes on the role of criminal as well as that of sick person.

Redlick[24] believes that the sex therapy–client role is not the classic sick role, but it does share some similar components. The sick person is not blamed for his sexual variance, and he is subjected to considerable societal pressure to conform to sexual norms and thus to seek treatment. The cultural value of physical and mental health and maximally optimum functioning can be translated into most forms of nonpsychoanalytic sex therapy that value sexuality as a natural and healthy function and teach techniques and procedures to achieve that goal. Pleasurable and adequate sexual function is equated with physical and mental health. These general values of sex therapists, especially those following the Masters and Johnson model, are assumed also to be the values of those seeking therapy. Are the values ethically correct, incorrect, or neutral? Is good physical and mental health a goal that has an ethical component, or is it a matter of personal preference only? Is it ever wrong to want to be sick, and is it sick to be sexually deviant? One cannot engage in a discussion of these questions without acknowledging the fact that the language itself used to describe the dilemma is value laden and has ethical components of its own. The only possible stopgap in this seemingly endless and circular dilemma is to compare the values of the therapist and the client. If the therapist-client relationship is begun with fully informed consent, values will probably be clearly understood. If values are similar, therapy is more likely to be successful, and ethical pitfalls can be more easily avoided. If values differ widely, the participants will encounter serious ethical and psychologic trouble.

One further note should raise an alarm about the ethics of sex therapy. In a 1973 survey of medical students, Kardener et al. found that 25% of the freshman class felt it to be appropriate for therapists to have intercourse with their clients if the therapist is "genuine and authentic."[25] Some of these 1973 students are probably now practicing therapists.

SEXUAL ETHICS IN HISTORY

Probably no other area of human endeavor better illustrates the conflict between ethical relativism and ethical absolutism than does sexuality. Trends, fashions, and acceptable conduct in sexuality change almost as frequently as clothing fashion, and some believe with about the same degree of capriciousness. Louis XIV indulged in sexual activities of all kinds in the presence of a full court (he was even given enemas while he conducted France's business!). Ladies and gentlemen of Victorian England would have fainted in horror at such goings-on (in Victorian upper-class homes the books of male and female authors were placed on separate library shelves). Only a century and a half, which is an instant on the continuum of recorded time, and a small body of water separated these two widely diverse sets of acceptable standards. It should also be noted that not everyone in France at that time copied the behavior of the Sun King, and that there was much licentious sexual behavior during the reign of Queen Victoria. Is public lewdness ethical or not? Should an ethical value be placed on it, or is it again a matter of personal preference? Is the question important to consider from a moral standpoint, or should it remain only a matter of changing fashion?

It is interesting first to look at some historical ideas about sex and sexuality before concerning ourselves with the moral content of these ideas. Early civilization ascribed magical, spiritual, and mystical qualities to sexuality; drawings and other artifacts represented these connections. Ancient mythology is filled with stories of sexual couplings between humans and gods who appeared to people in various human, animal, and chimera forms. Sexuality was an important aspect of polytheistic religious rites: female virgins were often ritually deflowered in public; great ceremonial fuss was made over male puberty; and temple prostitution, both male and female, was common. Adultery, however, was one form of sexuality that was almost universally taboo. When monotheism first appeared among ancient Jews, sexual practices became more rigid, and the list of taboos grew to include masturbation, celibacy, prostitution, and homosexuality. Pleasure was still associated with sex when it was permitted to occur, but monotheism also saw the beginning of sexual repression of women. Menstruation was considered one of the most unclean of human phenomena, and a man was considered to have sinned grievously if he touched his wife, even in a nonsexual manner, while she was menstruating.

The rise of Greek civilization was accompanied by a more liberated attitude toward sex. Sexual activities were conducted with joy, sensuality, and a great degree of cultural approval. Bisexuality among men was widespread and accepted, and female homosexuality, although mostly ignored in ancient Greece, traces much of its history to the poet Sappho who lived with women on the island of Lesbos (hence the term lesbian for a female homosexual). Sexual violence was a criminal offense in ancient Greece.

The Romans carried the sexual joyfulness of the Greeks to an extreme, and sex became more deliberate and purely physical with fewer mystical qualities; it was carried out with an intensity of concentration that is almost paradoxic to the nature of sexuality. No controls existed in regard to permissible forms of sexuality, and excesses soon turned to violence. Rape (heterosexual and homosexual), pederasty, and sadism were common. Sexual exploitation of other human beings seemed to mirror the Roman political and military exploitation of other nations.

From the fall of the Roman Empire to the Renaissance, a period known as the Middle Ages, sexual mores were controlled by the Catholic church, which held a generally rigid and moralistic view of sexuality. Universal acceptance of the Church's view of sexuality did not exist, and the Renaissance saw a bursting forth of anti-Catholic fervor. Art in all its forms blossomed, with emphasis on the beauty and sensuality of the human body. The erotic power of Renaissance art is strong, sometimes blatantly evident. Life mirrored art, and sexual license was again almost unrestricted. Women, however, continued in their subordinate role and were divided into two categories: whores (or courtesans if they were beautiful and catered to the upper classes) and wives, who were expected to remain chaste until marriage and then faithful and obedient to their husbands.

The seventeenth and eighteenth centuries saw the beginning of modern scientific and philosophic thought and were among the most exciting times in human history. Rational, anticlerical thought dominated the philosophy of Locke, Hume, and Berkeley, while Descartes, Galileo, and Newton were proving scientific theories. Shakespeare portrayed joy and playfulness in sex, but a pocket of Puritanism in the midseventeenth century created a grim, procreative, and obligatory view of sex. This soon gave way to the licentiousness of the Restoration and the personal rational sexuality of the Age of Reason.

Sexuality continued to fluctuate for the next two centuries, from severe repression and social (and even legal) censure of overt sexuality to more tolerant attitudes, outright bawdiness, and encouragement of the joy of sex for its own sake. Throughout this period women were, and still remain, sexually repressed in a variety of ways such as the constant danger of rape if they venture out without a man's protection, wifely obligations to fulfill sexual duties toward their husbands no matter what feelings exist, contraception that is haphazard in its safety and effectiveness, almost total legal responsibility for illegimate offspring, and the general feeling that women's sexual needs are less important than men's.

After a generation of the twentieth century had passed, attitudes toward sexuality had changed again but for different reasons. Freud increased human knowledge about psychosexual development; women received the right to vote and slowly began to think of themselves as full persons with strong sexual needs of their own; increases in technology and communication made dissemination of information about sexual attitudes and behavior available to the masses; and somewhat safer and more effective contraception became available. The last generation of the twentieth century is one of sexual openness, freedom, and almost total sexual license, which in many respects rivals the activities of the Roman Empire, especially in regard to sexual violence. If we use history as a guide, there is no reason to believe that a swing back to Puritanism is not on the horizon.

Has the morality of sexual behavior changed through the centuries, or has it remained constant with varying degrees of obedience to sexual moral codes? Morality involves some degree of sociocultural overlay on a basic system of ethics; this is how morality differs from ethics. Thus it is evident that morality has indeed changed, but the ethics of sexuality do not change. Those principles that dictate correct rules of behavior that human beings should follow as they relate to each other do not fluctuate with the tides of sexual fashion. Let us use the principle of nonmaleficence (the obligation to do no harm) as an example. In every period of history, including our own, people harm each other sexually in many ways: participation in general sexual licentiousness is harmful to individuals who wish to be more sexually discreet and private; repression of women's natural desires is harmful; creating a climate in which sex can be engaged in only in certain prescribed times and ways is harmful; exploiting women's childbearing capacities is harmful. The examples could go on forever, but the principles remain the same. Whether society is going through a period of sexual Puritanism or licentiousness, doing harm is morally wrong. All other ethical rules and principles described in Chapter 1 can be applied to sexuality in much the same way as nonmaleficence.

This is the ethical absolutist view. An ethical relativist would disagree by claiming that an ethically correct belief, particularly as it pertains to sexuality, is what the vast majority of persons in a given society at a given time believe to be correct. More people subscribe to ethical relativism than to absolutism.

Farley[26] notes several factors that tend to influence sexual ethics.

1. Ethical norms are grounded in human nature and are subject to a double standard of application, a procreative or scriptural standard vs. a sensual or pleasurable one.

2. New knowledge about the physical aspects of sexuality has an effect on ethics. For example, the rear-entry position for intercourse was considered immoral because some animals copulate in that fashion; however, it has been shown that conception is more likely to occur when the rear-entry position is used. Therefore critics who forbade it as animalistic must now approve it if the basic reason for sex is procreative. Research has shown that sex practices formerly considered unnatural (oral sex, homosexuality, masturbation, and the like) are common in many forms of animal life and must thus be considered part of nature.

3. Sexual deviation is highly dependent on culture.

4. Surveys of sexual behavior, such as those conducted by Kinsey and Hunt, have taught people to be skeptical of stated sexual norms, that is, people frequently do what they want to do regardless of cultural mores. This cannot help but raise questions about the morality of teaching certain sexual attitudes.

5. The women's movement has begun to free women from some of the repression to which they have been traditionally subjected. It has helped women to regard with suspicion many of the strictures and taboos placed on their sexual behavior. Rationality is beginning to supplant fear and oppression.

6. Psychoanalytic theory, Freudian and others, has provided individuals with information about the meaning and importance of sexuality in their lives. More important, sexual deviance or variance is more often seen as a result of psychologic illness or failure of psychosexual development than as a moral sin or evil. Psychoanalytic theory can, however, spawn myths and taboos of its own, which can be almost as detrimental to enjoyment of sex as can irrational, mystical, or religious beliefs.

7. Philosophic thought has had a profound influence on sexual ethics, both by reinforcing religious views and by opposing them.

Formation of a contemporary sexual ethic must combine general principles of human behavior with some degree of attention paid to prevailing social customs. A sexual ethic must be moved from the irrational image of sex as sinful bodily defilement into the rational sphere of human beings communicating and interacting with each other on a psychoemotional and physical level. There must be emphasis on respect for persons, the role of sexuality in their lives, and the degree to which each person is permitted to function autonomously. If sex is regarded as natural human expression, a sexual ethic that develops from this point of view will be more humane and therefore less likely to be affected by the tides of moral fashion. If sexuality is seen as an enhancement of human life, as are art, music, knowledge, and other pursuits, then it can be creatively channeled, disciplined, and controlled to attain heights of sensual refinement that have been rare in past history. Sex is not the primordial and all-consuming drive that Freud thought it was; neither is it an inexhaustable power that controls human life. It is a form of expression, a language perhaps, that grows richer and more flexible as it is defined and disciplined by those who use and control it.

Religious views

Religion has had a notoriously great deal to say about sex, much of it negative or qualifiedly neutral. Early Judaism, at the time of its formation, viewed sex as something less than sacred, but stringent laws were established prohibiting adultery, incest, rape, public nakedness, and other forms of sexual behavior. As Judaism developed, its sexual ethics derived solely from the Biblical injunction to marry and bear children. The divine command to procreate and the patriarchal nature of Jewish life led to the centuries-old belief that a woman is the property of her husband and is to be protected along with his other chattel (adultery can thus be seen as disrespect for property, not persons). But in addition to the double sexual standard that favored men, women benefited from the law against polygamy and the strong taboo against divorce, particularly if the woman was barren. Thus the marital relationship took precedence over the command to procreate. There is an interesting Talmudic law that requires a man, at the beginning of each Sabbath when evening prayers are concluded, to return home and sexually satisfy his wife.

Modern Jewish theology views the sacredness of marriage to be supremely important; therefore sex is viewed as a means of expressing love and reaffirming vows. Contraception is permitted if pregnancy would be harmful to the woman *or* to the marriage, and abstinence is regarded with suspicion because it cuts off a channel of happiness and communication and because it is unnatural. Other sex acts are considered unnatural and demeaning because they undermine the meaning of intercourse; those commonly mentioned are masturbation, homosexuality, and bestiality. Reform Judaism is reassessing sexual ethics in light of two major social changes: the sanctity of marriage appears to be decreasing in importance, and the patriarchal system of Judaism has been somewhat weakened by the women's movement. Orthodox Judaism is doing nothing to change ancient sexual ethics, but the Conservative branch is moving toward liberalism, although very slowly.

The Christian view of sex differs markedly from the Jewish one. Jesus and his followers said almost nothing about sex, and the New Testament offers contradictory values: marriage and procreation are sacred but so is celibacy; internal beliefs about sex are as important as external actions; sex is imbued with a sacred symbolic meaning, yet it has a great potential for evil and defilement. Those foundations are the basis for Christian sexual ethics, which have been both reaffirmed and challenged throughout history.

When Christianity emerged from the Hellenistic Age, it was still strongly influenced by Stoicism, which valued rational detachment of the mind from all forms of passionate desire, but it viewed intercourse as the vehicle for procreation. Early Christians saw intercourse as both praiseworthy (but only within the sacred matrimonial bond) for its procreative function and sinful because of its concentration on worldly passion. Fecundity and virginity were simultaneously worshipped.

Saints Augustine and Aquinas had an enormous influence on the developing Christian sexual ethic. The former held a generally negative view of sex because of its tendency to encourage evil; the only positive purpose for sex was procreative, and even that role was acknowledged grudgingly. Although love and companionship in marriage serve to strengthen the sacred bond, sex was not seen as another means to that end. Augustine believed that sexual desire was a part of original sin and that intercourse always interferes with rationality, reason, and will. These three phrases were defined by Augustine in terms of their use in serving God, not in the more modern context of objectivity and autonomy. Although there was dissent, the Augustinian view held sway until Thomas Aquinas began writing in the thirteenth century. Aquinas did not differ in substance from Augustine, but he clarified Christian morality in regard to sex, especially as it was perceived as evil. Aquinas did not acknowledge the *intrinsic* evil of sex but believed evil to be a result of moral choice; therefore sex could be used for evil means, but it did not exist by itself *as evil*. Aquinas reemphasized the procreative function of intercourse as its only purpose and prohibited forms of sexual activity that were used for pleasure only, that is, everything other than intercourse. As male orgasm is necessary for procreation, and female orgasm is not, the theology of Aquinas further underscored repression of women's sexuality.

The Protestant Reformation, led by Martin Luther, challenged traditional Christian (Catholic) sexual ethics by declaring that sexual desire is part of human nature and could be used as a force for good if it were channeled through marriage and viewed as part of the structure of life. John Calvin believed that marriage and sex perpetuated the human community but that sex could provoke individuals to engage in acts of lust and dissolution. No one denied the power of the sexual drive: Christian theologians merely disagreed on the way it was to be channeled. The desire for sex could be overcome through meditation, prayer, and devotion to God; it could be used as a vehicle for procreation, and to a lesser degree, as an expression of marital love and communication; or it could be a source of evil, lust, licentiousness, and greed. Almost nowhere in early Christian teaching were joy, affection, or sensuality mentioned in connection with sex.

In the midtwentieth century Catholicism recognized that sexual pleasure and procreation can be separated (hence the acceptability of the rhythm method of contraception) and that sex has a purpose uniquely its own in furthering human love and communication. After the Reformation Protestantism split into a number of separate communities, but

> Overall, Protestant sexual ethics is moving to integrate an understanding of the human person, male and female, into a theology of marriage that no longer deprecates sexual desire and sexual pleasure as primarily occasions of moral danger.[27]

Sexual intercourse should still ideally take place within the marital bond, according to most modern Christian theologians, but other forms of sexual pleasure in other contexts are no longer automatically discounted as immoral. Protestantism is opening itself to the naturalness of human sexual diversity.

SUMMARY

Psychosexual development is the phenomenon that causes us to be what we are sexually, how we think and behave about sex. It is composed of an interdependent combination of biologic, anatomic, sociocultural, and emotional factors. Failure of adequate psychosexual development almost always results in sexual dysfunction of some kind, although the individual may not perceive it as a dysfunction and consequently may not seek treatment.

Biologic and anatomic factors of psychosexual development are fairly immutable, but forces of culture and tradition are not and play a major role in attitudes about sex and in the kinds of sexual activity individuals prefer. The strong sexual repression of women, which has existed throughout history and is only now beginning to wane, stems from cultural and religious interpretations of the nature and function of women.

The sexual revolution is the result of technology (leading to personal privacy and greater affluence) and communication; it has changed, perhaps irrevocably, the sexual mores of Western civilization. Two comprehensive post–World War II surveys of sexual attitudes and behaviors indicate that Americans engage in more frequent and widely varied sex than most people would have believed. Male-female social relationships strongly influence sexual attitudes and ethics and have reinforced the repression of women. Social relationships are a direct result of psychosexual development and affect sexual behavior.

Definition of "normal" sexual behavior is an almost impossible task, one that depends on belief about the purpose of sex, sociocultural views, and personal preference. By and large, a line of normalcy can be drawn at the point where physical or emotional harm result from sexual behavior, although this line is by no means clear and precise.

Sex research is carried out by means of surveys, the participant-observer method, and direct observation. Ethical issues in sex research include confidentiality, the design and purpose of the research, the population to be studied, and the appropriateness of the research. Some of these same issues, and others as well, surround sex therapy, which has as its goal the relief of sexual symptoms and dysfunctions. The term *dysfunction* itself can be controversial and has a variety of ethical overtones, including differences in goals between therapist and client, appropriate modes of therapy, and the competence of the therapist. The question of whether sex therapy is ever morally obligatory or should be made mandatory in some instances has developed on both sides of the issue, particularly when the sexual variance to be treated is also criminal behavior.

A historical look at sexual ethics reveals that the pendulum of permissiveness has swung from Puritanism to bold licentiousness and back again so many times in the past 8000 or so years that it would be foolhardy to believe that it will not swing as vigorously in the future.

Notes

1. Money, J., & Ehrhardt, A. A. *Man and woman, boy and girl: the differentiation and dimorphism and gender identity from conception to maturity*. Baltimore: Johns Hopkins Press, 1972.
2. Hogan, R. *Human sexuality: a nursing perspective*. New York: Appleton-Century-Crofts, 1980. p. 39.
3. Woods, N. F. *Human sexuality in health and illness* (2nd ed.). St. Louis: The C.V. Mosby Co., 1979. p. 252.
4. Kaplan, H. S. *The new sex therapy*. New York: Brunner/Mazel, 1974.
5. Solomon, R. C., & Sanders, J. R. Sexual identity. In W. T. Reich (Ed.), *Encyclopedia of bioethics*. New York: The Free Press, 1978.
6. Money & Ehrhardt.
7. Kinsey, A. C., et al. *Sexual behavior in the human male*. Philadelphia: W. B. Saunders Co., 1948.
8. Deutsch, H. *The psychology of women* (Vol. 1.). New York: Grune & Stratton, 1944.
9. London, P. Sexual behavior. In *Encyclopedia of bioethics* (Vol. 4.), p. 1566.
10. London (Vol. 4), p. 1567.
11. Kaplan, pp. 122–136, 155–172.
12. Kaplan, p. 127.
13. Solomon & Sanders (Vol. 4.), pp. 1592–1595.
14. Solomon & Sanders (Vol. 4.), p. 1594.
15. Solomon & Sanders (Vol. 4.), p. 1595.
16. Kolodny, R. C. Ethical requirements for sex research in humans: informed consent and general principles. In W. H. Masters, V. E. Johnson, & R. C. Kolodny (Eds.), *Ethical issues in sex therapy and research. Proceedings of a conference sponsored by the Reproductive Biology Research Foundation*. Boston: Little, Brown & Company, 1977.
17. Kolodny, p. 58.
18. Murray, T. H. Learning to deceive. *Hastings Center Report*, 1980, *10*(2), 13.
19. Kelty, M. F. Ethical issues and requirements for sex research with humans: confidentiality. In Masters, Johnson, & Kolodny, p. 87.
20. Kelty, pp. 101–102.
21. Kaplan, p. 121.
22. Money, J. Issues and attitudes in research and treatment of variant forms of human sexual behavior. In Masters, Johnson, & Kolodny, p. 123.
23. Money, pp. 125–126.
24. Redlich, F. The ethics of sex therapy. In Masters, Johnson, & Kolodny.
25. Kardener, S., et al. A survey of physicians' attitudes and practices regarding erotic and nonerotic contact with patients. *American Journal of Psychiatry*, 1973, *130*(10), 1077–1081.
26. Farley, M. A. Sexual ethics. In *Encyclopedia of bioethics* (Vol. 4), pp. 1583–1585.
27. Farley, p. 1583.

Bibliography

Aufhauser, M. C. Sexual development. In W. T. Reich (Ed.), *Encyclopedia of bioethics*. New York: The Free Press, 1978.

Deutsch, H. *The psychology of women* (Vol. 1.). New York: Grune & Stratton, 1944.

Engelhardt, H. T., Jr. The disease of masturbation: values and the concept of disease. In T. L. Beauchamp, & L. Walters (Eds.), *Contemporary issues in bioethics*. Belmont, Calif: Dickenson Publishing Company, 1978.

Farley, M. A. Sexual Ethics. In *Encyclopedia of bioethics*.

Friedman, S. S., et al. *A woman's guide to therapy*. Englewood Cliffs, N.J.: Prentice-Hall, Inc., 1979.

Fromer, M. J. *Ethical issues in health care*. St. Louis: The C.V. Mosby Co., 1981.

Hiltner, S. Theological perspectives on the ethics of scientific investigation and treatment of human sexuality. In W. H. Masters, V. E. Johnson, & R. C. Kolodny (Eds.), *Ethical issues in sex therapy and research. Proceedings of a conference sponsored by the Reproductive Biology Research Foundation*. Boston: Little, Brown & Company, 1977.

Hogan, R. *Human sexuality: a nursing perspective*. New York: Appleton-Century-Crofts, 1980.

Hunt, M. M. *Sexual behavior in the 1970s*. Chicago: Playboy Press, 1974.

Kaplan, H. S. *The new sex therapy*. New York: Brunner/Mazel, Inc., 1974.

Kelty, M. F. Ethical issues and requirements for sex research with humans: confidentiality. In Masters, Johnson, & Kolodny.

Kinsey, A. C., et al. *Sexual behavior in the human male*. Philadelphia: W. B. Saunders Co., 1948.

Kinsey, A. C., et al. *Sexual behavior in the human female*. Philadelphia: W. B. Saunders Co., 1953.

Kolodny, R. C. Ethical requirements for sex research in humans: informed consent and general principles. In Masters, Johnson, & Kolodny.

London, P. Sexual Behavior. In *Encyclopedia of bioethics*.

Lowry, T. S., & Lowry, T. P., Ethical considerations in sex therapy. *Journal of Marriage and Family Counseling*, 1975, *1*(3), 229–236.

Martin, L. L. *Health care of women*. Philadelphia: J. B. Lippincott Co., 1978.

Money, J. Issues and attitudes in research and treatment of variant forms of human sexual behavior. In Masters, Johnson, & Kolodny.

Money, J. & Ehrhardt, A. A. *Man and woman, boy and girl: the differentiation and dimorphism and gender identity from conception to maturity*. Baltimore: The Johns Hopkins Press, 1972.

Murray, T. H. Learning to deceive. *Hastings Center Report*, 1980, *10*(2), 11–14.

Redlich, F. The ethics of sex therapy. In Masters, Johnson, & Kolodny.

Solomon, R. C., & Sanders, J. R. Sexual identity. In *Encyclopedia of bioethics*.

Woods, N. F. *Human sexuality in health and illness* (2nd Ed.). St. Louis: The C.V. Mosby Co., 1979.

CHAPTER 3

HOMOSEXUALITY

DEFINITIONS

There are several ways to define homosexuality, many of them carrying overtones of mental illness or reprehensible behavior. The definition of a homosexual that is most accurate and carries no judgmental weight is a person who feels a strong erotic attraction to persons of the same sex, who has the ability to be sexually aroused by members of the same sex, and who prefers to engage in sexual activity with members of the same sex.

It should be noted that this definition makes no mention of the existence of sexual activity itself, although it is not precluded, nor does it venture into the realms of causes, theories, or morality. One need not engage in sexual activity to consider oneself a homosexual, although most homosexuals, like most heterosexuals, are not celibate. Homosexuality need not indicate an exclusive preference for members of the same sex, although the definitive line between a homosexual who occasionally makes love with a person of the opposite sex and a bisexual is difficult to draw. Many homosexuals are married, and even though they engage in sex with their spouses, they still consider themselves homosexual.

Many believe that the definition of homosexuality depends, at least to some extent, on the repetitiveness of the behavior. A few experimental forays into homosexuality does not mean that a person *is* homosexual; the behavior needs to be repetitive and deliberately sought. Here the definitions begin to move away from the purely descriptive and into the judgmental and qualitative. Another definition of homosexuality is that it is a psychologic, some even go so far as to define it as pathologic, condition in which normal psychosexual development somehow failed, and the person is unable to relate sexually to members of the opposite sex. This places a negative cast on homosexuality, that is, that the homosexual is forced to resort to sexual activity with members of the same sex because he *cannot* become aroused by members of the opposite sex. This is vastly different from the definition that homosexuality is a chosen preference for the same sex, a choice consciously made by the homosexual person. Probably there are elements of natural proclivity, conscious choice, and aversion to the opposite sex, in varying proportions and degrees, in almost all homosexual behavior. That homosexuality may be a psychologic condition is a hotly debated issue in both psychiatric and homosexual communities. There has been some speculation and research that homosexuality can be defined in purely physical terms, not in differences in anatomic and physiologic structure and function, but in terms of genetic codes and perhaps hormonal concentrations, as in the tendency to be fat or thin or the fact of having green eyes or dark hair. Little concrete evidence exists for this point of view because of the haphazard familial incidence of homosexuality. But by the same token, enough people state that they have "always known" that they are homosexual, even from earliest childhood, that some possible credence must be given to the genetic definition.

Up to this point definitions of homosexuality have not taken gender into account. Can male and female homosexuality be defined differently, apart from their obvious gender differences? Descriptions of life-styles can be vastly different; ways of relating to each other within the homosexual relationship differ, sometimes widely, and perhaps there are even differences in views and feelings about the opposite sex. But it is not entirely clear whether these differences result from differences in male and female homosexuals or differences in men and women as persons who happen to be homosexual. It is abundantly clear that heterosexual men and women are different from each other in ways that transcend the purely physical; thus it seems reasonable to assume that there might also be great differences between male and female homosexuals. But because this book is about ethics, which is concerned with the way people treat each other as *persons*, the differences between male and female homosexuals will, for the most part, be put aside unless there is a specific reason to differentiate.

All the physiologists, psychologists, and laypersons who have studied homosexuals and homosexuality seem to agree that it is a phenomenon that almost defies definition and description. When two persons of the same sex engage in sexual activity with each other, it can be agreed that a homosexual act is taking place, but are the two persons necessarily homosexuals? One or both may be bisexual; one may be a heterosexual who is "trying out" a homosexual act for the first and only time; or one or both may be adolescents who have not yet settled into a heterosexual, homosexual, or bisexual mode. The diversity of homosexual acts, behaviors, and life-styles makes homosexuality difficult to define. An important consideration, however, in defining homosexuality, no matter how and by whom, is inclusion of the concept of personhood; that is, a homosexual is a person who always, sometimes, or occasionally feels a sexual attraction to members of the same sex and acts on those erotic feelings.

SOCIETAL INCIDENCE

Because of the essentially covert nature of homosexuality (the necessity for which will be discussed later in this chapter), it is difficult to estimate the number of homosexuals in society. Kinsey and his associates, in their 1948 survey of male sexual behavior and in the 1953 study of females, found that 13% of women and 37% of men[1,2] had had at least one homosexual experience, but this did not necessarily mean that all those persons considered themselves homosexual. In a survey undertaken two decades later, Hunt estimated that about 20% to 25% of males and 10% to 15% of females had had homosexual experiences.[3] These experiences, again, do not necessarily indicate that the person is an active homosexual. The best informal estimate, gathered from a variety of literature on homosexuality, is that about 10% of the population lead homosexual life-styles. Of this estimated 10%, about 6% are male and 4% are female, and only 1% are admitted "open" homosexuals, that is, homosexuals who do not make a conscious effort to hide their homosexuality. About 2% to 3% are exclusively homosexual, that is, they *never* engage in sexual activity with members of the opposite sex.

One of the most recent studies of homosexuality was done in 1978 in San Francisco with 979 subjects participating.[4] It must be noted at the outset that San Francisco, more than any other city in the United States, is an openly gay city, where the tolerance of homosexuals and homosexuality is exceptionally high; fewer homosexuals feel compelled to hide the fact, and homosexuals are more integrated into the general social, business, and political life of the city than anywhere else. For these reasons, it makes sense to study San Francisco homosexuals, but it must be remembered that their attitudes and experiences are not an accurate representation of what can be expected in the rest of the country. In this San Francisco study, Bell and Weinberg found that far more homosexuals were covert about their lives than were admittedly gay, even in San Francisco, and no generalizations could be made about the amount of sexual activity engaged in by homosexuals (it is as varied as heterosexual activity). Public cruising is engaged in more frequently by men than women, and the most popular place is the gay bar. *Cruising* is the term used when a person strolls through public places actively looking for a sex partner (heterosexuals also do it—in singles' bars). Homosexual men had more sex partners over the course of a lifetime than did lesbians, but more men than women regretted the fact of their homosexuality. More women than men had considered stopping their homosexual activities. Although the study did not speculate why this should be so, it seems likely that women might consider quitting their homosexual life-style more for social and economic reasons than for reasons of sexual preference, that is, the desire to find a husband for economic support.

In terms of nonsexual life, no significant differences were found between homosexuals and heterosexuals; job satisfaction and career mobility were about the same, and general happiness and social adjustment were similar. Homosexuals were no more dissatisfied with life than were heterosexuals, although homosexuals who are psychologically distressed *because of* their homosexuality seemed more unhappy than heterosexuals who are psychologically distressed because of a variety of life circumstances. Homosexuals have about as many problems involving sexual dysfunction as do heterosexuals, and the two groups probably experience a similar degree of psychologic distress because of it. This may be caused in great measure by the severe social and political oppression of homosexuals rather than by the fact that the person *is* homosexual.

Weinberg and Williams[5] studied male homosexuals in the United States, in the Netherlands, and in Denmark to determine how they adapt to the fact of homosexuality in a heterosexual world. They found that although younger men engaged in sexual activity more frequently than older men, the latter were no worse off than the former in terms of psychologic adaptation. Class consciousness is as evident among homosexuals as it is among heterosexuals; an upper-class homosexual felt a stronger affinity toward an upper-class heterosexual than he did toward a lower-class homosexual. Also the higher the job status of the homosexual, the more covert he was about his life-style. After the guilt, shame, and shock of the first homosexual experience wore off, the religiosity of most homosexuals was not affected by the fact of homosexuality; most felt they had not violated the precepts of their religion and felt no sense of sin in the religious sense about being homosexual. Blacks expected and experienced less discrimination as a result of homosexuality than did whites; this is understandable in view of the fact that their first, and probably stronger, experiences with discrimination were based on race rather than sexual preference.

Homosexuals exist in every stratum of society; the phenomenon cuts across racial, cultural, religious, and socioeconomic boundaries. Homosexuals are in all businesses and professions, and they come in every imaginable variety of physical appearance. Some homosexuals look and act "the part"; that is, they behave in a stereotypical manner, but the vast majority do not. Homosexual subcultures exist, with varying degrees of formal structure (political and social organizations; bars and community centers; churches and synagogues; circles of lovers, friends, acquaintances; etc.), but not all homosexuals are part of this subculture. Many major cities have areas where homosexuals tend to congregate, but many homosexuals never go near them and spend most of their lives almost completely integrated in the heterosexual world. Few, if any, assumptions and generalizations can and should be made about the incidence, distribution, and activity of homosexuals. Those who make them are usually wrong.

HISTORY

Homosexual history parallels and is integrated throughout the history of all humanity and is characterized by fear, oppression, and persecution. Jonathan Katz begins his book on the history of homosexuality in the United States with the following:

> During the four hundred years documented here, American homosexuals were condemned to death by choking, burning, and drowning; they were executed, jailed, pilloried, fined, court-martialed, prostituted, fired, framed, blackmailed, disinherited, declared insane, driven to insanity, to suicide, murder, and self-hate, witch-hunted, entrapped, stereotyped, mocked, insulted, isolated, pitied, castigated, and despised. (They were also castrated, lobotomized, shock-treated, and psychoanalyzed. . . .) Homosexuals and their behavior were characterized by the terms "abomination", "crime against nature", "sin", "monster", "fairies", "bull dykes", and "perverts".[6]

This is an ugly picture of what 90% of the population can do to the 10% who exhibit different sexual attitudes and activities. Hundreds of other groups of human beings have been and are being oppressed simply because of who they are, but few groups have experienced the history and consistency of oppression that homosexuals have.

I shall make no attempt to delineate a complete history of homosexuality, but a few vignettes from Katz' book should serve to illustrate the ways in which homosexuals have experienced American life and how Americans have experienced homosexuality. On June 23, 1629, while on a voyage to New England aboard the ship *Talbot*, the Reverend Francis Higgeson recorded the following in his diary:

> This day we examined 5 beastly Sodomitical boyes, which confessed their wickedness not to bee named. The fact was so fowl we reserved them to bee punished by the governor when we came to new England, who afterward send them backe to the company to bee punished in ould England, as the crime deserved.[7]

At the time, sodomy (usually defined as buggery, which meant anal intercourse) was punishable by death in England. In 1655 the New Haven colony published a series of laws dealing with sexuality. They differed from the codes in most of the other early colonies in that the people of New Haven stated that lesbianism was specifically prohibited and punishable by death[8] (female homosexuality was not usually mentioned in legal codifications, probably because female sexuality as a distinct entity, different from her role as sex partner to a man, was not acknowledged; the fact that two women might prefer to make love with each other was so foreign an idea to men that it was usually simply ignored).

Thomas Jefferson and other Virginia liberals in 1776 and 1777 reformed many laws concerning sexuality. Homosexuality had been punishable by death; now "Whosoever shall be guilty of Rape, Polygamy, or Sodomy with man or woman shall be punished, if a man, by castration, if a woman by cutting thro' the cartilage of her nose a hole of one half inch diameter at the least."[9]

In 1846 a New York City policeman, Edward McCosker, was accused of having made sexual advances to other males while on police duty. He was brought to a hearing in front of the mayor of New York and then denied the charges. The hearing took place just 1 year after New York's police department was founded. Various witnesses testified to McCosker's "lewd and indecent conduct," although another policeman did attest to McCosker's good character (while affirming his homosexuality) but to no avail. McCosker was dismissed from the police force.

> The charges against McCosker must be seen in the context of an antihomosexual society in which examples of homosexual misconduct are more likely to be recorded and labeled as such than equivalent heterosexual acts. How many heterosexual policemen, for instance, made advances toward women without finding this behavior used as grounds for serious complaint, much less for dismissal—and had their cases documented for posterity?[10]

Homosexuals used to be counted in the United States Census when it distinguished criminals from noncriminals in the population. In 1890, 224 were counted as having been convicted of "crimes against nature" (those crimes were homosexuality and bestiality—no distinction between the two was made in the criminal code).[11]

By the midnineteenth century the erroneous stereotype of the male homosexual dressing and acting as a woman had become widely believed. In 1896 an article "Sex and Art" appeared in the *American Journal of Psychology* that defined male homosexuals as "peculiar societies of inverts" who dressed in women's clothing and met for tea parties and sewing circles.[12] In 1914 Dr. Magnus Hirschfeld, a German sexologist and homosexual emancipation leader, described what he saw as homosexual life in America. He described it as fairly hidden even in the major cities of Philadelphia and Boston, although he found a great deal of male transvestism. When the fact of homosexuality was discovered, a man usually resigned from his job in disgrace and was considered a social outcast. Certain fields, however, were open to homosexuals and indeed seemed to attract them, most notably the creative and performing arts. Turkish baths were described as meeting places for homosexuals, as were areas around military installations. Hirschfeld found that homosexuals were found at universities as both faculty and students and were generally poorly tolerated. One further observation made by Hirschfeld was that Americans tended to blame one or another minority ethnic group for the existence of homosexuality.[13] The next year Havelock Ellis, the famous sexologist, wrote a similar account of what "inverts" do in dance halls. He also noted that red neckties were the badge of the homosexual and that any heterosexual venturing into public wearing a red tie risked derision and disgrace.[14]

In 1913 Margaret Otis published an account of coerced lesbianism in reform school that occurred between black and white girls. The account is not specifically homophobic, but it does carry a patronizing and racist air.[15] Katz selected several accounts of lesbianism in prisons, which were written in what must have been a factual and observant style for the time, although they appear biased and judgmental to the modern reader. Based on the accounts, it seems that if a woman were unlucky enough to be sent to prison, she could not escape the homosexual advances of other prisoners.

The history of homosexuality as portrayed in literature has been singularly negative. The judgments of evil or sickness always accompanied a homosexual character, and by the end of the work the person so afflicted usually meets one of two ends: death, usually by suicide, or conversion to heterosexuality. It is interesting to note that some of the most famous homosexual writers (Tennessee Williams, Gertrude Stein, Oscar Wilde, for example) rarely wrote about homosexuality as a literary subject or created many major homosexual characters.

During the 1950s when anticommunism was elevated to an almost religious zeal in the United States, homophobia followed a similar path; in fact, communism and homosexuality were linked by Senator Joseph McCarthy in an almost cause and effect relationship. Known homosexuals were not permitted to serve in the military, nor were they allowed government jobs, even those that did not require security clearance. If military personnel were found to be homosexual after they had entered the service, they received a less than honorable discharge, sometimes even a dishonorable one, which at the time was a serious stigma. Homosexuals were considered to be among the worst security risks because they were seen to be vulnerable to blackmail. The fact that the majority of government jobs involve no contact with secret information did not deter government agencies from refusing to hire homosexuals.

Less than a generation ago in 1966 and 1967 two women in Louisiana were convicted of "unnatural carnal copulation" and sentenced to 30 months in prison. They were solicited and entrapped by a police officer who paid them to perform cunnilingus and other sex acts in a motel room. The trial judge refused to consider the fact of entrapment because there was no evidence of it. The women were not convicted of homosexuality but of specific sex acts, but it seems obvious that the trial would not have taken place without the issue of homosexuality.[16] Civil and criminal oppression of homosexuals will be discussed in more detail later in this chapter.

If this account of the history of homosexuals appears bleak and depressing, it is. There is every reason to believe that individual homosexuals experienced joy and love in relationships with each other, that they were not constantly miserable and hunted by the rest of society, and that not every heterosexual American was homophobic. But in general it is safe to say that during the course of American history, homosexuals have been rejected more often than accepted, hated and ridiculed more often than tolerated, punished and discriminated against more often than left alone, and feared more often than understood. Homophobia (defined as fear and hatred of homosexuals) was and still is a common but poorly understood phenomenon that has strong psychologic overtones. If homophobia involved *only* fear and hatred of homosexuals, there might be no moral dilemma to discuss because it would then fall solely into the realm of personal preference. However, homophobes take action on their fear and hatred, and an ethical issue is created. Whatever action a homophobe takes will result in some type of unhappiness, oppression, and discrimination for homosexuals. The utilitarian would, as always, calculate total happiness produced as a consequence of an action. We can assume that homophobia will always result in unhappiness for homosexuals, but since they are in the minority, a happiness calculation might still add up to the permissibility of homophobia. However, the assumption can be made that discrimination, oppression, and persecution are acts that do not produce happiness for the actor; they are not generally considered pleasurable activities in the usual sense of the ways in which people derive pleasure or happiness. Consequently, the total amount of happiness resulting from homophobia would be minimal. The deontologist could not condone homophobia because it violates all basic moral rules and principles. No social or individual good ever comes from persecution of any group of people; only harm occurs. One has only to look at history to see that persecutors are also frequently harmed, although the harm might be delayed and is of a different nature than the harm done to the victims. There is surely no justice in homophobia, and a person who is being persecuted, no matter how "benign" the oppressive action, is being denied autonomy. A Kantian could not condone even the mildest form of homophobia because it could never be considered a universalizable maxim. It seems safe to say, then, that homophobic action is an absolute evil, as is any form of oppression of any minority group.

SOCIAL AND CULTURAL ASPECTS

This section should begin with a brief overview of the theories of the causes of homosexuality. The word *theory* should be stressed because to date no social, psychologic, or physical research has pointed conclusively to any specific cause of homosexuality, or even a reason why it exists at all. There is not even much agreement about the nature of the phenomenon. Those who have studied homosexuality cannot agree whether it is a social, psychologic, or purely physiologic occurrence.

The most traditional view is that homosexuality is an acquired psychologic condition (strong traditionalists call it an abberation or illness) resulting from some failure or error in psychosexual development. Freudian theory, which is the most prevalent, points to disturbed parental relationships, although the number of homosexuals who have had perfectly ordinary childhoods (and the number of heterosexuals who are the product of severely disturbed parent-child relationships) tends to detract from the reliability of this theory. Another common explanation is that homosexuals fear the opposite sex to the extent that they are unable to engage in heterosexual activity. The *vagina denta* myth is popular, that is, the fantasy that a vagina has teeth, and intercourse with a woman will result in predictably dire consequences (the absurdity of this myth becomes obvious when one thinks about what fellatio is). Some psychiatrists believe that homosexuality is a result of lingering infantilism, that is, the reluctance to accept the social and psychologic role of a mature adult, which these psychiatrists believe to be mating and reproduction. This view cannot account, however, for the many heterosexuals who do not marry or who marry and remain childless.

According to Kanoti and Kosnick,[17] physical causes of homosexuality cannot be ruled out. Few scientists would say that the cause of homosexuality is purely physiologic, but these physiologic variables cannot be ignored. Some areas of the brain are intimately tied to sexual behavior.

Anthropologists and sociologists have questioned the psychosexual developmental explanation of homosexuality by pointing to the wide variety of sociocultural reactions to the existence of the phenomenon and to the fact that some persons engage in homosexual activities only in certain situations, for instance, when imprisoned or while on a long military expedition. There is also the matter of the existence of homosexuality in nonhuman animals, particularly primates, to further refute psychosexual causes. There is some beginning research into the correlation between early gender identity and later sexual orientation, but the process is so poorly understood that not even early conclusions can be drawn.

Finally, there is the explanation, ascribed to by many homosexuals, that there is no explanation, that homosexuality just *is*. Some people prefer vacations that are filled with shopping and sightseeing; others would like to do nothing but lie on the beach for 2 weeks. Some people are tall and thin; others are short and fat. Some people are optimists; others are pessimists. Some people are heterosexual; others are homosexual. This explanation may sound easy or facetious, but there is no reason to believe that it is any more or less credible than the explanations discussed previously.

Homosexual society and culture is as varied as heterosexual society and culture. The gay bar may be a distinctly homosexual phenomenon, but it is no more out of the ordinary in homosexual society than is the singles' bar in a straight society. Homosexuals do have community centers where they meet, talk, and plan political and social activities. A trip to a community center for the heterosexual elderly will reveal similar activities. A homosexual recognizes the fact of his homosexuality in the same way as other self-knowledge takes place; action on the recognition may occur immediately, or it may be delayed for varying periods of time. One woman said she realized she was unhappy in her present career at about the same time she acknowledged her sexual attraction to other women. She acted on both pieces of knowledge in a way that was uniquely hers: she thought about and assimilated the feelings and then changed those parts of her life-style to ones that could produce both greater career satisfaction and sexual fulfillment.

Female homosexuality is generally studied less than that of males and as a result is more poorly understood (this may reflect the heterosexual belief that female sexuality in general is less important than male), but the women's movement surely has played a definitive role in lesbianism. One view of the movement's effect on lesbianism is that it has helped women to free themselves of male domination and to enter into relationships with women with diminished fear of approbation and rejection by other women. The movement also opened new career avenues and somewhat improved the economic status of women so they were less dependent on men as means of support and could turn to each other for emotional and sexual satisfaction. Many women have for many years felt that male sexuality was too brutal, too aggressive, and lacked sensual passion. The women's movement has helped women to acknowledge those feelings and to reject heterosexuality if they choose to do so. The women's movement has probably not *created* a greater number of lesbians than would have existed without the movement; what it has done is to create an atmosphere of freedom in which women can act on their homosexual inclinations. In that it has prevented a great deal of both internal and external sexual repression, the women's movement has been a liberating force.

Both male and female homosexuals enter into relationships that mirror and parallel heterosexual relationships. A permanent homosexual relationship might be likened to heterosexual marriage in the truest sense of the word. A strong commitment to the love, well-being, and happiness of the partner exists, and sexual fidelity is a given. Although homosexual marriage is not permitted in any of the 50 states, many couples do exchange formal vows at a ceremony presided over by a member of the clergy and attended by friends and acquaintances. There are varying points of view about the strength of a homosexual relationship as compared with that of a heterosexual marriage. The former is held together mainly by the desire and commitment of the partners, but there is also a strong communal support system, particularly among homosexual women. Heterosexual marriage is, however, sanctioned by law, traditional social custom, and formal religion. The homosexual union is not bound by legal barriers or the presence of children that result from that particular union, although many homosexuals are parents, and their children live within the homosexual family.

The other extreme of homosexual relationships is the casual sexual encounter where a couple may stay together for one night, or even for only an hour or so. These encounters are much more common among men than women, and in any major city the number of male gay bars (where the encounters frequently begin) will far exceed the number of female bars. Most homosexual relationships, however, fall somewhere between these two extremes, lasting anywhere from a few months to several years. Homes are often shared, but sometimes the couple lives apart. Living together usually signifies the intent to establish permanence, and because there is a sharing of resources and property, the bonds forged are more difficult to break.

It must be stressed that homosexual society is not at all completely distinct and separate from heterosexual society. Homosexuals eat in restaurants, work at jobs, buy and rent homes, shovel snow, shop for groceries, and wait in line at the motor vehicle bureau with exactly the same frequency as heterosexuals. They cheat on their taxes and help old ladies across the street with the same badness or goodness of character as heterosexuals. Everyone knows at least one homosexual, although they may not be aware of the fact. Most homosexuals do not appear or act in a stereotypical manner and therefore are indistinguishable from the rest of the population. Homosexual society and heterosexual society are inextricably intertwined.

Common myths

Any group of persons that is different in some significant way from other persons, especially those who are hated and feared, is the source of a wide variety of myths. Some are silly and are more or less, although never completely, harmless. Some are pernicious and have caused incredible suffering and persecution. The following are some of the most commonly believed myths about homosexuals, along with their refutation.

1. In homosexual relationships one partner plays the role of a man and the other the role of a woman (the terms *butch* and *femme* are used, regardless of the gender of the person described). The myth generally extends to both sexual and social spheres; that is, the partner who takes out the garbage and mows the lawn is also the more sexually aggressive. Actually in most homosexual relationships partners do what they like to do and what they have a talent for doing. Most of the time sexual roles have to do with personal preference or the mood of the moment, not with stereotypical roles expected by heterosexuals. Many homosexuals feel that they have an advantage over heterosexuals because they are relatively free of societally imposed sex-role stereotypes. Most homosexual relationships are more egalitarian, in bed and out, than most heterosexual relationships. One lesbian said, "If I wanted to make love to a man, I'd find a real one." She was attracted to her female lover *because* she is a woman, not a pseudoman.

2. Homosexuals really want to be the opposite sex and try to act like them. This is simply not true. Lesbians, as well as straight women, may envy the political, economic, and social power of men and may want some of that power, but that is not the same as wanting to *be* a man. Homosexual men may envy the softness and gentility of women and may desire some of those characteristics for themselves (as do many heterosexual men), but that is not the same as wanting to *be* a woman.

3. Homosexuals hate the opposite sex, probably because of an unfortunate or painful romantic experience. This is both untrue and illogical. Homosexuals are homosexual because they are attracted *to* the same sex, not *away from* the opposite sex, and both male and female homosexuals have close friendships with members of the opposite sex. The faulty logic of this myth is evident; if every time a heterosexual person had an unhappy romantic encounter, he turned to homosexuality for solace or as a permanent change of life-style, there would soon be no heterosexuals left in the world. By the same token, homosexuals have painful romantic experiences, yet they do not suddenly become heterosexual. Homosexuality may be caused by any one or a combination of factors, but a broken heart is not necessarily one of them.

4. Homosexuals are preoccupied with sex. Everyone thinks about sex a great deal, but homosexuals spend no more time thinking about it than anyone else. Homosexuals spend about the same proportion of time in sexual activities as does the rest of the population.

5. Homosexuals have a strong desire to seduce children. This is flatly untrue and has been the source of much persecution and discrimination. The FBI's Uniform Crime Report of 1979 (the last year for which statistics are available) states that the vast majority (95%) of persons arrested for the sexual molestation of children are heterosexual men who assaulted little girls. Although gay men have been known to sexually molest little boys (pederasty is almost nonexistent among lesbians), the incidence of this behavior is far less than is believed. When sexual molestation of children occurs, it is seen as far more perverted, evil, and damaging to the child if it is homosexual than heterosexual, although there is no empirical evidence to show that this is true. Most childhood homosexual experiences take place between peers in the course of such games as "house" and "doctor" and occur mostly out of a sense of experimentation and adventure.

6. Homosexual teachers want to "recruit" children to their ranks and are therefore poor role models for children. This is as illogical as it is untrue. The overwhelming majority of teachers, straight or gay, want nothing to do with their students as sex partners. Because teachers do not bring their sex lives into the classroom, being a sexual role model has nothing to do with what transpires between student and teacher. Russell Baker, a columnist for the *New York Times*, once pointed out in a column about the issue, that if teachers were life-style role models for students, he would now be a nun! By the same token, homosexual students are not "recruited" to a straight life-style by heterosexual teachers.

7. Homosexuals can always spot each other and have a sixth sense or "radar" that always attracts them to each other. Although homosexuals sometimes behave in a stereotypical manner and deliberately make their preferences known, most times the fact of homosexuality remains as hidden as any other sexual preference. In fact, because of society's homophobia, many homosexuals are careful to blend into the rest of society and to act and dress in such a manner that does not call attention to their homosexuality. Homosexuals have no distinguishing physical characteristics.

8. Homosexuals are unhappy and unfulfilled as persons. Homosexuals are as happy or unhappy as the general population and are about as neurotic or adjusted as anyone else. Most homosexuals who seek some kind of psychologic counseling do so because they are experiencing problems that are human problems: relationships with other people; difficulties at work; feelings of loneliness, isolation, and alienation; and the entire gamut of emotional trauma. They usually see homosexuality as a fact of their lives, not as a cause of the problem. If they perceive themselves

to be having difficulty adjusting to living in a straight world, the perception is probably realistic and the problems well founded because it is difficult for a homosexual to function if he must constantly fear being found out. These observations are made after a number of personal interviews with both male and female homosexuals. There was general agreement that society had more of a problem reacting and relating to their homosexuality than they did. One lesbian said she thought it was easier to be a gay woman than an unmarried straight woman in our society because of the strong community support system that lesbians have established.

9. The homosexual can be "cured" of homosexuality by a satisfying sexual relationship with a person of the opposite sex. Can a heterosexual be changed into a homosexual by a satisfying relationship with a person of the same sex? The only further comment that needs to be made about this myth is that many homosexuals do have sex with members of the opposite sex, occasionally or even frequently, and still remain homosexuals because they choose to do so.

RELIGIOUS ASPECTS

Before the advent of monotheism or in societies that did not accept monotheism (for instance, ancient Greece and Rome, which were in full flower long after the beginning of monotheism), homosexuality was not as thoroughly condemned as it was in monotheistic religions.

> In some cultures (including some North American Indian tribes) homosexuals were regarded as representatives of the deity and were credited with powers of divination and of magic. In other cultures, homosexual and heterosexual practices formed part of the religious cult by which the divinity was worshipped.[18]

Except for these few instances, although there is a lack of accurate historical data, it is safe to say that homosexuality has been condemned at various times throughout history.

No such doubt exists in monotheistic religions. Both Judaism and Christianity explicitly condemn homosexuality and punish it by death, the harshest penalty usually reserved for the gravest sins.

After one has acknowledged that Judaism and Christianity consider homosexuality a major sin, one would wonder what other religious aspects exist, but all Biblical injunctions are open to interpretation, and in Western culture today only a handful of the most homophobic persons believe that homosexuals should be executed. It is worthwhile to examine the Biblical passages responsible for the severity of religious attitudes.

The passage quoted most frequently is Leviticus 18:22, "Thou shalt not lie with a male as one lies with a woman; it is an abomination." It should be noted here that many lesbians claim that only male homosexuality is prohibited by this passage, and that may be true, but for the purpose here we shall consider that all homosexuality is prohibited. Possibly this passage means that a man should not lie with another man while pretending that he is with a woman or treating the other man like a woman, thus negating his personhood as a man. This is not a view shared by many, however, and we shall assume that Leviticus clearly and simply prohibits all homosexuality.

Almost the entire book of Leviticus deals with laws and commandments relating to the conduct of life. There is almost no detail of existence that is not commented on in Leviticus, which is probably as it should be for a people who were creating a new society after just having escaped from Egyptian bondage. The idea of worshipping one God was the most radical thing to have happened in history at that time. It is reasonable that rules of conduct should be carefully delineated, and the historical context in which homosexuality is considered an abomination and punishable by death must be taken into account.

Laws and commandments mentioned in Leviticus are stringent in matters other than homosexuality. Chapter 2 of the book is concerned entirely with how to present a meal offering, detailed down to the choice of flour, oil, and frankincense—with or without salt. Chapter 11 specifies exactly what foods may be eaten and which are forbidden (this is the basis for the laws of *kashruth* [literally, clean]). Chapter 11 goes on for several pages and discusses only food. Chapter 13 details exactly what should be done with rashes, discolorations, or swellings of the skin. When we arrive at Chapter 18, which deals entirely with sexual conduct, it is no surprise that homosexuality would be mentioned and considered an abomination. There are 17 specific sexual abominations mentioned in this chapter, many of which concern respect for persons, (for example, "Do not uncover the nakedness of your brother's wife; it is the nakedness of your brother.") and some of which carry extremely harsh penalties.

Most modern Biblical scholars, although they do not generally approve of homosexuality, temper their condemnation with knowledge of psychosexual development, with the belief that many Biblical injunctions resulted from cultic practices and not because the specific act prohibited was necessarily sexually improper or an affront to God, and with the knowledge that in Biblical times if sexual activity and procreation were not closely linked, a tribe or even an entire nation would die. Masturbation was also forbidden by the Old Testament and punishable by death, perhaps for the same reasons—procreation did not occur.

Many other practices and acts were severely punished in the Old Testament by death or exile, for example, touching or eating unclean flesh, failure to observe the Sabbath, and the worship of graven images. Modern practitioners of religion (both lay and clergy) choose which Biblical laws and commandments to obey and which to ignore, or at least to obey in a somewhat relaxed manner. Jews who work on Saturday or Christians who do not attend church on Sunday do not expect to be executed for their behavior. More important, they do not expect to be morally castigated by their friends and colleagues. The Christian who goes fishing with his friends on Sunday but condemns homosexuality for religious reasons is behaving inconsistently. His sin, that of not observing the Sabbath and keeping it holy, is equally forbidden in the Old Testament, and his preference not to observe the Sabbath is no more or no less morally blameworthy than is the homosexual's preference to break a particular commandment that deals with sexual behavior. (Actually the commandment to observe the Sabbath is the more important of the two because it is mentioned in the Ten Commandments.) Those Jews who ride in cars on Saturday, which is forbidden, while proclaiming the unnaturalness of homosexuality are being equally inconsistent. It is true that homosexuality is specifically forbidden in the Old Testament, but so are a great many other human actions. One must obey every single Biblical command in order to morally criticize homosexuality as a sin.

Homosexuality has received an enormous amount of unwarranted "bad press" from the story of Sodom (Genesis 19:1-29). The city of Sodom is associated with sexual sin of such horrendous proportions that God felt compelled to destroy it. The story of Sodom is the story of two angels in the form of men, who arrived in Sodom to carry out God's command to destroy the city. They were persuaded to spend the night in the home of Lot, who lived there. After the angels had eaten, but before they had retired for the night, a group of men came to Lot's house and wanted the two men/angels to come out "that we may be intimate with them" (sexual intimacy was not specified). Lot implored the angels not to go outside and offered his two virgin daughters to the men in place of the men/angels. Lot apparently offered his daughters in their stead because the men/angels were guests in his home and to have permitted them to have been disturbed would have been an act of gross inhospitality. Lot may have done the wrong thing, though, because the angels were so angry that Lot offered his daughters that they blinded the men milling about and told Lot that they had indeed been sent by God to destroy the city.

When dawn broke, the angels saved Lot, his wife, and his daughters from the destruction of the city (because of Lot's act of hospitality the night before) by leading them outside the city. Lot begged to be allowed to seek safety in the nearby small town of Zoar, which the angels permitted him to do.

Nowhere is homosexuality specifically mentioned in the story of Sodom, except in the oblique reference to the townsmen wanting to be "intimate" with the men/angels. Intimacy in this sense can be as easily interpreted as comradery and revelry as sexuality. The two worst sins in the story were Lot's offering his daughters to the townsmen and the general inhospitality of the townspeople, yet ironically it was Lot who was saved from the destruction of Sodom.

It is difficult to know why the story of Sodom is used as a metaphor for the evil of homosexuality; perhaps it was the presence of general licentiousness and the aura of sexual permissiveness that pervaded the city and the totality of its destruction by sulfurous fire from heaven. But from the story comes the word sodomy, which has been defined in various ways and which is an act that is practiced by *both* homosexuals and heterosexuals.

The story of Sodom has greatly influenced the formulation of both religious and civil law.

> The Code of Theodosius and the Code of Justinian, for example, prohibited all sodomistic practices under pain of death by fire. . . . The sixth-century Code of Justinian had considerable impact on both the ecclesiastical and civil laws of the Middle Ages and indirectly on civil law in the West. . . .[19]

The philosophic rationale for believing homosexuality to be unnatural and immoral stems mainly from the belief that all sexuality must be primarily procreative in nature and intent.

In the New Testament the Epistle of Paul the Apostle to the Romans (1:26–27) states that homosexuality was forbidden as a sin "against nature." Those who committed such sins would not be permitted to enter into the Kingdom of God and were "worthy of death." For the first time female homosexuality is specifically mentioned (verse 26), where women change natural use (of sexuality) to that which is unnatural. This and other New Testament prohibitions had given rise to the Christian concept of natural law, which has been debated by philosophers and theologians ever since. Natural law has often been confused with the laws of nature and will be discussed in greater detail in subsequent chapters. Suffice it to say for the present that laws of nature are descriptive and concern the way the physical world works (both human and nonhuman). An example of a law of nature is the female menstrual cycle. A natural law is prescriptive and concerns itself with what persons ought to do about laws of nature. An example of a natural law is the prohibition against touching a menstruating woman. A law of nature is morally neutral; a natural law has a moral value.

Even though religions are generally negative about homosexuality, many homosexuals are unable or unwilling to reject religion or to live without that important spiritual component. For this reason homosexual religious groups have been founded, and many major religions have a strong national network of groups that function in the same way as heterosexual churches and synagogues, with one important exception. The exception is that in almost all instances the gay groups do not have the support of the religious organizational hierarchy, and in many cases the existence of the gay religious group is simply not acknowledged.

The Metropolitan Community Church (MCC) is a huge national network of nondenominational gay Protestants. It was founded in Los Angeles and has branches in every major city, and each branch functions as a separate church (for example, MCC, Philadelphia) with strong ties to the parent organization. The name of the Catholic national organization is Dignity, and the Episcopalian group is called Integrity. They each function in much the same way as MCC. The International Congress of Gay and Lesbian Jewish Organizations stretches from the United States across Europe to Israel and Australia. It is composed of individual synagogues, each with a different name and each of which sends representatives to an annual conference. Some of the American synagogues are even recognized by and are a part of the mainstream Reform Jewish national organization.

Attendance at religious services and social functions vary, but religious holidays usually mean a packed house—exactly the same phenomenon as occurs in straight churches and synagogues. These are not "underground" organizations; they are simply separate from the mainstream, mainly because of the strong negative feelings that homosexuals experience in straight religious congregations.

ETHICAL ISSUES

The reader is referred to Chapter 2 for a discussion of the purpose of sexuality in general as a basis for the ethical issues inherent in homosexuality. Obviously a procreative function cannot exist for homosexuality, but there is no reason to preclude any of the others.

> Apart from the question of the meaning of sexuality, the ethical and moral questions raised by homosexuality do not differ substantially, if at all, from the ethical and moral questions raised by heterosexuality, since the question of the normative aspects of the interpersonal and intersocial behavior are the same for homosexuality as for heterosexuality.[20]

This is an important statement to understand because by making it the authors have declared that homosexuality per se is morally neutral. This position appears to be the only acceptable one from any theoretical point of view. Any moral condemnation of homosexuality as a phenomenon (this does not apply to specific sexual and nonsexual acts engaged in by homosexual persons) will necessarily involve homophobia and resultant acts of repression and persecution, and we have shown that homophobia is immoral from both the utilitarian and deontologic views. One is not necessarily obligated to like homosexuality, or to even approve of its existence, any more than one is obligated to like or approve of any other sexual activity. Homosexuality is neither good nor bad. It exists in life and is practiced by people who are as good or bad as any other people.

Kanoti and Kosnick[21] discuss three approaches to the ethical analysis of homosexuality: the integrist, the recreational, and the relational. The integrist view sees homosexuality as completely immoral because it negates or denies the interrelationship of sexuality and reproduction and is therefore unnatural. The integrist does not accept empiric evidence in making normative decisions; the only sources used are religious teaching, tradition, or philosophic concepts of nature and the order of things. In this rejection of facts and empiric evidence, the integrist is irrational. The integrist condemns homosexuality by insisting that a homosexual act frustrates the purpose of sexual organs and must therefore be judged unnatural. Whatever is unnatural is a disruption of the order of nature and thus thwarts the will of God.

The recreational view holds that not only is homosexuality natural, empirical evidence proves it. All mammals exhibit homosexual behavior, and it has existed in all human cultures. Therefore it cannot be considered unnatural. Almost all societies consider homosexuality to be a deviation from the majority, but it continues to exist and to be practiced by significant numbers of persons whether the society suppresses homosexual behavior, actively encourages it, legally regulates it, or does nothing at all. The happiness and general well-being of homosexuals can be affected by societal attitudes; the existence of homosexuality cannot. "The extent of homosexual behavior in all levels of mammalian creatures and the nondeleterious effects of such behaviors on the lives of the participants constitute a new source of information which challenges the assumptions upon which the integrist view builds its analysis of homosexuality."[22]

The relational understanding has developed to a great extent as a result of the personal experience of homosexuals and the existence of empiric data based on psychologic and sociologic research. The relational view is that homosexuality is morally neutral and holds the same normative value as heterosexuality. The ethical quality of relationships is based, not on the nature of the sexual contact between partners, but on the nature of the relationship of the *persons* involved. The rejection of the naturalistic approach is a rejection of the view that the sexual act itself is the primary source of moral value.

The integrist view seems to be losing ground in numbers of advocates, and those philosophers who write about the ethics of homosexuality appear to take some or all of the following into consideration: the etiology of the phenomenon, its impact on society, the relationship between private behavior and public policy, the meaning of sexuality, empirical evidence, and traditional religious and philosophic thought.

CIVIL, CRIMINAL, AND SOCIETAL REPRESSION

There are few groups in American history (with the notable exception of blacks) that have been as consistently oppressed and have had as many human rights abrogated as have homosexuals. Although homosexuality itself is not against the law in any state, all states have laws pertaining to sexual behavior that have been used to discriminate against homosexuals. Although arresting a homosexual for a practice that a heterosexual would be permitted to practice with impunity (for example, sodomy, which is illegal in many states) is blatant discrimination, other forms of homosexual oppression run the gamut from equally as blatant to very subtle and insidious. The following are some examples of ways in which homosexuals have been and are discriminated against:

1. Although the United States Constitution upholds the right of freedom of speech for all citizens, and although all homosexual citizens enjoy that right and cannot be arrested for publicly espousing gay rights or otherwise publicly talking about homosexual issues, a federal court of appeals upheld the right of a state university to refuse to employ a homosexual as head of the university's library cataloging division because the man had applied for a license to marry another man.[23] The university's refusal to hire the man was based on his publicly stated views that homosexuals should be entitled to the same civil rights (marriage is a civil right) as heterosexuals. The man was not refused a job, according to the university, because of his homosexuality, but because of his public espousal of gay rights. Thus his First Amendment rights were abrogated.

2. Private employers may legally discriminate against homosexuals solely on the basis of their homosexuality. No federal or state laws exist to prohibit this kind of discrimination, although increasing numbers of cities have local ordinances that guarantee equal employment rights to homosexuals. However, to achieve legal redress based on these ordinances, the homosexual must prove that it was his homosexuality that cost him his job or job opportunity. Most employers will not voluntarily admit this, and the homosexual must engage in a civil suit that can prove long, costly, and emotionally draining. Most people do not have the resources or stamina for such a fight; employers know this, and discrimination continues. Moreover, if a homosexual were to win such a suit and then moved to another city, he would likely have to fight the battle all over again.

3. Occupational licensing laws are often administered in such a way as to further restrict the employment opportunities of gays. While the purported justification of such laws lies in the public's asserted interest in ensuring that people in certain occupations are duly qualified, in practice such laws have often been used as vehicles for enforcing majoritarian social and political views.[24]

In *Dent v. West Virginia* (1899)[25] the Supreme Court held that the power of the state to provide for the welfare of the people authorized it to prescribe such regulations with regard to certain occupations, that it deemed necessary to protect people against ignorance, incapacity, deception, and fraud. Inherent in this ruling is that occupations may themselves decide what activities will be prohibited to protect the general welfare, and the courts have been reluctant to interfere in regulations pertaining to the granting of occupational licenses. State licensing boards use their power to discriminate against homosexuals in a variety of ways. Many occupations will not license a person (or will revoke an existing license) who has been convicted of a criminal offense, even a misdemeanor such as loitering (a common charge levied against cruising homosexuals). This in itself is not necessarily discriminatory *if* all misdemeanors are deemed equally sufficient cause for nonlicensure (for example, shoplifters may not lose a license while a homosexual loiterer will). Many occupations require that the practitioner demonstrate "good moral character" or that they refrain from "moral turpitude." These phrases then are not specifically defined and are open to interpretation by members of licensing boards who may be homophobic to varying degrees.

4. Homosexuals are not permitted to serve in any branch of the United States military services. If they are accused of homosexuality while in the service, and if the charges can be proved, a general discharge is usually the result. On January 16, 1981, the Department of Defense issued revised policy guidelines in regard to homosexuality in the military. In Volume 37, Section 41.13 of the Code of Federal Regulations, the policy is spelled out.

> Homosexuality is incompatible with military service. The presence in the military environment of persons who engage in homosexual conduct or who, by their statements, demonstrate a propensity to engage in homosexual conduct, seriously impairs the accomplishment of the military mission. The presence of such members adversely affects the ability of the armed forces to maintain discipline, good order, and morale. . . .

The regulations further define "homosexual" as "a person, regardless of sex, who engages in, desires to engage in, or intends to engage in homosexual acts."

These regulations are highly discriminatory, and it is surely conceivable that heterosexuals who make a chance remark about the physical attractiveness of a person of the same sex could be accused of "desiring" a homosexual act. A heterosexual who had a homosexual friend could also place himself in jeopardy.

5. An alien who is a homosexual may be prohibited from obtaining a United States visa or even from entering the United States.[26] The Supreme Court, when it made this decision, did not clearly define homosexuality, nor did it distinguish between a person with a "psychopathic personality" and a "sexual deviation."

6. There are no legal protections for homosexuals against discrimination in housing except in rare instances where the federal government is involved in a housing program and if protection against homosexual discrimination is specifically mentioned in the federal regulations. All the Civil Rights acts that have protected blacks and other minorities from housing discrimination have not affected homosexuals. A landlord is legally permitted to inquire about a perspective tenant's sexual preference before he agrees to rent the property.

7. The law clearly discriminates in favor of monogamous, heterosexual marital relationships. An elaborate body of law has developed with respect to the benefits, rights, and privileges of persons who commit themselves to such relationships. Marital partners have advantages in income, gift, and estate-tax rates. They may inherit from one another without a will; they may own property in tenancy by the entirety; they may run businesses at lower cost in taxes; each may recover for the wrongful death of the other; they may adopt children more easily than singles; and they may lawfully have sexual relations. All of these and other benefits are denied to those who elect not to marry, or who are not permitted to marry. Private organizations such as airlines, insurance companies, and banks offer their goods and services on terms that discriminate in favor of married persons.

No state has ever upheld the right of two people of the same sex to marry, even though this is clearly government interference in the right of privacy in personal matters guaranteed by the Supreme Court in several instances[28,29] and is protected by the First Amendment.

8. On June 28, 1980, at a memorial service at the Tomb of the Unknown Soldier in Arlington National Cemetary, the Gay Activist Alliance (GAA) paid tribute to homosexuals who had died in service to their country. A floral wreath was contributed. During the service the word "gay" was blocked from the ribbon by rearranging the flowers, the name of the GAA was not mentioned during the service, and the wreath was removed from the tomb immediately after the service. The service was distinctly different from ones held for other organizations that always mention the name of the organization holding the service and leave the wreath in place until the flowers wilt.[30]

The list of acts of discrimination against homosexuals could continue almost indefinitely. In the past decade or so, homosexuals have been taking social and political action to protect themselves against civil and criminal oppression. The gay liberation movement has spawned many organizations that fight for gay rights and provide counseling and professional services for homosexuals. As a result of these actions, some forms of discrimination have diminished, but by and large the gay rights movement has not had the social and political impact of the women's movement. There are several reasons for this: male hatred of women is not as strong or as widespread as heterosexual hatred of homosexuals; the fact of being a woman is not in itself seen as immoral, while the fact of homosexuality is in many instances; women are not considered mentally ill, while homosexuals often are. It must be noted that the gay liberation movement is a civil rights issue in the same way as is the drive to secure full legal equality for women and blacks. The purpose of the movement is not to encourage more people to be homosexual or to insist that homosexuality is better than heterosexuality; it seeks only to end discrimination against homosexuals.

The Wolfenden Report

In 1967, after more than 10 years of debate in Parliament and elsewhere, the principles of the Wolfenden Report were enacted into law in Great Britain. In effect, homosexuality was decriminalized, and persons could not be criminally prosecuted for sexual acts between consenting adults, regardless of the sex of the participants. The committee that wrote the Wolfenden Report stated, in part, that the function of criminal law was to protect persons from the exploitation and corruption of others, particularly those who are in some way physically or mentally vulnerable. Since private sexual acts between consenting adults do not criminally exploit or endanger anyone, there is no reason for them to be subject to criminal prosecution. The report also emphasized the importance of a society granting freedom of choice in matters of private morality. The government has no business equating the concept of crime with the concept of sin as long as harm does not occur and the acts in question are done privately.

The Wolfenden Report was hotly debated before it was enacted into law. Of course not everyone approves of the decriminalization of homosexuality. Those persons who disapprove of the decriminalization base their opinions on the belief that the law must reflect the moral principles of a majority of members of a society. This is a strongly ethical relativist view and has to do with the differentiation between public and private morality where law is used as a weapon to enforce the morality of the majority on all members of society. It is also concerned with instances when private acts can be regulated or prohibited by law.

The relativist will agree that because a majority of persons believe an act to be wrong does not necessarily mean it *is* wrong; what they do advocate is that the collective judgment of society has a bearing on what private behavior is and is not permitted by law. The view that a public morality exists (not all agree that it does) is expressed in the view that a society is a community of ideas, both in terms of politics and the way people behave and live. The community of ideas is known as morality, which may or may not, in whole or in part, be ethical. This is the problem with application of the relativist view; when and if the community of ideas is unethical, should it be discarded as such, or should it be embraced simply because it is the result of the community morality?

Sir Patrick Devlin,[31] in opposing the Wolfenden Report, stated that if a society does not have the right to make judgments about morals, then the law must find a justification for entering the realm of morality. If homosexuality is not in and of itself wrong, then the legislator must find a way to justify the exceptional treatment of homosexuals. That justification can be based on society's right to make a moral judgment about particular acts. Society may use the law to safeguard the collective moral judgment in the same way it uses the law to protect anything else it considers essential to its existence. Society then has a right to legislate for or against morality in the same way it has the right to legislate about matters of public health and safety. "There are no theoretical limits to the power of the State to legislate against treason and sedition, and likewise I think there can be no theoretical limits to legislation against immorality."[32]

Sir Patrick's linkage of treason and sedition with homosexuality seems a bit excessive, but he is not alone in believing that homosexuality should not be publicly condoned (although the Wolfenden Report did not specifically condone homosexuality, its decriminalization has that effect in the eyes of many). Malcolm Muggeridge believes that homosexuals at the higher levels of the civil service have a greater propensity for treason than do heterosexuals because they are more vulnerable to blackmail. It is interesting to note that if homophobia did not exist, neither would the likelihood of blackmail because homosexuals would not feel compelled to hide the fact of their homosexuality.

When philosophers repudiate the liberal point of view concerning governmental interference in private consensual behavior, they usually make their attack on liberals from the position of either divine or natural law. Sir Patrick does neither; he bases his opinion on the collective feelings of the average person, a kind of morality by popular demand, a Nielson rating of ethical behavior. These are insufficient and incorrect grounds on which to base a rational moral judgment (refer to Chapter 1). Thus this judgment cannot be correct because it is based on an illogical premise.

H. L. A. Hart agrees that in some aspects of the criminal law consensus is necessary for enforcement, such as regards laws against murder, theft, and rape. But he just as emphatically states that not all areas of morality are of equal importance to society, "nor is there the slightest reason for thinking of morality as a seamless web: one which will fall to pieces carrying society with it, unless all its emphatic vetoes are enforced by law."[33] There is no reason to believe, because there is no demonstrable proof, that permitting private consensual activity to continue without criminal punishment will cause an increase in any other forms of behavior that people believe to be immoral. Because homosexuals are not prosecuted does not mean that society will have to endure more murders, burglaries, and rapes. One class of actions has nothing to do with the other; to compare them in terms of morality or criminality is not rational.

Hart also makes another important distinction in reasons why a particular action is considered immoral, even by a majority of persons. He asks us to consider whether general morality is based on ignorance, superstition, or misunderstandings and whether there is a false belief, on the part of those condemning an action, that the action is somehow hostile or dangerous to society, and "whether the misery to many parties, the blackmail and other evil consequences of criminal punishment, especially for sexual offenses, are well understood."[34] In other words, is it worth it to put homosexuals through the misery of criminal prosecution, with its possible evil consequences, for acts that harm no one and cannot be construed as dangerous to society? If homosexuals are not causing harm, then society has no right to harm them. If decisions about criminality are matters of politics, then political power should surely be in the hands of the majority in a democratic society. However, when the majority uses that power to subjugate a minority, or when it behaves in a way that loses sight of the limits of power, the democratic society is destroyed and replaced by totalitarianism. Britain has tried, in part, to prevent that state of affairs by decriminalizing homosexuality as recommended in the Wolfenden Report.

SUMMARY

Homosexuality is difficult to define because many definitions are value laden. The definition that carries the least moral weight is that a homosexual is a person who feels strong erotic attraction to persons of the same sex and who prefers to engage in sexual activity with persons of the same sex. Other definitions are concerned with the repetitiveness of homosexual behavior, sociocultural and psychologic causation, and various degrees of moral overtones.

Homosexuality occurs in all cultures and strata of society, and it cuts across all religious and socioeconomic boundaries. It is impossible to know exactly how prevalent homosexuality is, but a fairly accurate estimate is that about 10% of the adult population of the United States lead active homosexual life-styles. There are more male than female homosexuals. Studies have shown that in comparison to the general population, homosexuals are no more or less happy nor more or less psychologically adjusted than other persons.

The history of homosexuality is characterized mainly by fear, repression, criminal prosecution, and even execution, although surely all homosexuals are not and were not always in fear. Repression of homosexuals stems from the phenomenon known as homophobia, which is fear and hatred of homosexuals and which leads to their subjugation and persecution. Although homophobia is a common heterosexual experience, it is shown to be unethical on the basis of both utilitarian and deontologic moral theories. It is as unethical as any other form of persecution of minorities.

Several theories have been advanced about the cause of homosexuality, for example, a failure of, or error in, normal psychosexual development; fear of the opposite sex; physical causes, such as unusual endocrine balances or abnormal chromosomal configurations; correlation between early gender identity and later sexual orientation; and the cause of "no cause," that is, homosexuality simply exists as do other human characteristics and sexual preferences.

Although some homosexuals do function sometimes as part of a subculture, they are also highly integrated into heterosexual American life, and it is safe to say that everyone associates with homosexuals on the job or socially, even though they may not be aware of that fact. Homosexual interpersonal relationships function in the same way as do heterosexual relationships, although there are no formal marital bonds because homosexual marriage is not recognized or permitted in any of the 50 states.

All Western religions strongly condemn homosexuality, and both the Old and New Testaments insist that homosexuals be put to death. However, Biblical passages that forbid or appear to forbid homosexuality can be interpreted in a variety of ways, and many modern theologians are taking a more enlightened approach toward the condemnation of homosexuality, although no religion advocates it as a positive way of life.

Ethical issues in homosexuality depend mainly on one's view of the purpose of sexuality in general. If sexuality is seen as only reproductive in nature, then homosexuality will be considered unnatural and therefore immoral. If the purpose of sexuality is purely pleasure, then any sexual activity, including homosexuality, that provides pleasure is permissible.

Civil and criminal oppression is common, and it is clear that the civil rights of homosexuals are violated more frequently than those of heterosexuals, just as the civil rights of blacks and women are violated more frequently than those of whites and men. A variety of gay liberation groups has sprung up to counteract this oppression, and in Great Britain homosexuality was decriminalized in 1967 as a result of the Wolfenden Report, which stated that private consensual behavior is not properly a matter for governmental interference.

Notes

1. Kinsey, A. C., et al. *Sexual behavior in the human male*. Philadelphia: W. B. Saunders Co., 1948.
2. Kinsey, A. C., et al. *Sexual behavior in the human female*. Philadelphia: W. B. Saunders Co., 1953.
3. Hunt, M. *Sexual behavior in the 1970s*. New York: Playboy Press, 1974.
4. Bell, A., & Weinberg, M. *Homosexualities*. New York: Simon & Schuster, 1978.
5. Weinberg, M. S. & Williams, C. J. Male homosexuals: their problems and adaptation. In M. S. Weinber (Ed.), *Sex research*. New York: Oxford University Press, Inc., 1976. pp. 246–57.
6. Katz, J. (Ed.). *Gay American history*. New York: Avon Books, 1976. p. 17.
7. Francis Higgeson's journal In S. Mitchell (Ed.), *The founding of Massachusetts*. Boston: Massachusetts Historical Society, 1930. p. 71.
8. Katz, p. 36.
9. Jefferson, T. *The papers of Thomas Jefferson* (Vol. 2). J. P. Boyd (Ed.), Princeton, New Jersey: Princeton University Press, 1950. p. 325.
10. Katz, p. 46.
11. United States Department of the Interior, Census Office. *Report on crime, pauperism, and benevolence in the United States at the eleventh census: 1890* (Pt. 1). Washington, D.C.: U.S. Government Printing Office, 1896.
12. Scott, C. Sex and art. *American Journal of Psychology*. 1896, *7*(2), 216.
13. Hirschfeld, M. *Die Homosexualität des Mannes und des Weibes* (J. Steakley, trans.). Berlin: Louis Marcus, 1914. pp. 550–554.
14. Katz, p. 81.
15. Otis, M. A perversion not commonly noted. *Journal of Abnormal Psychology*. 1913, *8*(2), 113–16.
16. Katz, pp. 194–195.
17. Creson, D. L. Homosexuality: clinical and behavioral aspects. In W. T. Reich (Ed.), *Encyclopedia of bioethics*. (Vol. 2). New York: The Free Press, 1978. p. 669.
18. Kanoti, G. A., & Kosnick, A. R. Homosexuality: ethical aspects. In *Encyclopedia of bioethics* (Vol. 2). p. 671.
19. Kanoti & Kosnick, p. 672.
20. Kanoti & Kosnick, p. 673.
21. Kanoti & Kosnick, pp. 674–675.
22. Kanoti & Kosnick, p. 674.
23. *McConnell v. Anderson*, 451 F 2nd 193 (8th Cir. 1971), *cert. denied*, 405 U.S. 1046 (1972).
24. Boggan, E. C., et al. *The rights of gay people: an American civil liberties union handbook*. New York: Avon Books, 1975. p. 33.
25. *Dent v. West Virginia*, 129 U.S. 114, 122 (1899).
26. *Boutilier v. Immigration and Naturalization Service*, 387 U.S. 118 (1967)
27. Boggan, p. 103.
28. *Griswold v. Connecticut*, 381 U.S. 479 (1965); *Eisenstadt v. Baird*, 405 U.S. 438 (1972).
29. *Roe v. Wade*, 410 U.S. 113 (1973).
30. Chibbaro, L., Jr. GAA seeks apology from Army secretary. *The Blade*, July 10, 1980, p. 4.

31. Devlin, Sir Patrick. Morals and the criminal law. In J. R. Burr, & M. Goldinginger (Eds.), *Philosophy and contemporary issues* (2nd ed.). New York: Macmillan Publishing Co., Inc., 1976. p. 237.
32. Devlin, p. 239.
33. Hart, H. L. A. Immorality and treason. In Burr & Goldinger, p. 248.
34. Hart, p. 250.

Bibliography

Bell, A., & Weinberg, M. *Homosexualities*. New York: Simon & Schuster, 1978.

Boggan, E. C., et al. *The rights of gay people: an American civil liberties union handbook*. New York: Avon Books, 1975.

Clark, D. *Loving someone gay*. Millbrae, Calif.: Celestial Arts, 1977.

Creson, D. L. Homosexuality: clinical and behavioral aspects. In W. Reich (Ed.), *Encyclopedia of bioethics*. New York: The Free Press, 1978.

Devlin, Sir Patrick. Morals and the criminal law. In J. R. Burr, & M. Goldinger (Eds.), *Philosophy and contemporary issues*. New York: Macmillan Publishing Co., Inc., 1976.

Friedman, S. S., et al. *A woman's guide to therapy*. Englewood Cliffs, New Jersey: Prentice-Hall, Inc., 1979.

Hart, H. L. A. Immorality and treason. In Burr & Goldinger.

Hogan, R. *Human sexuality: a nursing perspective*. New York: Appleton-Century-Crofts, 1980.

Hunt, M. *Sexual behavior in the 1970s*. New York: Playboy Press, 1974.

Jay, K., & A. Young (Eds.). *After you're out*. New York: Link Books, 1975.

Kanoti, G. A., & Kosnick, A. R. Homosexuality: ethical aspects. In *Encyclopedia of bioethics*.

Katz, J. (Ed.). *Gay American history*. New York: Avon Books, 1976.

Kinsey, A. C., et al. *Sexual behavior in the human male*. Philadelphia: W. B. Saunders Co., 1948.

Kinsey, A. C., et al. *Sexual behavior in the human female*. Philadelphia: W. B. Saunders Co., 1953.

Martin, D. & Lyon, P. *Lesbian woman*. New York: Bantam Books, Inc., 1972.

Weinberg, M. S. & Williams, C. J. Male homosexuals: their problems and adaptation. In M. S. Weinberg (Ed.), *Sex research*. New York: Oxford University Press, Inc., 1976. pp. 246–57.

Woods, N. F. *Human sexuality in health and illness* (2nd ed.). St. Louis: The C.V. Mosby Co., 1979.

CHAPTER 4

CONTRACEPTION

HISTORY OF ETHICAL THOUGHT

Women have been trying to prevent conception since they first connected the act of intercourse with pregnancy; and physicians have been prescribing potions, contraptions, herbs, and even incantations to help women achieve their goal. A series of papyri that date from 1900 to 1100 BC depict physicians prescribing application of crocodile dung, acacia tips, and dates in a variety of mixtures to block sperm.[1] In some cultures the power of prayer was thought to be a sufficient contraceptive. Around 300 BC the Tantras in India believed a true yogi should have sufficient self-control to have intercourse without emitting semen. Approximately 400 years earlier, it was believed that if a man said (during intercourse), "With power, with semen, I reclaim the semen from you," the woman "comes to be without seed."[2] The former Indian method could be interpreted as coitus interruptus; the latter surely cannot. Tantric thought was, however, considered heresy by Hindus because male descendents were essential to help perform death rites for parents; thus procreation was extremely important in Hinduism (this necessity to procreate will be explored more fully in Chapter 5 in connection with overpopulation in India and in other countries.

Potions were commonly used in ancient Greece and Rome; some were drunk (particularly those containing copper distillates), and some were poured on the woman's body "where the seed falls." Physicians of the Hippocratic school determined when they thought a woman was most likely to become pregnant (mostly they were wrong), and Herodotus wrote of men having anal intercourse with their wives to avoid conception. Contraception was widely practiced in the ancient world by rulers who wished to wait for auspicious astrologic conditions before conceiving, by slaves who did not want to bear more children for their masters, by prostitutes who did not want the inconvenience of pregnancy, and by all women because they already had too many children or wanted to hide adultery or preserve their youth and beauty.

Because conception and contraception are so closely allied with religion and spirituality, a history of ethical thought as it relates to contraception must take ancient religious belief into account. In ancient Judaism childbearing took on an aura of supreme importance because of the divine command (Genesis 1:27–28) to increase and multiply. Ancient Jewish law did not specifically condemn contraception, but it became a traditional taboo because fertility was so highly valued. Onan (Genesis 38:10) was slain by God because he refused to impregnate his dead brother's wife, which was a law at that time. Although Biblical interpretation finds several reasons why God struck down Onan, the practice of coitus interruptus became "the way of a wicked man" and was considered a serious sin. Although there were limited circumstances in which it was permissible to prevent conception, the practice of contraception was generally condemned in ancient Judaism.

In the Greco-Roman world there was little interest in the morality of contraception. Hippocrates, although he was specific in prohibiting abortifacients, said nothing about contraception, and Plato, in his *Republic*, envisioned an ideal world in which people did not have too many children. There was controversy about the practicality of contraception in much of the ancient world, especially among the Romans who were particularly militaristic. The security of a state often depended on population, and armies could not function without a constant supply of manpower. The Stoic school of philosophy was opposed to contraception because the Stoics believed that the sole purpose for intercourse was procreation, and anything that thwarted that goal was unnatural and therefore wrong. Philo, an Alexandrian Jew, combined Judaism with classical philosophy to approximate the Stoic distinction between marital intercourse for procreation and intercourse only for pleasure. "A man acted evilly, he taught, if he married a woman known to be sterile. 'Those persons', Philo added, 'who made an art of quenching the life of the seed as it drops stand condemned as the enemies of nature.'"[3]

Early Christianity took a position on the morality of contraception that melded ecclesiastic doctrine (love of God and love of neighbor) and the beliefs of other Mediterranean people. There were five basic themes in early Christian sexual ethics, as follows: (1) the superiority of virginity, (2) the institutional goodness of marriage, (3) the sacred character of sexual intercourse, (4) the goodness of procreation, and (5) the evil of extramarital intercourse and homosexuality.[4] It is easy to see that early Christians could have become confused about these inconsistencies, but a balance was struck by permitting two ways of life—that of celibacy, which emulates the example of Jesus' virginity, and that of marriage, in which intercourse occurs for the purpose of procreation. All contraceptive and abortifacient drugs and devices were denounced as sinful. "As Christianity permeated the Mediterranean world, it entered a society in which women were widely regarded as objects of pleasure; prostitution, particularly of slaves, was widespread; divorce and sexual infidelity were common."[5] It is possible that the Christian view of contraception might be, at least in part, a reaction against treating women as mere things, as sex objects, in today's parlance. It should be noted, however, that early Christianity, in its efforts to counteract the inhumane treatment of women by nonChristians, by denying them contraception did not further the position of women as full persons. If women did not have the power to control their reproductive capacities (limited and haphazard though that control would have been at the time), they could not be considered fully autonomous persons. Therefore although both ancient Judaism and Christianity protected women in some ways, they repressed and enslaved them in others.

In the fourth century AD as Christianity spread throughout the Roman Empire, an underground religion called Manicheanism sprang up, after the prophet Mani who had been executed in Persia. Manicheanism was based on the following central myth: human beings originated through lustful intercourse between princes and princesses of darkness after they had devoured the sons of the King of Light. Particles of light remained imprisoned within all humans and always struggled to be free. Manicheanism held that procreation was the worst of sins because all the alienated lights sought to return to earth. Intercourse was not forbidden but procreation was, and of course contraception was highly favored. The Catholic Church outlawed Manicheanism, and by 444 AD Pope Leo the Great had successfully driven its followers out of Rome.[6]

The existence of Manicheanism, which was an important cult at the time but now is of interest primarily to Biblical scholars, would not ordinarily be mentioned in a book of this kind except for the highly significant fact that Augustine was a Manichee from the age of 18 to 29. By the time the Manichees had been expelled from Rome, Augustine had joined the Catholic Church, and his personal reaction against his former beliefs was extraordinarily significant for all of Christian ethical thought, especially as it related to the ethics of sexuality because Manicheanism was based on a highly sexual central myth. Augustine became a convinced and aggressive foe of contraception. He believed that if marital intercourse was to be entirely free of sin, not only must contraception not take place, but offspring must result. Every act of intercourse had to have a procreative intent; without it, sex turns "the bridal chamber into a brothel." To compound the evil of nonprocreative intercourse, Augustine believed that original sin was transmitted through intercourse, with or without procreative intent; hence all offspring were necessarily born with original sin.

Augustine exhibited the kind of fervor of belief that is common to many converts and may have carried his procreative zeal to unnecessary lengths. "Augustine's synthesis of personal experience and reaction, Old and New Testament, anti-Manicheanism, and Christian sacramental theory was to constitute the strongest ethical case against any form of contraception."[7]

The development of Islam followed that of Christianity, and by the seventh century it was the dominant religion in the Middle East and North Africa and remains so today. The Koran, which is the central book of Islamic laws and commandments, does not specifically forbid contraception, but Islam to some extent adopted the cultural mores of the people already living in the Middle East, especially as they applied to increasing population as a defense against the ever-present variety of conquering marauders. In eleventh century Damascus the famous physician Avicenna wrote a comprehensive text, *Canon of Medicine*, in which he listed a pharmacopoeia of contraceptives, most of them plants. He also distinguished between contraceptives and abortifacients, although the latter were not specifically prohibited.

Medieval Europe was strongly under the influence of the Catholic Church, which expressly forbid contraception, both for the reasons already cited and because sexual intercourse without the purpose of procreation was closely associated with pagan magic and other forms of antitheistic beliefs. In addition to classifying contraceptive acts as sinful, inquisitional detection methods were developed, as was punishment in the form of penances. There was, however, opposition to the Church's view. Catharism became organized as a church and by the eleventh century had become firmly established in southern France and northern Italy. The doctrine of Catharism opposed sexual intercourse that led to procreation because it was thought that the devil had given "seed to the children of the world." Each time a woman conceived, she was thought to be housing Satan in her uterus and was refused the Cathar sacraments. Catharism was similar to Manicheanism and was viewed as a threat to the Catholic Church because it endangered the institution of marriage and the goal of perpetuating the species. The spread of Catharism developed into an ecclesiastic crisis.

> The Dominican order was founded to convert them. The Inquisition was used to discover them. The Fourth Lateran Council in 1215 encouraged a holy crusade against them. The Hail Mary, with its key words 'Blessed are you among women; and blessed is the fruit of your womb', became a popular prayer, prescribed to counter Cathar sentiment.[8]

Canon law thus drew heavily on Augustinian teaching, which condemned contraception and contraceptive marriage.

In addition to Catharism, other anti-Catholic views regarding contraception found favor in Medieval Europe. Avicenna's *Canon of Medicine* was translated into Latin and was the standard medical text for the next 500 years. Because most contraceptive techniques were ineffective (and some actually dangerous), it is difficult to know the extent of actual contraceptive practice, but Chaucer mentions three methods in *Canterbury Tales* ("The Parson's Tale"), and Catherine of Sienna had a vision in which contraception was widely practiced among the bourgeoisie. Some Christian theologians interpreted the doctrine of St. Paul ("Let the husband render to his wife what is due her, and likewise the wife to her husband" [1 Corinthians 7:3]) as a marital duty or debt. Fulfillment of the debt was virtuous in itself, and procreation was secondary to the marital obligation. The Church also permitted those who were incapable of procreation (the sterile and those past the age of childbearing) to marry; thus procreation was not necessary for marriage. Presumably these marriages were to be consumated; thus certain acts of intercourse that did not involve procreative intent were permissible. Christian theology was also beginning to develop the idea of universal religious education. Inherent in this concept of education for the good of offspring is rejection of the growth of population for its own sake and the promotion of a better educated community of Christians.

Although the Protestant Reformation shook the foundations of the Catholic Church, it had minimal effect on marital conduct and contraception. Martin Luther patterned both his theology and morality on Augustine, and in his *German Catechism* he taught that the purpose of marriage was for husband and wife to be fruitful, to beget children, to nourish them, and to raise them in the glory of God. John Calvin was even more opposed to contraception than Luther and characterized the sin of coitus interruptus as "doubly monstrous." The Reformation eventually led to a rivalry between Protestant sects. The number of people who belonged to a sect greatly increased its chances for societal and religious supremacy; therefore contraception as a sin was preached with even greater vigor. Another reason why changes in sexual and contraceptive ethics did not occur during and as a result of the Reformation was that sex was imbued with a sense of mystery, and although it was known that intercourse resulted in conception, the anatomy and physiology of the process was not well understood and thus was viewed as controlled by God. One did not interfere with God's creative powers without risking severe consequences; therefore most sexual acts and all contraceptive acts remained sinful. During the Reformation no major numbers of people nor any societal institution demanded changes in traditional taboos; therefore none occurred.

The eighteenth century saw the development of rational, logical thinking about contraception. In 1798 Thomas Malthus, an English theologian, wrote *Essay on the Principles of Population*, which warned of the dangers of a geometrical growth of population while resources grew arithmetically. That essay remains the theoretical basis of many of today's advocates of population control, which will be discussed in more detail in Chapter 5. The economist Jeremy Bentham, who is most famous for the development of utilitarianism, advocated the use of "sponges" (presumably inserted into the vagina to soak up semen) to reduce the population growth of the poor. (Utilitarians are, of course, strong advocates of both individual contraception and large-scale population control.) In the United States the first published advocacy of contraception and birth control methods was a book by Robert Dale Owens titled *Moral Physiology: or a Brief and Plain Treatise on the Population Question*, in which he advocated coitus interruptus as a technique well tested by the French. During this time scientific theories began to be developed, and empiric evidence about the nature of the physical world increased. As sexuality and procreation are part of the physical laws of nature, it is not unusual that matters of sexuality came to be part of the general desire to control nature.

A backlash to these ventures into fertility control soon appeared, and theologic, medical, and government institutions remained even more strongly adamant in anticontraceptive stances. France was seen to be economically doomed because of its shrinking population, and in England in 1877 Annie Besant and Charles Bradlaugh were prosecuted for distributing an imported American text on contraception, *The Fruits of Philosophy*, by Charles Knowlton. In 1873 the United States federal government enacted the Comstock Law, which forbade the mailing or import of contraceptives, and most American states had laws forbidding the sale and advertisement of contraceptives.

By the end of the nineteenth century the birth control movement had gained strength in Western Europe and in America, and new and effective methods were developed. In 1880 Wilhelm Mensinger invented the diaphragm, and by 1935 there were over 200 mechanical contraceptive devices (usually barriers) and spermicides in use.[9] During this period the medical profession came to accept contraception, mainly because of the humanistic climate created by economists, sociologists, and women themselves who, in the wake of advancing knowledge about reproductive control, wanted the technology made available to them. Since the mid-1930s contraceptive technology has advanced rapidly, as have the social conditions that made it possible. The last vestige of government control of contraceptive practices disappeared in 1965 and 1972 with the Supreme Court cases of *Griswold v. Connecticut*[10] and *Eisenstadt v. Baird*.[11] In the former the Court declared Connecticut's statute against the use of contraceptives unconstitutional; the latter struck down as unconstitutional a Massachusetts law forbidding the selling of contraceptives to unmarried persons.

Modern religious thought has changed from ancient views, especially since rulings frequently must be made about specific contraceptive techniques. Ortho-dox Judaism forbids any device or practice, such as coitus interruptus or the condom, that interferes with the act of sexual intercourse. The diaphragm, the intrauterine device (IUD), and oral contraceptives are permissible because their use is removed from the act of intercourse. Conservative and Reform Judaism permit all forms of contraception.

Non-Catholic Christian ethicists slowly began to change their views in the twentieth century. In 1930 the bishops of the Anglican Church voted to permit contraceptive methods "other than abstinence" (presumably the rhythm method is not preferred because it relies solely on abstinence during the time of a woman's greatest fertility). By the middle of this century no Protestant American church forbade contraception to married couples, although its use was hoped to be only temporary. Childbearing was still considered a major function of marriage, but each act of intercourse was not required to have a procreative intent.

Modern Catholic theology has been shaken to its foundations by the exist-ence of relatively safe and inexpensive birth control and by the growing number of individual Catholics who practice contraception regardless of direc-tives and encyclicals from Rome. At the end of 1930 Pope Pius XI issued the famous encyclical *Casti Conubii*,[12] which stated, in part, "Any use whatever of contraception in the exercise of which the act by human effort is deprived of its natural power of procreating life, violates the law of God and nature, and those who do such a thing are stained by a grave and mortal flaw." The strength of language left little doubt in anyone's mind where the modern Church stood on contraception.

Then in the late 1950s the contraceptive pill was developed, and some Catholic theologians began to examine the Church's stance on contraception. It is interesting to note that it was only this piece of technology—development of a contraceptive method that has nothing to do with the act of intercourse and that does not physically come into contact with the genitals—that prompted new theologic inquiries. After much urging by Catholic theologians and publi-cation by some Church officials of books and articles condoning some forms of contraception in some circumstances, Pope John XXIII appointed a commis-sion to study the contraceptive pill in relation to Catholic doctrine. Because there had been in the Catholic hierarchy a gradual erosion of belief that every act of intercourse must have a procreative intent, part of the moral underpin-nings of the anticontraceptive stance had been removed. The rhythm method of contraception had been allowed by the Church for many years; therefore it could be said that Catholicism is not opposed to contraception per se but only to certain ("artificial") methods, that is, some method that uses a mechanical and/or chemical barrier to prevent union of sperm and ovum. The next step in loosening the strictures was to determine if there was positive value in non-procreative intercourse. (Augustine, whose views on the subject held sway for many centuries, believed such an act to be sinful.)

The Second Vatican Council (1963–1965), which was held during the reign of Pope John XXIII, decreed that, "Love directed from person to person was singularly expressed and perfected by the proper work of marriage."[13] Another step had been taken. The majority of Catholic theologians, many Catholic priests, and an overwhelming number of laypersons believed that the Church should change its conservative stance on contraception. Pope Paul VI, however, did not agree, and in 1968 he issued the encyclical *Humanae Vitae*,[14] which reiterated the 1930 encyclical of Pope Pius XI. Catholics responded to the letter in various ways. Church officials in England, Ireland, Italy, and the United States accepted it without question. Other officials, such as those in Belgium, Canada, France, Germany, Indonesia, and particularly the Netherlands, still permitted Catholics to practice contraception. In other words, they ignored the letter for all intents and purposes. "The discussion did remain open. Paul VI's authoritative but fallible statement of Catholic doctrine has not closed debate; in practice many Catholics adopted a different rule."[15]

The debate has grown more heated than ever. Pope John Paul II has stated his intentions not to change the Church's anticontraceptive position, but with increasing knowledge of what unchecked population growth can mean to the future of the human race, more and more Catholic theologians are publicly opposing the Church's view. It is safe to say that the debate will continue with increased fervor as the population problem worsens.

CURRENT ETHICAL ISSUES

Noonan[16] believes there are several issues that will have a bearing on future discussions of the ethics of contraception.

1. By 1970 a new American trend had become evident; 2.75 million couples of childbearing age had chosen to be sterilized, either by vasectomy or tubal ligation. Noonan questions whether the commitment to contraception has not caused many couples to make a premature decision to give up a "basic human good."
2. A strong public policy favoring contraception may have led to a dependence on abortion as a contraceptive method, particularly if and when other methods have failed.
3. It is sometimes difficult to determine the difference between a contraceptive and an abortifacient, or even to prove that differences exist, as in the intrauterine device.
4. The voluntariness of contraception is clearly in jeopardy in certain

segments of the American population and to an even greater extent in other countries, particularly those of the Third World.

5. Government-aided contraception in the United States may have strong racist overtones. In other countries where society is more formally divided into classes or castes, accusations of racism (some even go so far as to use the word genocide, although no empiric evidence of this exists in regard to contraceptive practices in the United States) may have even greater validity.

6. Marxist philosophy, while not holding that contraception is intrinsically evil, sees the efforts of capitalist countries to control economic conditions, in part, by controlling the size of the world's population to be another method of capitalistic plunder of underdeveloped countries. Marxists urge Third World countries to resist the efforts of the United States and other capitalist countries to use population control as a principal means to achieve economic growth and stability.

Public policy

When discussing public policy in terms of individual contraceptive practices, it is sometimes difficult to separate policy that applies only to individuals and that which applies to entire populations, or at least to significant segments of populations. Population policies and practices are intertwined with individual beliefs and practices. One area of endeavor that unites the two is contraceptive research—policies that direct the amount of money available and the direction the research will take.

There is a wide variety of contraceptives available, but all have major drawbacks to their sustained use. The more effective the method the more dangerous it is likely to be (the reader is referred to any one of several contraceptive manuals for statistics on contraceptive safety and effectiveness), therefore the more ethical dilemmas inherent in its use. There is no existing contraceptive that is completely safe, highly reliable, uncomplicated to use, and inexpensive. It is obvious that one is badly needed, but questions of public policy surround the nature of the research; that is, by what basic method should conception be prevented? Should the method be designed for use by men or women, and how and on whom should the research be carried out? Public and private funding for contraceptive research is not forthcoming; in fact, the amount of research money has remained relatively stable since 1973.

> Pharmaceutical companies, once heavily involved in contraceptive research, are finding it increasingly unprofitable to develop new products which, after up to ten years of very expensive animal testing and clinical trials, can be marketed only a few years before their patents expire.[17]

Moreover pharmaceutical companies may be loathe to invest in contraceptive research because of their past experience with the pill, which when first developed was believed to be as perfect a solution to control of reproductive capacities as was humanly possible. Then when the side effects, some of them very serious, came to be known, the cost to the pharmaceutical companies, both in decreased sales and loss of public confidence, was enormous. Government funding for contraceptive research is increasing, although it is still small in comparison to money spent on diseases that result in death or disability. Moreover, the mood of Congress recently has been to deemphasize contraceptive research, and the proposed Family Protection Act would outlaw the prescription or sale of contraceptives to minors. In the current political climate there is little public pressure to view the inability to control reproduction as a major health problem.

Although members of Congress are strongly influenced by groups such as the Moral Majority and the New Right, there has been another factor affecting government decisions to fund contraceptive research. Some ethnic minorities have made accusations that federal and state policies in contraceptive research and services are racist; that is, more blacks, Hispanics, and other minorities are encouraged to practice birth control than are whites. Certainly health professionals have the same kind and degree of racist tendencies as do other persons, and they put their beliefs into practice with the same degree of frequency and enthusiasm as others, but there is no existing proof that government policies are specifically racist in theory or in practice. In fact, in today's social climate of liberation groups and political lobbies for all minority groups (those concerned with sexual orientation, age, occupation, gender, and national origin, as well as ethnic background), it seems likely that health professionals would bend over backwards to avoid charges of racism and thus to remain as neutral as possible when providing contraceptive information and advice to ethnic minorities.

Although contraceptive research funding is not flowing as freely as it should, the financial wellspring is not completely dry. The following are some avenues that contraceptive research will take in the next several decades[18] and some ethical questions that should be asked about the research methods and the contraceptive techniques themselves:

1. Long-acting drug-release implants consist of a series of miniature tubes or capsules injected under the skin to release a variety of steroids over a long period of time, usually 3 to 5 years. One would wonder if it is ethically permissible to ask a woman to commit herself to a surgically implanted contraceptive device for so long a period of time. Surgery would also be required to remove the implants when the woman wished to conceive, or they would have to be replaced with fresh ones if she wished contraception to continue. Control for making the decision to stop contraception will be far outside the power of

the individual woman, and personal autonomy will decrease. There would be many opportunities for coercion, and health professionals could control the reproductive capacities of large numbers of women.

2. The IUD for postpartum insertion has a biodegradable protrusion that dissolves in the body over a period of time (the IUD does not dissolve; the method for keeping it in place does). IUDs inserted immediately after delivery or abortion have had a high expulsion rate. The biodegradable method of attaching the protrusion to the cervix will likely result in a significantly decreased expulsion rate. Researchers believe that the advantage of this new type of IUD is that women are already in contact with health professionals during delivery or abortion and thus will not have to return 6 to 8 weeks later for IUD insertion. This method might also imply a high probability of coercion. A woman who has just delivered or undergone an abortion may not be in the appropriate frame of mind to make a contraceptive decision, and therefore informed consent could not be said to exist if she gives permission for IUD insertion at that time.

3. Prostaglandin suppositories can be used for "menstrual regulation" or for very early abortion. Prostaglandins, used in sufficient doses to have an effect on fertility, are known to have a high incidence of serious side effects, and the ethical issue rests on whether the benefits are worth the risks. There is also the problem of differentiating contraception and early abortion (early abortion in such instances usually refers to the period after conception has taken place but before the fertilized ovum has been implanted on the endometrial wall, a time span of about 7 to 14 days). For those opposed to abortion at any time and in any form this difference is significant.

4. A Silastic vaginal ring that gradually releases progestin and estrogen is inserted by the woman. The advantages over the current contraceptive pill are that the woman does not have to remember to take a pill every day and there is a decrease in the number and severity of side effects because the hormones will bypass the digestive system. Ethical questions are similar to those that exist now for contraceptive pills: Is the benefit worth the risks?

5. Chemical sterilization involves pellets containing the drug quinacrine being inserted through the cervix into the uterotubal junction, which causes permanent scarring and closure of the fallopian tubes. Other drugs are also being tested for the same purpose. There are already many known risks inherent in this method, such as the increased chance of ectopic pregnancy, and frequently several applications of the pellets are required to achieve the desired results. Because tubal ligation is such a relatively uncomplicated surgical procedure, one wonders why chemical sterilization would be an improvement. Risk is greater when a foreign chemical is introduced into the body than when uncomplicated surgery is performed. Danger of damage to nearby genital

organs is considerable, and the possibility of systemic absorption of the chemical cannot be ignored. The risk to benefit ratio of this procedure appears particularly precarious.

6. Male contraceptive drugs temporarily inhibit sperm production. To date all drugs tested have had an unacceptably high rate of serious side effects, and the possibility of the irreversibility of the contraceptive effect is as likely in males as it is in females. A major ethical question about research on male contraceptives exists; should males be as responsible for contraception as females, given the fact that they have a lesser degree of "vested interest" in the results? There are two possible views in examining the question. Since parenthood is an activity that is, or should be, shared equally by both the mother and the father except for the 9 prenatal months, the responsibility for contraception should also be equally shared. The other view is that, although one may believe in the equality of parental roles, the physical fact of pregnancy happens only to women; therefore there is no reason for a man to expose himself unnecessarily to the risk of chemical interference with sperm production (the condom or other extremely low-risk methods do not enter into this debate about male contraception).

7. Reversible female sterilization is the process by which a plug can be inserted into the uterotubal junction or a fimbrial cap applied that can then be removed when the woman wishes to become pregnant. This is highly delicate surgery that requires special physician training. The ethical question that comes immediately to mind is whether women will be so anxious to submit to this technique that they will fall prey to improperly trained physicians. One must also wonder about the ethics of asking women to submit to two surgical procedures to achieve a contraceptive goal.

One of the most interesting issues of public policy, and the story of contraceptive research in microcosm, is the history of Depo-Provera. The contraceptive qualities of Depo-Provera were discovered by accident by a Brazilian physician who was using it in clinical trials to prevent premature labor. He noticed that the women who took the drug did not become pregnant again for as long as a year after taking it. The Upjohn Company tested Depo-Provera and began clinical trials (on humans) in 1963. Upjohn applied to the Food and Drug Administration (FDA) in 1967 for permission to market Depo-Provera. Permission still has not been granted for reasons based on conflicting ethical and social values.

Depo-Provera is widely used in Europe, in the Middle and Near East, and in South America as a contraceptive. It is not approved for contraceptive use in the United States (although it is used legally as a palliative treatment for advanced endometrial cancer, and studies are now being done to use Depo-Provera to reduce testosterone levels in men who have been convicted of sex crimes) because the number and severity of side effects were considered unacceptable and the risk of further unknown side effects too great. Several Congressional subcommittee hearings have taken place, and lobbies for the Upjohn Company have fought furiously to have the drug approved.

The drug is now supplied to Third World countries by means of a roundabout, and some believe highly unethical, route. American drug companies cannot legally export drugs that are not licensed for use in the United States, nor can an agency of the federal government buy a nonlicensed drug for the purpose of distributing it abroad. Therefore the United States Agency for International Development (AID), which is the principal supplier of contraceptives to the Third World, is prevented from foreign distribution of Depo-Provera. However, there is no law against an international agency distributing any drugs anywhere it chooses. Thus the International Planned Parenthood Federation (IPPF) and the United Nations Fund for Population Activities (UNFPA), both of which are supported in part by American funds, buy Depo-Provera from Upjohn, which is not legally prohibited from selling an unlicensed drug to an international agency, and distribute it widely throughout the Third World.[19] Although the letter of the law is obeyed, its spirit is flagrantly abused.

There are several ethical issues inherent in the use of Depo-Provera and in its distribution to Third World countries. Is it ethical to knowingly provide a drug, whose risks and side effects are seriously questioned, to persons who may not have the opportunity or capacity for fully informed consent? Is it ethical to establish a double standard for a drug's use: one for American women and the other for those of the Third World? Because the risks are so unknown (and controversial), is it possible to give informed consent for use of this drug? Even if informed consent could be developed, those women in both the Third World and in the United States who are educationally disadvantaged would have difficulty understanding the consent, which would necessarily be complex because of the complexity of the drug itself. A double standard would still exist.

Questions of values and risk to benefit ratio are also part of the Depo-Provera dilemma. There are many drugs currently licensed for use in the United States that carry an extremely high risk. However, the uses for which they are intended carry proportionately high import, for example, saving life or preventing the spread of cancer. Is prevention of pregnancy worth the risk of severe side effects, especially when other contraceptives exist?

> The purpose of the drug is not to treat disease but to prevent pregnancy. Is that goal so crucial to the lives of those patients for whom Depo-Provera might be recommended that the risks ought to be discounted? This is an arguable point; however, those who are arguing that contraception is paramount are not the women themselves but those who claim to speak for them—family planners, medical professionals, program administrators. Depo-

Provera is now more attractive to these people, since sterilization is more closely regulated under DHEW's new guidelines.

   Although Upjohn vehemently denies the allegations made by women's health groups, health activists, and others that Depo-Provera is intended for poor women, or for "second-class citizens", it is difficult to avoid the conclusion that the drug's target in the United States would be those or similarly vulnerable groups, such as institutionalized mentally ill women, and the mentally retarded.[20]

The FDA's advisory committee made public the potential users of Depo-Provera if the drug were to be licensed in the United States. They are persons who have been made aware of and accept the fact that they might not be able to become pregnant even after Depo-Provera is discontinued; persons who refuse or are unable to accept the responsibility demanded by other contraceptive methods; those who are incapable of or are unwilling to tolerate the side effects of conventional oral contraceptives; and persons in whom other methods of contraceptives are contraindicated or have failed.[21] The intentions of the FDA, if it chooses to license Depo-Provera, and of the manufacturer are clear—Depo-Provera will be used on the women who have little or no choice in the matter.

   This kind of public policy regarding contraception is highly paternalistic; thus one can seriously question its morality. From the utilitarian point of view the use of Depo-Provera might be permissible, for example:

A woman is borderline mentally retarded, that is, her intellect is not sufficient to allow her to complete more than a low-level education, but she is able to function in the community and holds a job as an assembly line worker in a factory. Contraception, however, is a problem. She cannot remember to take a pill every day, and the complexities of diaphragm preparation and insertion are too much for her. She once had an IUD inserted, but the consent was not fully informed because when she found the plastic string in her vagina she became frightened and pulled—hard. The cervical lacerations that resulted were a physical and emotional trauma for weeks. She cannot master the technique of using the foam inserter, and it would be unreasonable to expect that she insist that her sex partner use a condom. She has had two abortions already and is still only 22 years old. The abortions were paid for by her mother, and although she (the retarded woman) signed the consent form, she did not really understand what was happening and was extremely distressed during and immediately after the procedure, although she appeared to recover quickly. No one is happy with this state of affairs. Her mother is threatening to refuse to pay for the next abortion, and the clinic physician is totally frustrated and wants her to be sterilized, but the current federal guidelines prohibit this. The woman herself is unhappy because people are angry with her, and she has faced pain and psychologic upheaval several times and knows it to be the result of her sexual activity. She is an "excellent" candidate for Depo-Provera, which can be administered as a long-acting, time-released injection. Her mother would take her to the clinic every 6 months or so, and public funds would be used to pay for the contraceptive (they will not pay for an abortion). The physicians would feel they had a successful user of contraception, and the woman herself could enjoy as much sex as she wanted without risking the trauma of continued abortions. And "best" of all, the state would be spared the expense of providing financial and other resources for a child if this woman (or her mother) ever decides to continue a pregnancy to term. The total amount of happiness for all persons concerned will be increased immeasurably as a consequence of giving this woman Depo-Provera. Therefore the utilitarian would see it as a morally correct action.

The utilitarian view is seductive because at times it is so eminently sensible and practical, but as has been noted in Chapter 1, it is also easy to justify clearly immoral acts by applying utilitarian theory. This example is likely to be one of those instances; thus we must look at the action from a deontologic view. The Kantian would surely note that the woman is being used as a means only to achieve other people's ends: society, her mother, and the physicians. Although she might indeed benefit as a result of receiving Depo-Provera, the major purpose for doing so would be to use her to reach goals that ultimately have little to do with her *as a person*. The goal is to prevent pregnancy in retarded women, not necessarily to contribute to *this* woman's benefit or well-being. In addition, placing her on Depo-Provera without her fully informed consent (it must be assumed that her degree of retardation forever prohibits informed consent in this matter) is not an action that can be universalizable because it is unethical in other situations to provide drugs or treatments for persons who have not consented. Therefore this action can be seen as morally impermissible.

On the other hand, providing this woman with Depo-Provera could be directly beneficial to her. She is unhappy now and is likely to continue having sexual intercourse. Therefore if she used a contraceptive for which she had to take no responsibility, she could continue the pleasures of sex without the trauma of further pregnancies. In this instance the risk of side effects and the provision of the drug without her fully informed consent *might* be justifiable.

Kantianism alone would be sufficient to make this action wrong from a deontologic view, but we should examine some other principles that apply to this type of dilemma. It is confusing to use the principle of autonomy because one could say that it would be overridden by giving the woman Depo-Provera, but it is also questionable whether she has the capacity for sufficient autonomy *in regard to this particular situation*. If a decision were to be made, perhaps by a court, that she is incapable of making a decision about contraception, would it be ethical to extend the state's paternalistic power to this woman and override whatever autonomy she does have? To begin to examine that question, we must also use the principles of beneficence and nonmaleficence. What good and what harm are inherent in the proposed action, *not* the consequences of the action? The retarded woman will surely be harmed if she is given a drug without informed consent, thus betraying the trust she has in her mother and the physicians, but is there any benefit at all? Surely being able to enjoy sexual activity without the fear of an unwanted pregnancy is a benefit, *but* we really do not know if she really wants to prevent pregnancy. Everyone has so far assumed that pregnancy is not desirable for this person, but she has not yet expressed her own preference. (The matter of whether she *should* be allowed to become pregnant in view of her retardation is another, not unrelated, matter that will be discussed in Chapter 12.) This brings us back again to the principle of autonomy. If she is prevented against her will from becoming pregnant, harm will have been done, no matter what the social consequences of that pregnancy might be.

This is an excellent example of how principles conflict in an ethical dilemma and why it is sometimes so difficult for a deontologist to make a moral judgment. The majority of philosophers will agree that the principle of nonmaleficence is higher than the principle of beneficence; that is, it is more important to refrain from doing harm than it is to engage in doing good. Therefore when the two principles conflict, as they do in this instance, if harm will be done by an action, and if that harm has no direct causal relationship to a benefit, then the action is morally impermissible. (An example of a harm having a direct causal relationship to a benefit is causing a person pain for the purpose of treating an illness or disease, as in any kind of surgery; the postoperative pain is considered morally permissible because the condition that required the surgery has been alleviated, and the person benefits.)

This example has been used to illustrate the ethical problems inherent in public policy and contraception because it incorporates all the elements of the dilemma: How are individual persons affected by society's need to control population growth and by their own requirements for safe, effective contraception? The woman in this example happened to be retarded, but the principles involved in the public policy dilemma remain the same no matter where the persons live, what their intellects are, and what others believe should be done about their reproductive functions.

Abortifacients as contraceptives

An abortifacient is any device or substance that produces abortion, and technically the term can be used to apply to those procedures used in all abortions, regardless of the term of pregnancy. However, the term is used almost exclusively to refer to those substances that prevent the fertilized ovum from implanting on the endometrial wall and is sometimes used synonymously with the word contraceptive, although the two are not precisely the same. A contraceptive, by definition, prevents the joining of sperm and ovum. There are two commonly used abortifacients: the IUD (although the precise mechanism by which an IUD has its desired effect is not known, the best theory is that it causes small wavelike contractions of the uterus, thus making implantation impossible; therefore the IUD is classed as an abortifacient), and the "morning after pill," which is a series of high doses of estrogens taken after intercourse has occurred. The morning after pill, however, has extremely unpleasant side effects. It was usually used for women who had been raped, but its use has now fallen into disrepute.

There can be, depending on one's view of personhood, a distinct ethical difference between a contraceptive and an abortifacient. A contraceptive, although it destroys individual sex cells or causes them not to be used, affects only individual cells. However, an abortifacient destroys a group of cells that is undoubtedly a potential person simply because it is not potentially anything else. Those who view abortifacients as morally permissible see this group of cells as just that—a number of undifferentiated cells that just happened to join as a result of sexual intercourse. At this point in the development of the blastocyst, each cell is simply a cell; it has no specific human function, nor has it been "assigned" to a body organ or system. Destruction of this group of cells is morally no different from destroying individual sex cells.

Those who view abortifacients as morally impermissible see the group of cells as a potential person because it has a full complement of the genetic characteristics of the person it will become if left to develop on its own. The issues of personhood and potentiality as they relate to abortion will be discussed in more detail in Chapter 6; suffice it to say for the purpose here that there may be an ethical difference, and the woman who is using a contraceptive should be aware of that difference. In fact, if she has not been told that her contraceptive is indeed an abortifacient, informed consent has not been given.

There is some research currently being conducted on new abortifacients to be used by the woman herself. Many substances that are termed *menstrual regulation* drugs are in fact abortifacients. The term *menstrual regulation* can be misleading, and its use has serious ethical overtones. A woman who misses a menstrual period and receives an injection from a physician, while being told that the injection will "bring on" her period, is being lied to by the physician. *If* she were pregnant (and a pregnancy test would not ordinarily be done in such circumstances), he would have chemically aborted her. If she were not pregnant, it might be asked why a menstrual period should be artificially begun.

Self-administered abortifacients can carry serious risks and therefore raise ethical questions. An abortifacient would of necessity be a more potent combi-

nation of hormones or other substances than are in conventional contraceptive pills. The risk to the woman *might* be greater than the risk involved
in an early mechanically induced abortion, even though an abortifacient pill
or suppository might mean increased personal convenience and privacy and
surely lower cost.

> The existence of such simple abortifacient methods as a backup would also
> allow greater dependence on more traditional barrier methods and a move-
> ment away from systemic drug-related methods, whose extended use may be
> inadvisable for certain categories of women. Even if the potential side effects,
> discomfort, or inconvenience associated with a new abortifacient drug proved
> to be greater than those of existing methods of contraception—pills, IUDs,
> spermicides, and injectibles—many women might still find the abortifacient
> more acceptable since its use would be limited to single occasions as needed to
> bring on a missing period.[22]

The logic of this statement seems somewhat faulty. No proof exists that an
abortifacient, even used on single occasions, contains less risk than continued
use of conventional contraceptive pills. Moreover a woman who knows that a
self-administered abortifacient is always available might become increasingly
careless about using the traditional barrier methods and would rely more and
more heavily on the abortifacient, perhaps even aborting herself every month,
and thus expose herself to increasingly greater risks. Again the phrase "certain
categories of women" is troublesome; one wonders which categories King is
referring to and why it would be more appropriate to expose certain women
rather than others to unknown side effects. The statement appears suspiciously
discriminatory.

STERILIZATION
Methods and definitions

The process of sterilization is the process of rendering a person incapable of
reproducing. The most common method is to prevent, usually surgically, the
transport of the sperm or ovum to the site where it unites with its opposite
number. In the male the procedure is known as bilateral vasectomy, where the
vas deferens (sperm ducts) are cut or occluded by cauterization. Complete
sterility does not occur for several weeks because viable sperm are present in the
distal ducts for up to 2 months. Microscopic examination of semen is the
assured proof of sterility following vasectomy. Although research is now being
done on the reversibility of vasectomy, much of it successful, the man who
submits to sterilization should do so with the idea that it will be permanent.

The procedure in the female is bilateral partial salpingectomy, or more commonly, tubal ligation, in which the fallopian tubes are cut and tied in such a way that when the sutures are absorbed, the ends of the tubes are covered by the peritoneum, thus providing total occlusion. Access to the tubes is gained through either the vagina or the abdomen. The morbidity rate for the former is somewhat higher; therefore it is used only infrequently. When access is gained through the abdomen it is done by means of either a conventional surgical incision or by laparoscopy in which a laparoscope is inserted via a tiny incision near the umbilicus, the abdomen filled with compressed air to better visualize the reproductive organs, and the fallopian tubes cauterized. For a while the laparoscopic procedure was the most common, but lately it has fallen into some degree of disrepute because of increasing incidence of risk, such as cauterization accidents in which organs other than fallopian tubes are burned and uterine or bowel perforations with subsequent hemorrhage or peritonitis. The laparoscopic procedure is more technically difficult for the surgeon, but because there is no major incision, it is done on an outpatient basis with considerably less cost to the woman. Tubal ligation also must be considered a permanent procedure, although research has shown that possibilities for reversibility are good in some instances. However, it should be noted that a man or a woman who intends to be sterilized, while seriously considering reversibility, should not be sterilized until such time as a decision for future permanence is made.

Ethical issues

Lebacqz[23] states that sterilization is done for five major purposes—therapeutic, contraceptive, eugenic, social, and punitive—and that these purposes are not necessarily mutually exclusive. Therapeutic sterilization usually indicates that a reproductive organ(s) is removed to save the life, or to significantly improve the health of the person. The only circumstances in which one sees the term *therapeutic sterilization* used today is when the principle of double effect is invoked (refer to Chapter 1 for an explanation of double effect) by the Catholic Church to remove the uterus or fallopian tubes of a woman still in her childbearing years or the penis or testes of a man. The term *clear and present danger* refers to a life-threatening condition, such as cancer, when therapeutic sterilization is then permitted. Some Catholic theologians, however, have broadened the scope of instances in which therapeutic sterilization is permissible to include a badly damaged or scarred organ that might likely result in a pathologic condition. This is referred to as clear and future danger.

Many modern Catholic theologians approve of limited contraceptive sterilization if proportionately grave reasons for it exist, for example, if a marriage is seriously threatened by continued fertility and other contraceptive methods are inappropriate or if a woman's health would be seriously jeopardized by bearing more children. In condoning sterilization in certain grave instances the Church again demonstrates inconsistency about the permissibility of contraception itself vs. the means used. "In condoning the 'rhythm' method of contraception, the Church opens the door to other means of contraception (including sterilization) since there is no obvious moral difference between temporal and spatial barriers to procreation."[24] Church officials would, of course, argue that there is a distinct moral difference.

Most Protestants believe that there is no moral difference between kinds of contraception, and some theologians would even go so far as to maintain that a method that interferes least with the act of sexual intercourse is preferred.

Traditional Jewish law has been opposed to both male castration and female sterilization because they interfere with God's command to be fruitful and multiply. Leniency is sometimes allowed for a woman if she is in great fear of the pain of childbirth or if pregnancy and childbirth would place her in physical jeopardy. Modern Conservative and Reform Jewish theologians apply no strictures to contraceptive sterilization. In fact, if the only other choice of contraception is abstinence, sterilization would be the favored method because the function of sexuality is so important to marriage.

Most theologians would argue against totally unlimited contraceptive sterilization, although this view has its inconsistencies when an attempt is made to draw a line between limited and unlimited and permissible and impermissible sterilizations.

> Spokespersons from the Judeo-Christian tradition do not generally accept the notion that one's body is one's own to control completely. Although such representatives might share a concern for population limitation, they are therefore reluctant to support unlimited sterilization as a means to that end.[25]

Feminists would disagree with this view by stating that *only* by gaining total control over one's own body can women escape the political and economic subjugation under which they have suffered.

Eugenic and social sterilization always contain elements of coercion, no matter how seemingly benign. Eugenic sterilization is seen by some ethicists as justifiable in some circumstances, such as if the person is so mentally diseased that he is believed to be a menace to the state, if a mental or physical disease is proved hereditary, or if a mentally ill or retarded person exhibits such intractable (sexual) behavior that sterilization is seen as the only means of controlling behavior. All these justifications have strong inherent contradictions. For example, if a person is so mentally diseased that he is a menace to others, an appropriate action might be to prevent him from coming in contact with those he would be likely to harm; his reproductive capacity is irrelevant to the likelihood of his committing acts of violence. Another inconsistency is that sterilization might be paradoxic in that if the fear of pregnancy can be somewhat of a deterrent to sexually promiscuous behavior, and if the deterrent is removed, promiscuity could increase. Those female inmates of hospitals who are so retarded or emotionally disturbed that they are easy sexual prey for male attendants and inmates might become even more tempting targets if they were sterilized. It should be noted that when eugenic or social sterilization is discussed, it is almost always in terms of female sterilization. Mentally ill and retarded men who are sexually promiscuous are almost never sterilized. The most common justification for this discrimination is that females are the ones who become pregnant; therefore it is practical to sterilize only them. If, however, the reasons for sterilization have to do with the desire to prevent future persons from suffering from certain forms of genetically caused retardation, then it would be equally practical to sterilize males.

There is little empirical evidence to show that eugenic sterilization would materially affect the social quality of life in any significant way; therefore it is difficult to find eugenic sterilization morally acceptable from even a utilitarian view. Compulsory sterilization for eugenic purposes must be viewed as a violation of individual rights, although possibly there are reasons why it could be justifiable to sterilize someone involuntarily .

The social and political mood of the United States has been moving to a more conservative position in recent years with a resultant impatience with the increasing amount of public funds being spent supporting children of persons who cannot or will not support them. Bills have been introduced into several state legislatures (Louisiana, Arkansas, Alabama, and others) calling for compulsory sterilization of women on welfare who have had a certain number of children and who show no interest in becoming self-supporting. Proponents justify the bills on the grounds that they will reduce welfare payments and lower the rate of illegitimate births. Those who oppose these bills point out that no reason exists for the belief that fewer illegitimate children will be born (and furthermore the marital status of the mother is no business of the state) and that compulsory sterilization of a few will not materially affect the social welfare of the majority. Moreover, the laws tend to be extremely racist in both theory and practice, and there is no possible justification for abrogating the basic human right of reproduction. Those who point to the fact that it is unfair to children to bring them into a world of poverty, misery, and severely curtailed opportunity ignore the fact that not only is it impossible to predict with absolute certainty what kind of life any particular person will have, but it is equally unfair to force a woman to be sterilized on the basis of what the future for her and her children *might* be.

Punitive sterilization is used almost exclusively for those who have committed violently antisocial acts, usually rape and sex crimes. The justification is partly Biblical (the "eye for an eye" theory), partly emotional, and partly practical; a man who is castrated will not be able to rape again. However, there is almost no practical, theologic, or philosophic support in favor of punitive sterilization (punitive sterilization for a man implies castration, not vasectomy). A rapist is a man who commits an act of violent aggression against another person using his penis as the instrument of aggression. If he is castrated, he may simply use another, perhaps deadly instrument. Many also believe that punitive sterilization is perverting the role of the physician whose healing art should not be turned to punishment.

There are several reasons to believe that involuntary sterilization is unethical. First, control over one's body is a matter of personal privacy, and the exercise of the decision-making function is the exercise of autonomy. If one has the legal and moral right (and that right does exist) to control what substances are introduced into the body or surgically excised from it, then it would be inconsistent to remove reproductive control, and it is therefore a morally incorrect action. Second is the matter of ethics related to culture. Women have almost complete responsibility for rearing children (changing trends still are not socially significant in most parts of the world) and they have had and will continue to have, at least for the foreseeable future, total responsibility for bearing children. Therefore women should control reproductive technology. Because the medical and scientific establishments are controlled by men, the closest women can come to managing reproductive technology is to control their own reproductive capacities; therefore involuntary sterilization would be unethical.

There had been in the United States a sufficiently large number of documented cases of coerced involuntary sterilization, especially of the mentally retarded, racial minorities, the poor, the uneducated, and others who were disenfranchised in some way, to alarm those who saw sterilization abuse as a dangerous and continuing trend.[27] In 1976 the General Accounting Office discovered that 3000 sterilizations of American Indians had occurred over a period of 4 years in which the consent form used was not in compliance with federal regulations for informed consent.[28] The practice of performing hysterectomies on minority women by resident physicians who "needed the practice" was commonplace, and there were many physicians who denied gynecologic care to some women unless they agreed to be sterilized. Because of the increasing amount of sterilization abuse, the Department of Health, Education and Welfare in 1977 established guidelines to ensure voluntariness and noncoercion in sterilization.[29] A summary of the guidelines follows:

1. Voluntary informed consent must be obtained using a standardized consent form in the client's preferred language.
2. The person may not be threatened with loss of welfare or Medicaid benefits as a result of nonconsent.

3. Consent may not be obtained during labor, before or after an abortion, or while the person is under the influence of drugs or alcohol.
4. The distinction between contraceptive and noncontraceptive (therapeutic) sterilization must be abolished for the purpose of the federal regulations.
5. Hysterectomy for contraceptive purposes is prohibited in federally funded programs.
6. There must be a 30-day waiting period (which can be waived in the event of an emergency) between consent and sterilization procedure.
7. The person must be provided, also in the preferred language, with complete information regarding the risks, side effects, and irreversibility of sterilization.
8. A moratorium was called on all federally funded sterilizations of persons under age 21 and those involuntarily institutionalized or declared legally incompetent.
9. A federal audit of sterilization programs was to take place in the 10 states where the highest number of federally funded sterilizations occur.

As might be assumed, there was some vigorous opposition to these guidelines. In New York City a group of obstetricians and gynecologists charged that the regulations violated both the individual client's "right to choose" and the physician's First Amendment rights. Both charges are absurd. There is nothing in the guidelines to prevent a person from voluntarily choosing sterilization, and First Amendments rights do not provide the right to coerce another human being to engage in any action. Opposition to point number 8 revolves around the belief that sterilization of the mentally retarded and others declared incompetent will provide a "rehabilitation" service, that is, make these persons "fit" to function in society, and that this fitness should take precedence over individual choice and over exploitation of a few individuals. The objection to the 30-day waiting period is usually couched in pragmatic terms—the woman will have to return to the hospital or clinic a month after she was already there for delivery or abortion, and she may have the added inconvenience of having to take time off from work and/or of arranging for childcare. Proponents of this view maintain that it is more practical and inexpensive to sterilize a woman while she is still available to health care personnel. This seems a thinly veiled disguise for the fear that a woman will "get away from" health professionals and might change her mind if sterilization is not performed immediately after she gives consent. The convenience of the woman or the health professionals cannot take precedence over the assurance of voluntariness.

Another serious objection to the guidelines is the charge of paternalism. There have been many instances of laws that were designed to protect the weak, vulnerable, and disenfranchised that have been used to discriminate against those people they have been designed to protect. It is sometimes difficult to distinguish between protective and paternalistic laws, for example, laws prohibiting women from working at particular jobs (or in entire occupations) or during certain hours. It could be charged that the DHEW guidelines might "protect" women out of unlimited access to sterilization and might prove paradoxic to autonomy. In discussing the charge of undue paternalism, Petchesky points out that the critical factor is the irreversibility of sterilization, that inconvenience is worthwhile when compared with the abuses that have occurred when there are no regulations. Charges that the number of sterilizations will decline as a result of the guidelines have not been born out, according to statistics released by the New York City Bureau of Maternal Services and Family Planning.[30]

> Whether or not fewer women choose sterilization as a result of the regulations, it is not *their* "right to access" that is really being defended, but rather the medical profession's privileged autonomy and the "right" of providers to process people through sterilization procedures as expediently as possible. Protection against sterilization abuse is justifiable protection, insofar as it provides a necessary condition for avoiding undue pressure and being able to deliberate carefully about an irreversible procedure. The thirty-day waiting period and the other requirements attached to informed consent do not prevent anyone who wishes to do so from undergoing a sterilization operation.[31]

The utilitarian will likely be opposed to many of the restrictions in the DHEW guidelines, while a deontologist will applaud them. Although the ethical issues of coercion and autonomy remain constant whether the dilemma at hand concerns sterilization, human experimentation, donation of organs for transplant, or any other biomedical issue, it should be mentioned that the argument over the DHEW guidelines is taking place against a social backdrop of the women's movement, the increasing political move to the right, abortion rights, federal funding for abortion, the rights of the retarded in relation to childbearing, and other discussions concerning that most private of human spheres—sexuality and reproduction.

Legal considerations

Compulsory sterilization is legal in 21 American states and in many other countries. In some states it is not only legal, the statute is so loosely worded that almost anyone could be caught in the net of legal permissibility. For example, in Oregon a panel of physicians and mental health workers is empowered to *order* the sterilization of any person who would produce children "who would have an inherited tendency to mental retardation or mental illness" or "who would become neglected or dependent children as a result of the parent's inability by reason of mental illness or mental retardation to provide adequate care."[32] In 1961 the Oregon Attorney General published a list of those persons who were candidates for compulsory sterilization. The list includes the feeble-minded, the insane, epileptics, habitual criminals, incurable syphilitics, moral degenerates, sexual perverts, and persons committing sodomy or "an act of sustained osculatory relations with the private parts of any person, or permitting such relations."[33] This list is so absurd that if the (then) Attorney General had had his way, the state of Oregon would soon be populated only by deer, chipmunks, and perhaps a few remote orders of celibate clerics.

The constitutionality of such state sterilization laws was first upheld by the 1927 Supreme Court Case of *Buck v. Bell*[34] and has not been overturned in the high court. Justice Oliver Wendell Holmes wrote the opinion in which he stated,

> It is better for the world, if instead of waiting to execute degenerate offspring for crime, or to let them starve for their imbecility, society can prevent those who are manifestly unfit from continuing their kind. . . . Three generations of imbeciles are enough.

The last phrase has become the rallying cry of those who wish to promote and maintain compulsory sterilization laws. Because *Buck v. Bell* has never been challenged in the Supreme Court, each state is free to declare the constitutionality of compulsory sterilization. During the more than 50 years since this decision, the Supreme Court has repeatedly upheld the right to privacy in matters of sexuality and reproduction, for example, *Griswold v. Connecticut* and *Eisenstadt v. Baird*. *Roe v. Wade* (1973) was the landmark case in which the state could not deny a woman a right to an abortion and was fought on the grounds of the right to privacy. In an interesting contradiction a United States federal trial court in 1974 held that "federally assisted family planning sterilizations are permissible only with the voluntary, knowing, and uncoerced consent of individuals competent to give such consent. . . . No person who is mentally incompetent can meet these standards."[35] The case *Relf v. Weinberger* (1974) did not state that compulsory sterilization was illegal, only that it could not be done with federal funds. It was also the impetus for the DHEW guidelines mentioned previously.

In the matter of the legality of voluntary sterilization, Friedman poses the following four major questions[36]:

1. Can an incompetent adult or child give consent for sterilization that is legally sufficient? *Relf v. Weinberger* appears to answer this question, but the problem lies in determining competency, particularly in borderline cases. A further safeguard might be to require that the person desiring sterilization requests it and understands the nature of the procedure's irreversibility. The most important factor is that the request arise from the person himself, not from a parent, spouse, or health professional.

2. Can a mentally competent minor give consent to voluntary sterilization that is legally sufficient? Three factors help to protect minors: *Relf v. Weinberger* declared minors to be incompetent, the DHEW guidelines declared a moratorium on all sterilizations of persons under age 21, and almost all states have statutes that prohibit sterilization of minors. No statute or guideline is immutable, however, but for the moment competent minors are fairly well protected by law in regard to sterilization.

3. Can the state or state-assisted hospitals proscribe sterilizations for mentally competent adults? Several foreign countries such as Turkey and Italy prohibit sterilization (Italy is heavily under Vatican influence, and Turkey is well known for its medieval attitudes about the sexual freedom of women), but in the United States no state actually prohibits voluntary sterilization, although individual physicians may refuse to sterilize an individual. However, hospitals are permitted to exercise a "religious belief" or "moral conviction" and thus refuse to perform sterilizations. This is not a problem in a large metropolitan area where a person can simply go to the next hospital to be sterilized, but it is a problem in small towns where there is only one hospital or in rural areas where the next hospital might be hundreds of miles away. It is unlikely that these conditions will change. In 1975 the United States Court of Appeals for the Ninth Circuit permitted a Roman Catholic hospital to refuse to sterilize a woman even though the hospital received federal funds and had the only maternity department in the city.[37] The Supreme Court refused to hear the appeal. Other courts of appeals have come to conflicting decisions, and the Supreme Court's inaction on the dilemma has resulted in a nationally uneven interpretation of what hospitals receiving federal funds are permitted to do or refuse to do in regard to requests for voluntary sterilization.

4. When voluntary sterilization is permitted, what conditions must be fulfilled before a competent adult can be sterilized? Almost all jurisdictions have a compulsory waiting period of 3 to 30 days, and all hospitals receiving federal funds must abide by a 30-day waiting period between consent and the procedure. In Denmark consent is automatically nullified if the person waits more than 6 months, and in some countries a woman will not be sterilized before she has given birth to a certain number of children. No such statute exists in the United States, but in some states childless women are subjected to longer waiting periods than are women who have had children.

Legal issues and debates surrounding sterilization concentrate on the voluntariness of the procedure, protection of those who are for some reason unable to give informed consent, and the state's paternalistic interference in personal reproductive privacy. The desire to be sterilized, the desire to sterilize someone else, and the fear of losing one's reproductive capacity have social, cultural, psychologic, and racial overtones. No matter what laws are passed, they will be seen as unfair to some group of people. Thus given the fact that the law is not a perfect instrument and that it is bound to err in some direction, it is better to err on the side of "too much" protection for the vulnerable rather than too little.

SUMMARY

The history of contraception began when people first discovered the sequence of events involving intercourse, pregnancy, and childbirth. Premonotheistic cultures had a variety of strongly positive and negative views about contraception, but as monotheism spread, the complexity of ethical thought increased. Although ancient Jewish law did not specifically condemn contraception, it became a traditional taboo because of the strong command to procreate, both for spiritual reasons and for more practical ones such as the need to increase population for self-defense. Early Christianity prohibited all forms of contraception, although various sects opposed that view from time to time, and as the Catholic Church spread throughout what had been the Roman Empire, the prohibition solidified and strengthened. The Protestant Reformation, although it shook the foundations of the Church in other ways, also forbade contraception and reiterated that the primary purpose for marital intercourse was procreation. It was not until the eighteenth century that rational thought about sexuality led to somewhat more permissive attitudes about contraception. Although theologic and lay attitudes from time to time slipped back to a more restrictive era, continued progress has been made in the freedom to use contraception as one chooses. Today only traditional Catholics strictly forbid contraception, and even there the prohibition is not absolute. Other theologians demonstrate a varying degree of liberality of attitude.

Current ethical issues are concerned mainly with matters of public policy. The amount of money available for contraceptive research and the direction that research will take are one of the major issues, especially as they relate to policies that could be interpreted as racist or discriminatory in some other way. All contraceptive research projects currently underway entail serious ethical questions relating mainly to the risk to benefit ratio. Another ethical issue is the differentiation between contraceptives and abortifacients. One's view of the moral difference between them will depend almost entirely on how one views the group of fertilized, but still undifferentiated, cells that is prevented from implanting on the endometrial wall by the abortifacient.

Sterilization is surgical contraception that is generally considered to be permanent, although research is now going on to determine ways to reverse the procedure. Both ethical issues and legal considerations focus on the voluntariness of sterilization. Because of the tremendous number of sterilization abuses, especially among women (men are almost never involuntarily sterilized) who are mentally retarded, emotionally disturbed, or members of a racial or ethnic minority, the federal government has interceded to protect persons who are to be sterilized in federally funded programs. There are, however, 21 states that permit compulsory sterilization, and the Supreme Court, after it condoned compulsory sterilization for certain categories of persons in 1927, has refused to hear all appeals in regard to the matter. As a result, there is great legal inconsistency about what may and may not be done, even in hospitals receiving federal funds.

Notes

1. Noonan, J. T., Jr. Contraception. In W. T. Reich (Ed.), *Encyclopedia of bioethics* (Vol. 1). New York: The Free Press, 1978. p. 204.
2. Noonan, p. 205.
3. Noonan, p. 206.
4. Noonan, p. 206.
5. Noonan, p. 207.
6. Noonan, p. 207.
7. Noonan, p. 208.
8. Noonan, p. 209.
9. Noonan, p. 211.
10. *Griswold v. Connecticut*, 381 U.S. 479 14L Ed 2nd 510 85 S. Ct. 1678 (1965).
11. *Eisenhardt v. Baird*, 405 U.S. 438 31L Ed 2nd 349 92 S. Ct. 1029 (1972).
12. Pius XI. Casti Conubii. *Acta Apostolicae Sedis* 22 (1930), pp. 539–592 (Translated as On Christian Marriage.). *Catholic Mind*, 1931 29, 21–64.
13. Noonan, p. 213.
14. Paul VI. Humanae Vitae. *Acta Apostolicae Sedis* 60 (1968), pp. 481–503 (Translated as Human Life.). *Catholic Mind*, September, 1968, pp. 35–48.
15. Noonan, p. 213.
16. Noonan, pp. 213–214.
17. Connell, E. B. Reproductive physiology and contraceptive research. In *Draper Fund Report*. No. 6. Summer, 1978. Washington, D.C.: The Draper Fund. p. 4.
18. *Draper Fund Report*. No. 6. Summer, 1978. Washington, D.C.: The Draper Fund. pp. 14–15, 18–19.
19. Levine, C. Depo-Provera and contraceptive risk: a case study of values in conflict. *Hastings Center Report*, 1979, 9 (4), 8–11. Reprinted with permission of The Hastings Center. © Institute of Society, Ethics and the Life Sciences, 360 Broadway, Hastings-on-Hudson, N.Y. 10706.
20. Levine, pp. 10–11.
21. Levine, p. 11.

22. King, T. M. Abortion and abortifacients. In *Draper Fund Report*, p. 28.
23. Lebacqz, K. Sterilization: ethical aspects. In *Encyclopedia of bioethics* (Vol. 4). p. 1609.
24. Lebacqz, p. 1610.
25. Lebacqz, p. 1611.
26. Petchesky, R. P. Reproduction, ethics, and public policy: the federal sterilization regulations. *Hastings Center Report*, 1979, *9* (5), 29–30. Reprinted with permission of The Hastings Center. © Institute of Society, Ethics and the Life Sciences, 360 Broadway, Hastings-on-Hudson, N.Y. 10706.
27. Petchesky, pp. 31–32.
28. Petchesky, p. 32.
29. *Federal Register* 43:217. p. 52147.
30. Petchesky, p. 36.
31. Petchesky, p. 36.
32. Oregon Revised Statutes, Section 436.
33. Opinion of the Attorney General of the State of Oregon, No. 5158, February 2, 1961.
34. *Buck v. Bell*, 274 U.S. 200 71L Ed 1000 s. Ct. 584 (1927).
35. *Relf v. Weinberger*, 372 F Supp 1196 (D.C. 1974).
36. Friedman, J. M. Sterilization: legal aspects. In *Encyclopedia of bioethics* (Vol. 4). pp. 1616–1617.
37. *Taylor v. St. Vincent's Hospital*, No. 75–759, 44 U.S.L.W. 3492 (1976).

Bibliography

Baltazar, E. R. Contraception and the philosophy of process. In *Contraception and holiness: the Catholic predicament*. New York: Herder and Herder, 1964. pp. 154–74.

Connell, E. B. Reproductive physiology and contraceptive research. *Draper Fund Report*, pp. 3–5.

Curran, C. E. Sterilization: exposition, critique and refutation of past teaching. In *New perspectives in moral theology*. Fides Publishers, 1974. pp. 194–211.

Donovan, P. Sterilizing the poor and incompetent. *Hastings Center Report*. 6 (5), pp. 7–8.

Draper Fund Report. Washington, D.C.: The Draper Fund, Summer, 1978.

Fagley, R. M. *The population explosion and Christian responsibility*. New York: Oxford University Press, 1960.

Feldman, D. M. *Birth control in Jewish ethics: marital relations, contraception, and abortion as set forth in the classic texts of Jewish law*. New York: New York University Press, 1968.

Ferster, E. Z. Eliminating the unfit—is sterilization the answer?" *Ohio State Law Journal*, 1966, *27*, 591–633.

Friedman, J. M. Sterilization: legal aspects. In *Encyclopedia of bioethics*. New York: The Free Press, 1978.

Fromer, M. J. *Ethical issues in health care*. St. Louis: The C.V. Mosby Co., 1981.

Hellman, L. M. Sterilization: medical aspects. In *Encyclopedia of bioethics*.

Kindregan, C. P. State power over human fertility and individual liberty. *Hastings Law Journal*. 1972, *23*, 1401–1426.

King, T. M. Abortion and abortifacients. *Draper Fund Report*, pp. 27–30.

Lader, L. (Ed.) *Foolproof birth control: male and female sterilization*. Boston: Beacon Press, 1972.

Lebacqz, K. Sterilization: ethical aspects. In *Encyclopedia of bioethics*.

Levine, C. Depo-Provera and contraceptive risk: a case study of values in conflict. *Hastings Center Report*, 1979, *9* (4), 8–11.

Martin, L. L. *Health care of women*. Philadelphia: J. B. Lippincott and Co, 1978.

Noonan, J. T., Jr. Contraception. In *Encyclopedia of bioethics.*

Petchesky, R. P. Reproduction, ethics, and public policy: the federal sterilization regulations. *Hastings Center Report*, 1979, *9* (5), 29–41.

Pilpel, H. F. Voluntary sterilization: a human right. *Columbia Health Rights Law Review*, 1975, *7*, 105–119.

Reuther, R. Birth control and the ideals of marital sexuality. In *Contraception and holiness.*

CHAPTER 5

POPULATION ETHICS

DEFINITION OF THE POPULATION PROBLEM

Significant portions of the world's population will starve to death within the next several decades or will die in other ways directly related to overpopulation if the current rampant growth of population is not brought under control. The population problem is essentially uncomplicated in its statement but almost impossibly complex in its solution. It is such that the rate of growth and/or distribution of population will, in certain parts of the world, continue to the point where it will not be possible to maintain or develop a necessary level of resources to prevent mass starvation. Severe famine will also result in high morbidity, epidemics, and many other sequelae short of death.

There is a finite number of ways to solve the problem, but each possible solution or combination of solutions creates an almost infinite number of ethical dilemmas. The four major categories of solutions to the population problem are as follows: (1) limit numbers of people, (2) increase the production of natural and other resources, (3) exclude some segments of the world population from sharing in the general supply of resources, and (4) require that each individual or population group be allocated a smaller share of the total available resources. This chapter will explore the ramifications of each of these four options.

There are several components to the causes of overpopulation. One is population distribution, defined as the way in which a population is distributed over a particular area. About 90% of the people in the world today live on about 25% of the land. Two major factors that influence population density are growth rates and migration patterns. Population tends to increase at a faster rate as density increases, and migration depends to a great extent on topographic and climactic conditions, as well as cultural, political, technologic, and economic factors. Some population planners believe that redistribution is a viable option to relieve some of the problems caused by dangerously high population density, such as deteriorating cities, increasing violence, pollution, mental illness, and crime. Redistributing significant numbers of people to effect noticeable change is not a popular idea and is far less workable than other proposed solutions. For example, Lucas and Ogletree suggest that vast numbers of people from underdeveloped, starving countries (e.g., India and many African nations) be moved to large countries with abundant resources and low population density, such as Canada and Australia. It is highly unlikely that any developed country would willingly accept hordes of starving refugees. One has only to remember the plight of the Cambodian boat people in 1979 and the wave of outrage and indignation that swept across many quarters of the United States when hundreds of thousands of Cubans sought refuge from Castro's regime in 1980. Almost every developed country has immigration quotas, usually based on the immigrant's natural origin, and the more developed the country, the stricter the quota system. International migration is not a practical option, but national migration might be an effective temporary stopgap. (Only a change in the ratio of resources to population will provide a permanent solution to the problem.) Forced national migration would not be as effective as less coercive means to significantly alter population density, such as government tax incentives, free land and/or housing, zoning and land use regulation, and government subsidies to individuals and businesses.

In addition to a general statement of definition of the population problem, it should be understood that there are elements of the problem that might be characterized as intermediate, that is, those aspects that cause severe human suffering without necessarily causing death by starvation. If left unchecked, all could have a direct causal relationship to mass death. The major intermediate elements can be summarized as follows:

1. On a worldwide basis the rate of illiteracy is rising sharply, and the countries with the highest birth rates usually have the least to spend on public education.[1] A high illiteracy rate in a country causes high rates of unemployment, a lower quality of life, and increased ignorance of people who can ill afford to be unaware of the world situation.

2. The more persons there are on earth, the more waste and refuse they produce. The pollution problem of human refuse ranges from disposing of both animal and human excrement to the waste produced by technologically advanced nations that are running out of places to dump their chemical and

nuclear garbage. The earth's air, land, and water can absorb only so much pollution before it will be irrevocably affected. Some scientists think we are fast approaching the saturation point, and some think we have already reached it.

3. The world inflation rate is reaching unmanageable proportions because demand for goods and services exceeds not only the supply but also the potential to increase supply in many places, for instance, in Israel where triple-digit inflation has existed for several years. The escalation of the price of petroleum, firewood, natural gas, soybeans, and many grains has had a profound negative effect on world economy.

4. A growing share of all illness and death in the world today is directly attributable to human changes in the environment. These changes stem from new technologies, population growth, and the need to produce ever more goods and services to satisfy human needs. Among the illnesses linked to environmental alterations are emphysema, stroke, parasitic infections, heart disease, and cancer.[2]

The greatest cause of this increase in environmental disease is the introduction of new chemicals into the ecosystem without providing a way for the system to either absorb them or to render them harmless. It is interesting to note that those who cause the environmental pollution are equally subject to its hazards as are the persons who have no control over environmental wastes. Corporate executives, who make the decisions, and members of government regulatory agencies, who choose not to enforce existing laws that may have been impotent in the first place, must breathe the same air and eat the same contaminated food as those who are powerless to control their actions.

5. Hunger is an all-consuming problem. Per capita consumption of grain has been steadily decreasing, and there are serious doubts that depleted grain reserves can be rebuilt.[3] Although demand for grain keeps increasing because of population gains, production has fallen in two of the major grain producing countries, the United States and Russia. This decrease results from geopolitical factors that are complex and not pertinent to this discussion. Much of the Third World is dependent on grain exports from North America. This is a precarious position in which to have to exist over a long period of time. World food production is decreasing, and those countries with the lowest production capacities also have the lowest purchasing power and often cannot buy food from countries that have a surplus. An example of the relationship between population and hunger is the comparison in development between North America and Latin America, two regions of approximately equal land mass. In 1950, the populations of North America and Latin America were approximately equal, but in the next 30 years the population growth of North America slowed considerably, while population growth in Latin America increased by 3% each year. There are now about 100 million more people in Latin America

than in North America, and one of the results of this phenomenon has been an increase in the number of hungry people on the former continent and an increase in the production capacity of the latter. One of the major sequelae of hunger, in addition to the more obvious ones of disease and death, is that malnutrition in infants and children causes irrevocable brain damage. If a sufficient number of children suffer such irrevocable damage, it is possible to speculate that future generations may not have the intellectual capacity to solve the inevitable social and economic problems. The obvious result would be a significant change in, and possibly a decline of, that society.

6. Ironically, as human population in underdeveloped countries increases, so does the livestock population. Animals are used for food, for transportation, for draft power, as financial security, and for bartering. Consequently as herds multiply, they overgraze the land, which leads to deforestation and soil erosion, making land useless for agriculture. Loss of topsoil is one of the major factors contributing to decreased food production.

> History provides us with graphic examples of human abuse of the soil. North Africa, once the fertile granary of the Roman Empire, is now largely barren and unproductive. The Fertile Crescent of the Tigris-Euphrates Valley may have supported more people in the pre-Christian era than it is able to support today. In North America, the Chihuahuan Desert in New Mexico and the Sonoran Desert in Arizona are now believed by some analysts to have been expanded by overgrazing in the few hundred years since the arrival of Europeans.[4]

7. Urbanization and crowding lead to death by violence, hunger, crime, disease, exposure to the elements, and possibly even to abnormally disastrous consequences of natural events. For example, in November 1970, 168,000 people who had crowded into the coastal areas of Bangladesh were killed by a tidal wave. Millions more were injured and left homeless. Crowding experiments done on laboratory animals such as rats show that when masses of them are forced to live in close proximity to each other, adverse behavior patterns result. Many sociologists and psychologists infer similar human reactions to overcrowding; there is a breakdown in normal social behavior; competition for resources grows fiercer; infant mortality increases; personal violent aggression increases in the form of rape and murder; and juvenile delinquency increases, as do all forms of violent and nonviolent crime. There are also psychologic responses to overcrowding such as increased adrenal activity leading to a shortened life span, hypertension, heart disease and stroke, and alcoholism. Although many animal studies have not been done under controlled conditions, and it is not always possible to predict human behavior from that of animals even if conditions are similar or the same, it seems reasonable to state, based on what we have observed in the laboratory and in nonlaboratory life, that all known effects of overcrowding are harmful, if not eventually lethal.

8. Decreased resources, with the inevitable desperation that results, leads to the increased likelihood of war.

9. Health services, which are now unavailable to hundreds of millions of people, will become even more scarce as ever more people grow ill and debilitated from the effects of overpopulation. And because health services will be less available, health problems will increase, resulting in a vicious cycle reaching fatal proportions.

Thus it becomes evident that the definition of the population problem cannot be restricted simply to a "head count" or even to a simple comparison of people to resources. The problem affects every area of human activity and endeavor, and there is no misery known to humanity that will not increase if population growth is not checked. Few population experts deny that the problem is reaching crisis proportions; the dilemmas arise in trying to find solutions.

Demography

A demographic picture of the population problem involves both the numbers and the distribution of people. Shifts in size, density, and migration of populations depend on the social, cultural, religious, and economic factors operating at a given period of history. For example, from the first appearance of human beings on earth until the beginning of early recorded history, it took about 35,000 years for the world population size to double. In contrast, during the period of 1650 to 1750 the rate of population increase was 0.3% (a doubling time of 240 years).[5] Since World War II the doubling time has steadily decreased.

During the latter half of the seventeenth and the first half of the eighteenth century world society underwent enormous social and economic changes. This was a time of increased urbanization, the beginnings of industrialization, and the dawn of scientific enlightenment (with subsequent decrease in the influence of the Church) including rapid advances in medical understanding that resulted in a sharp increase in life expectancy. These changes, just beginning to blossom in 1700, have accelerated in both speed and complexity so that today population is growing unchecked.

Most demographers classify all countries as either developed or underdeveloped (with a few in between labeled *developing* or *emerging*). The population problem increases in severity in inverse proportion to the development of a country. It should be noted here that a country's development is usually measured in technologic, scientific, and economic terms. Therefore Canada would be a more developed country than Chad, and the United Kingdom is more developed than Uruguay. Measures of a country's development are usually stated only in quantitative terms and do not take into account the desirability of life-styles or values. Thus for some, a country that functions on an agrarian tribal system might be a desirable place to live, but a country that is urban and industrialized will be considered more developed. Both birth and death rates are higher in underdeveloped countries than in developed ones, although the difference in death rates is smaller than that of birth rates. Thus population growth rates differ significantly between developed and underdeveloped countries, and the gap is constantly increasing. "The rich get richer and the poor get children" is an adage that is more than a cliché; it is a way of life in many parts of the world.

Migration is a demographic aspect of the population problem that tends to be less obvious than growth rates, although it has a profound impact. Internal migration (within a country), usually from rural to urban areas, significantly affects the growth rate as well as many of the intermediate problems mentioned previously. International migration played a large role in Europe and in the New World a few centuries ago but has in the present day become a less significant factor. International migration has slowed, and that which still continues usually takes place between countries that are similar in terms of population patterns. The number of people moving from country to country is statistically significant only when the country is physically small (Israel, for example) or sparsely populated (Australia).

Demography is concerned also with the interrelationships among fertility, mortality, migration, and socioeconomic factors. These interrelationships are poorly understood but are nonetheless hotly debated. For example, Coale[6] and others put forth the classic "theory of demographic transition" that holds that European fertility (as well as that of other industrialized countries) declined as a result of the social and economic upheaval resulting from the industrial revolution. In this way it is predicted that if greater industrialization is encouraged in underdeveloped countries, the population will then decline. In contrast to the transition theory are ones based on biologic factors such as changes in diet or genetic deterioration; that is, these factors will have a greater impact on population growth than will industrialization.

Demographic theories can be categorized as either Malthusian pessimistic or natural optimistic. The former position holds that natural checks on population growth have been eliminated for the most part, while the potential for food production has been so severely limited that it may have exceeded its capacity. Therefore if population is to achieve some sort of equilibrium (which many Malthusians doubt is possible), it must come about as a result of increased death rates rather than decreased birth rates.

The natural optimistic view holds that both society and nature are highly resilient and that catastrophes have been averted or overcome in the past. Thus emphasis is placed on varying ways of adapting to an admittedly serious problem.

Midway between these two views is interventionism, which holds that nature will not take care of these problems but that the Malthusians are unnecessarily pessimistic. The kinds of interventions called for range from highly coercive ones to those that are more or less voluntary. These interventions will be discussed later in the chapter.

It is impossible to demonstrate that a particular demographic theory is correct or will prove effective if applied to the solution of population problems. There surely is no sensible reason to believe, based on historical evidence, that nature will take care of itself without some human intervention, but neither is it necessarily true that all is lost and that inexorable processes cannot be reversed. Interventionism seems to be the most pragmatic position in theory, but the various sociocultural, political, and religious forces at work make application of theories extremely difficult.

The population growth rates of ethnic groups are different from each other and vary within a group from time to time. An important factor in assessing the effect of ethnicity on population is definition, that is, of which people is an ethnic group composed. Some groups do have ethnic characteristics, but they may not be relevant to population growth in terms of differentiating them and similar groups. For example, Jews are ordinarily considered an ethnic group; however, the population growth rate of Jews living in the United States is vastly different from that of Israeli Jews. The differences are mainly political and social even though there are strong ethnic similarities in the two groups that live in different hemispheres. Differences also exist among American Indians. Tribal customs and practices vary enormously, as do geography, location, and outside influences, which account for the great variety in population growth patterns. Interethnic population growth rates not only result in part from the sociocultural factors of the countries in which the groups live, but the rates also have a direct effect on social and political life. Witness the fact of the persecution of ethnic minorities or of civil war as a result of one group or another suddenly increasing population size (the recent history of Lebanon and its fluctuating proportion of Christians and Moslems is a good example).

Theories of population control

TRIAGE. Using the principle of triage (some use the phrase *social triage* to differentiate it from medical triage) to solve the problem of world hunger is a drastic step, one which many believe to be ethically insupportable. Triage is a process of selection or culling and can be used in a variety of contexts (for example, trappers use the term when grading the quality of fur pelts when they are grouped according to price), although the most familiar is a medical one that grew out of the necessity to assign treatment priority to the wounded on a battlefield or in a disaster. The process calls for division of the wounded into three groups as follows: (1) those who are expected to survive regardless of treatment, (2) those who are expected to die regardless of what is done for them, and (3) those who will die *unless* given immediate treatment. Obviously treatment priority goes to those who can be saved only if they receive immediate help.

The concept of triage was first devised in France around the dawn of the nineteenth century in reaction to the then common practice of leaving wounded soldiers where they lay until the battle was over. The military would then depart, and local townspeople were expected to attend to them as best they could. As a result, a great many soldiers died because immediate first aid was not available. In contrast, Medevac helicopters flying into the thick of battle to remove the wounded during the Vietnam war provided a clear example of the practice of triage. On the battlefield triage is used to best advantage when there are large numbers of wounded in one place; in natural and technologic disasters (the latter range from train wrecks to terrorist bomb attacks) the wounded also tend to be in a somewhat confined area, and triage can be carried out with some degree of precision.

Translation of the triage concept to a global locus and use of the principle on a large percentage of the population of an entire country is a much more complex and ethically questionable matter. In using triage to solve the world's overpopulation and starvation problem, countries are divided into three groups as follows: (1) those whose resources will be sufficient to feed the population regardless of whatever foreign aid is provided, (2) those whose population (or a significant part of it) will starve to death even if unlimited foreign aid is provided, and (3) those whose population can be saved *only* if aid is immediately forthcoming. The application of the principle suggests that countries in the second group should be left to sink or swim on their own and all foreign aid should be stopped. Massive efforts should be made to help countries in the third group, and countries in the first group should be helped on a voluntary basis if there is sufficient surplus after group three countries have been aided. Application of triage to the population problem rests on the following assumptions:

1. The populations that are starving (the vast majority of certain underdeveloped countries and even segments of developed countries) brought their plight on themselves by laziness, uncontrolled fecundity, and the like. If this were indeed true, only then would more advantaged countries be justified in deliberately letting them starve. There is no proof, however, that starving people have only themselves to blame.

2. Political circumstances, the greed of those in the ruling class, climactic conditions, and the history of a nation do not play a significant role in

the present plight. A history of the world will show that these and other factors all contribute to the problem.

3. Conditions of mass starvation (or the very real threat of it) have always existed; therefore whatever aid is given will be ineffective in the long run. It is undoubtedly true that throughout history groups of people have starved to death but not in the numbers seen today and not because resources are so drastically out of proportion to need. The future has never looked this bleak.

Although surely there are those people who will never move to help themselves regardless of how much is done to help them, and clearly there will always be greed, and the vagaries of the class system and severe weather that destroys (or prevents the development of) food resources, the population problem is so complex that these factors are only a portion of it. Many population planners who are now suggesting that triage be used to solve the problem live in countries that have contributed to the enormity of the differentiation between developed and underdeveloped countries. The rapid explosion of technology in industrialized countries following World War II created major social and economic changes, while in countries where technology did not blossom, there was no need for advancement. Thus the gap widened. Transportation and communication further increased the distance between development and underdevelopment. Moreover, the postwar boom in medical technology brought with it an enthusiasm to end infectious diseases, lower mortality, and generally create a healthier life for people in underdeveloped countries. However, wonder drugs and new surgical techniques can effect immediate change, but centuries-old customs and traditions remain as they always have been, thus creating conflict for both the providers and recipients.

> Immense loss of infant life, for example, was accepted as a way of life in many nations. With higher than average death rates for all other age groups, combined with a low life expectancy, it had become traditional and customary—indeed essential for survival—for these people to have very large families. In due historical course this reproductive pattern has become part of their culture. It was accepted as a good and necessary thing to have a large number of children both to help scratch a living from the soil and to act as an insurance against the needs of the later years of life.[7]

Thus population problems cannot be solved simply by representatives of the developed countries pointing out the "error of their ways" to people in underdeveloped countries.

Developed countries have contributed to the population growth gap in yet another significant way by forcing up the price of oil, causing a serious energy shortage and adversely affecting the farming practices of underdeveloped countries. Many poor, small agrarian nations have been using ancient farming techniques that involved animal labor to plow fields, draw water, and harvest crops. In the rush to spread modern technology around the world, representatives of developed countries encouraged use of machines for farming and high-grade fertilizers to improve the quality and quantity of crops. The beasts that pulled the plows were slaughtered for food, and now many of these farmers cannot afford to buy fuel for their tractors or fertilizer for their soil. In some countries today, such as Turkey and Pakistan, agricultural yield is lower than it was before the introduction of high technology.

Social triage, or the deliberate decision to aid some underdeveloped countries and to permit others to wither and die, involves both legal policy on the part of individual countries and binding international agreements. For it would defeat the intended purpose to have affluent country B step in to feed starving country X after affluent country A had decided to cut off funds and surplus food from X. Social triage also carries implications far beyond simply feeding or not feeding starving people.

> There are, unhappily, a whole multiplicity of hidden objectives and alternatives (for example, politics, economics, and a variety or nationalistic or egoistic priorities) which may motivate triage to be accepted as a reasonable and logical social policy (as revealed, for example, in the recent U.S. involvement with the Chilean coup). Countries which embrace "social triage" might be accused, for example, of political opportunism—of hoping that governments under the stress of famine might fall or that animosity might arise between neighboring countries to the end that situations and governments more favorable to their own might be established. We could be accused, that is to say, of neocolonialism of the most abhorrent variety.[8]

In arguing for the principle of social triage, Joseph Fletcher[9] states that charity and generosity are double-edged, that giving makes us feel good, and that we have a tendency to keep giving even if the consequences of the generosity are not totally beneficial. Fletcher maintains that the unabated flow of food, aid, and other resources to countries that demonstrate uncontrolled fertility will not solve the hunger problem. Some people, he holds, will be fed, but the basic problem of disproportion between production and consumption of resources will continue. Those who advocate the use of social triage make a case for the "tyranny of survival"; that is, that the ultimate survival of the human race is the summum bonum, the highest good, because without survival no other values have meaning, and charity, generosity, and all the other altruistic principles we are so proud of will be for naught. Fletcher sums up the basic ethical argument in favor of social triage as follows:

> We must presuppose that no responsible person would insist on sharing regardless of the consequences, whether in matters of food or anything else. Such a posture would be purblind and irrational. We ought not to enter upon

courses of action which foreseeably end in the negation of the good being sought. If it could be shown that the beneficiaries of our generosity would, on balance, suffer more than they benefitted, and if it is our proper business as moral agents to optimize the good, rather than blindly following a moral rule or value (virtue), then in such a situation to share the food would be immoral. We should give if it helps but not if it hurts. This reasoning has the most direct bearing on many problems of famine relief. It simply is not always true that is is "more blessed to give than to receive."[10]

The major thrust of Fletcher's argument is a utilitarian one, that the consequences of generosity should be the appropriate guide to moral actions rather than "blindly following a moral rule." This is quite consistent with his belief that the ultimate survival of the human race is of primary importance.

Garret Hardin is another proponent of social triage and coined the phrase *lifeboat ethics*.[11] He devised this analogy by asking us to imagine a scene following a shipwreck. Some people were lucky enough to find a place in lifeboats that are well equipped for survival (these are the image of developed, affluent countries), but some could not make it and are swimming around in the sea asking to be let onto one or another of the boats (underdeveloped, starving countries). The lifeboats can make room for a few extra passengers, but if all those swimming in the sea were to be taken aboard, the lifeboats would become overcrowded, and the likelihood is that they would capsize and everyone would drown. So too with the starving countries. If the affluent countries (which he states do not have the plentiful food surpluses commonly believed) take full responsibility for feeding the starving countries, they will eventually deplete their own resources to so dangerous a level that their citizens would be endangered. Hardin's lifeboat analogy is an oversimplification of the problem; realistically the sharing ethic would end in tragedy only if it is practiced with no critical limits whatever, as the boats would sink only if all the people swimming in the water were permitted aboard.

Social triage can be practiced in the following two ways: (1) complete withholding of aid and resources and (2) making aid conditional on certain actions of the recipient. The first would appear to be far more severe, and many would view the second to be a less than ethical form of generosity. Fletcher points out that those people who victimize their own children by bearing more than they know will reach maturity, thus condemning a percentage of their own children to certain death, may not deserve to be the recipients of the beneficence of others. The burden of responsibility for bearing children belongs to the parents of those children and to the society that condones and perpetuates such practices, not on total strangers who happen to be more affluent. High mortality is, of course, caused by factors other than lack of food, but this fact simply strengthens the position of proponents of triage. If high mortality will continue even with the provision of food, then the food should be withheld until other factors can be ameliorated to the point where the provision of food will be demonstrably beneficial. Without these conditions the generosity of affluent countries would be irrational.

A more drastic form of social triage is to simply turn one's back on those countries that are deemed to be in such trouble that no amount of help could reverse the trend toward mass starvation, much as the soldier who is mortally wounded in battle is left to die. If a miracle occurs and the soldier shows definite signs of at least cessation of the dying process, if not recovery, then he could be reclassified by the triage officer and given treatment. By the same token, if a starving nation could somehow reverse its slide into mass death, it would then become eligible for aid.

Even if one could agree wholeheartedly with social triage, pragmatic problems exist. In a disaster or in battle an experienced triage officer can make quick decisions about treatment priority with a high degree of accuracy. It is not so simple when an entire country is in need of "diagnosis." The complexities involved in deciding which country is hopeless and which is salvageable are so enormous that it seems unlikely that it could ever be done with any degree of accuracy or justification.

Those opposed to social triage (Shriver, Verghese, and others) base their opposition on humanitarian or deontologic grounds and raise several important issues that must be examined in the process of coming to grips with the conflict. The first is the meaning of existence or the chief purpose of humanity. Theologians of monotheistic religions respond by stating that the major purpose is to serve or glorify God, which implies a hierarchy of moral values. Somewhere near the top of that hierarchy (or at the top in some views) is belief in the preservation of life—not only life in the aggregate, as in humanity, but individual lives as well. Hundreds of thousands of lives, or even one life, cannot be sacrificed to save others, even a majority of others. Those who oppose triage acknowledge that whatever value system is chosen by a society, there must be a concomitant acceptance of responsibility for that value system. In other words, if triage is unacceptable as a means to control population, then members of a society (or the decision makers in that society) must either take responsibility for the consequences of rampant population growth or choose another means to control population.

The second issue is deciding which countries should be sacrificed. An assumption must be made (and one cannot guarantee that the assumption can be made) that some countries are beyond salvage, but even if some groups must be sacrificed, what principles can be applied to the choice? Would a group of social triage officers be equally willing to sacrifice members of their own society if the same criteria of social responsibility were to be applied? For example, would Americans, who are willing to let a nation of people who refuse to use birth control be sacrificed, also be willing to cut off all welfare payments and other forms of public and private aid to fellow Americans who refuse to use birth control? In other words, would they be willing to apply the same standards to themselves as they would to strangers? Part of the issue is a universalizability of standards and values, that is, those that can be sacrificed without regard to ethnicity, political boundaries, and other such factors. It is unlikely, in this highly pluralistic world, that such universalizability can be achieved.

A third issue, closely allied with the second, is deciding which countries should be the major producers for the world's consumers and which can be allowed to produce less than they require. Opponents of triage tend to view the carrying capacity of ecologic systems on a global basis, that is, how great a population load can be carried by the ecologic system before disaster strikes. If it is true that ecology is global, and all data seem to suggest that whatever ecologic conditions exist in one country or region will ultimately have an effect on the entire planet, then the responsibility for caring for ecologic systems should be globally shared. This means no one is sacrificed, especially by those who contribute significantly to the disruption of the global ecology. It also would mean, however, that everyone must contribute in some way.

At issue also is the question of justice. It is indeed true that life is frequently unjust, and it is often claimed that those who produce goods are the only ones who have the right to consume them and that a society can take from a system only that which it has contributed to it.

> But on the level of substantive ethical theory, the issue is whether or not justice must be defined strictly as an equal exchange of resources between equally able agents; or whether a qualifying "bias towards the weak" is a second, necessary principle. Biblical scholars have tried to find just that bias in the ethics of the Old and New Testaments.[12]

Opponents of triage accuse those who favor it of inhumanity toward the weak and helpless and maintain that a moral obligation of humans is to help the starving achieve independence, not sacrifice them in the hope that others will not follow in their disastrous footsteps.

There is also the issue of differing perceptions of the present situation and differing beliefs in what the future will hold. That is, how wretched does one's life have to be before it is considered not worth living, and how certain are we that science and technology will not be able to solve some major problems in the foreseeable future? Could we, for example, send a team of researchers to country X, where the population is on the brink of mass death by starvation, and take a poll of its citizenry to find out if they would agree to be sacrificed because of the misery of their living conditions? Imagine the worst possible scenario—a woman, whose husband was killed by bandits as they stole the loaf of bread he was carrying, sits by the lean-to that is her home (it is literally a lean-to, without walls and with only tattered canvas for a roof) surrounded by two living children and the corpse of the toddler who has just died in her arms. Two other children have also died. She has no work, no food, and no energy. She has nothing except her children and the knowledge of her existence. Why does she not kill herself and her children? If we can assume that she continues to live because she prefers life to death, then we must acknowledge that perceptions of what is tolerable in life differ because there are surely those who would view this woman's life as intolerable. Therein lies the most pressing issue: what ethical justification can be used to make the necessary decisions if the principle of social triage is to be put into practice, and, as always the question arises, who should make these decisions?

CONFLICTS AMONG ALTERNATIVE SOLUTIONS. All theories of population control can work in principle and can be made to work in practice if enough coercive measures are used. However, all aspects of each theory have characteristics that are more or less desirable, pragmatic, and ethical. There are also various beliefs about how much, if any, coercion is permissible. Potter[13] surveys the major sources of conflict among theories.

1. Ecologic limits may preclude increased development of resources. The earth cannot continue to be exploited at the present rate without significant permanent damage. Some resources are finite (for example, oil and coal) and some take so long to replenish themselves (trees, topsoil, etc.) that the rate at which they are consumed makes a critical difference. Therefore improving agricultural techniques and increasing crop yield per acre of land may not be the answer to the problem of overpopulation.

2. Liberty, autonomy, and freedom to reproduce as one wishes are seen by many to be a serious barrier to the implementation of certain theories of population control. The coercive factor inherent in any theory to change reproductive practices ranges from very mild to very strong. Liberty and coercion will be discussed in more detail in the next section.

3. Unless formal justice can be practiced on a global basis, which is an unrealistic hope, some people and societies will have less access to resources than others. Even without the deliberate institution of social triage, this inequality will in all likelihood continue. Ignoring this inequality can be seen as a kind of passive form of triage, analogous to not stopping to help accident victims who are obviously seriously hurt. The conflict lies not only in active or passive triage but also between maintaining the status quo, knowing that it will worsen, and taking active steps to alleviate the problem. Moreover, conflict exists in one's view of the root causes of the problem. On one hand, starving countries can be blamed for their own problems by seeing them as a matter of only uncontrolled fecundity. On the other hand, one can take into account all

the social, climatic, religious, and economic forces that contribute to the seriousness and complexity of the problem.

4. The conflict that engenders considerable emotional outrage is the suggestion that the affluent learn to moderate their perception of what they believe necessary for a desirable standard of living, thus increasing the ability of the nonaffluent to be consumers. The conflict is basically between a capitalist, free enterprise system and a Marxist one. There is, however, little empirical evidence to show that a significant decrease in consumption by one group of people would result in a significant increase by other groups. For example, in the United States agricultural surpluses have often been used for purposes other than feeding the starving in this and other countries. Many times surpluses have been destroyed to affect farm prices. In other words, the farmers, who in this country are free enterprise capitalists, would rather destroy surplus food to benefit themselves than leave market prices alone and give the food to others who are hungry. It is also unlikely that the very affluent, who are what they are because of a dedication to a certain socioeconomic philosophy, would willingly change that philosophy for the sake of total strangers who have no emotional impact on their lives. True, the giving of charity may be part of this philosophy, but the basic desire to continue one's own affluence is not generally affected by charitable actions.

ETHICAL ISSUES
Individual freedom of reproduction

The principle of justice, along with autonomy and nonmaleficence, can be applied to the conflicts inherent in the world population problem. Justice always has to do with the distribution of things, goods, services, access to those goods and services, and societal burdens. The population problem can be seen as a miscarriage of justice; that is, somehow the distribution of benefits became so unfairly skewed that the result was starvation and misery for a good deal of the earth's population. However, according to Brown, justice requires deciding who is entitled to what benefits.

> A variety of commonsense notions are normally advanced in answer to this question, including need, effort, contribution to society, etc. A contraceptive program could be just, for instance, if it provides similar contraceptive services or devices to those equally in need of them.[14]

On the other hand, high fertility rates among certain groups might be acceptable if they were viewed as being a reward of sorts for high community production or achievement.

If we were to take this concept of justice literally, we would still be faced with the problem of what constitutes need in a contraceptive program or how to define a highly productive member of society. Far better, one might be tempted to say, to distribute justice absolutely equally, regardless of any factor other than the personhood of the individuals affected. Justice implies rights, and in a system of global equality everyone would have the right to bear as many children as desired and would have the right to share equally in the consumption of resources. But justice and rights also imply responsibility, and here we run directly into the conflict between the freedom to reproduce at will and the responsibility not only to care for the children produced but to put back into society a measure of what one takes from it.

The right to reproduce without limitation is grounded in the principles of liberty and autonomy; that is, a free person should not be interfered with in the use of his own body; to do so in any way would be an impingement on his liberty. This concept is well understood by most readers and poses no major problems in theory. The opposite position, that is, the right of some people to restrict the reproductive practices of some other people, is a more complex issue and deserves some discussion. There are several reasons why it might be considered permissible to restrict one's reproductive rights.

1. If a claim can be made that the parents have sole (or at least the bulk of) responsibility for children, then the right to bear them can be forfeited if the parents do not have the means to feed, clothe, and house them. Society can then restrict reproductive freedom.

2. Entitlement to food and other societal benefits can generally be claimed only if one has contributed to the production of these benefits or if a person or society is in a position to trade benefits of relatively equal value. If a claim cannot be made on this basis, then one cannot be expected to be able to feed one's children, and the right to bear them can be forfeited.

3. If a person or society provides a constant source of food and benefits for another person or society and is not in turn the recipient of goods and benefits of similar or equal value, that society may put a price on the continuation of the provision of those goods and services in lieu of payment in kind. That price might be the restriction of reproductive freedom.

4. One who causes suffering to others can, by the mores of most societies, have some of their own rights and freedoms revoked. Therefore if the birth of too many children causes deprivation of the populace as a whole, individuals' reproductive freedom may be curtailed. This point

> turns on an understanding of the moral significance of inflicting injury on
> the innocent. The argument would have to go something like this: all else
> being equal, persons have a right not to be injured or made to suffer. To

put it another way, causing unjustified suffering to the innocent is immoral.
...it is an act of violence against free agents to subject them to suffering
or injury (or, for that matter to any state) without their consent. Such imposi-
tion would be a circumscription of freedom, and while future persons may be
presumed to consent to happiness, they cannot be presumed to consent to
pain.[15]

Thus in some instances it would seem that reproductive freedom can be
curtailed, but even in the unlikely event that everyone in a given society could
agree in principle to limit reproduction, certain other ethical problems would
immediately crop up. Whose reproduction would be limited: men or women,
the childless or those who already have children, only the poor or the affluent
as well? By what means would this restriction of liberty be accomplished:
enforced sterilization; various incentives such as food, money, or other tangibles;
or a voluntary program with education about contraceptives? For how long a
period and under what circumstances should reproductive freedom be limited:
should no couple ever have more than two children, or should reproductive
rights be tied to the gross national product or some other economic measure?
These problems are the ones that face population planners today, and it is the
method of population control, not so much the fact that control appears
necessary, that causes most ethical conflicts.

There are, however, those who maintain that freedom of reproduction
should not be restricted. This position is based in part on the rationale that
persons are valuable in their own right, that they are the highest value of all
things that exist, and that the more persons there are, the more value will exist
in the world. A second argument is that reproduction is a natural and inalienable right, akin to life and liberty, and therefore cannot be abrogated for
any reason.

Famine, starvation, and violence

Famine is both a Biblical and a modern phenomenon and is interpreted
by much of the world's population today as both a natural and unavoidable
event and as a punishment for the sins of humans. In the light of modern
knowledge and technology, this appears to be a rather fatalistic view, although almost everyone will acknowledge that the exigencies of climate
can cause severe drought or flooding with a resultant drastic destruction
of crops. Both the Old and the New Testament are filled with examples of the
anticipation of famine (for example, Genesis 12:10 and 37–50, Kings 19,
Luke 15:11–32, and Matthew 5:45) and the preparation for it by storage
of grain for the lean years, thus reducing to a minimum the number of deaths
by starvation. But the earth's population was far smaller then, it was confined

to a relatively small area, and people lived in tribal communities of manageable size.

Today most affluent countries are predominantly Christian, although there are notable exceptions such as Japan and some of the oil-rich nations of the Middle East. Many, although not all, of the underdeveloped countries are non-Christian. This may have a good deal to do with the way famine is perceived, the role it plays in people's lives, and what is believed can and should be done to prevent it.

> While Judaism and Christianity differ fundamentally over the question of the consummation of God's work in the world, both give large place to these promises of biblical religion. The promises indicate the authentic and true character of human life. Life is intended to be marked by wholeness, by peace, by possibilities for all human beings. Food, clothing, shelter, and opportunity for a meaningful existence are purposed by God for all. Famine, therefore, is not God's intention. Where famine exists, the purpose of life remains unfulfilled.[16]

Famine is thus seen by most Westerners as something to be feared, avoided, and deliberately prevented. Many Easterners and non–Judeo-Christian religions have a strong sense of karma, or fate, and view famine in the same way as they see some of the natural phenomena that contribute to it—as natural occurrences that cannot be controlled or prevented by humans. Because people believe that famine itself cannot be prevented, they take steps thought to thwart or circumvent its ravages, for example, bearing "extra" children that will serve as buffers against the loss of a large percentage of children that almost always occurs in underdeveloped countries. Thus the cycle of overpopulation and famine continues. There are, of course, other reasons besides the hoped for control of famine that people choose to have large numbers of children, such as the intrinsic value of children and the unavailability of or unwillingness to participate in abortion. But overpopulation remains a strong causal factor in increasing famine.

The problem of the ratio of resources to food can be stated, perhaps overly simply, in the following way: rich countries produce the most food and believe, for the most part, that they have ownership rights to that food. Poor countries, again in the main, do not have enough food nor the capability to feed their populace and thus are put into the position of supplicants. If the rich do not provide food (or the means to produce it) for the poor, the latter will continue to starve.

The fundamental ethical problem lies in the conflict over the right to ownership of food and resources. Again an analogy can be made to a shipwreck. After the wreckage has cleared and people are swimming about in the water (no lifeboats this time), one person spots a wooden beam that he can hang onto for rest and flotation. Others see what he has found and clamor to share a handhold. He flails at them and tries to drive them away, claiming that he saw the beam first and now deserves sole ownership. "Go find your own," he shouts in anger, fear, and frustration. Does he indeed have a moral claim to the entire beam, or is he obligated to share it with others? To answer the question requires an examination of how rights are claimed, which rights are legitimate, and what consequences to others are involved in the claiming of rights. (The reader is referred to Chapter 1 for a discussion of rights and of teleologic as compared with deontologic moral theories.) If one were to respond that the swimmer must share his beam with other shipwreck victims, then one would likely also claim that the rich nations are obligated to share food resources with poor nations to avert famine.

VIOLENCE. Violence is a fact of life in all parts of the world, and where conditions of overcrowding and mass starvation exist, it is reasonable to assume that the incidence of violence will increase.

> The relationship between crowding and physical violence is close. Animal studies have shown that crowding beyond certain limits, either in nature or in captivity, leads to a breakdown in social order, fighting to the death, cannabalism of the young, and severe alteration of certain reproductive processes. In this way the population of species of lower animals is controlled when it exceeds a certain density or passes a critical point in the survival of the species.[17]

There is surely evidence that overcrowding leads to violence in humans; any experienced police officer can cite case after case of murder that was caused in large measure by the fact that people live too tightly packed together. In the history of the world many wars have been waged over the effort to wrest resources from other countries; however, mass killing in the form of periodic wars is neither a practical nor an ethical solution to the problem of overpopulation. Civilized people decry the existence of violence and make efforts to contain it. Those efforts, however, have been for the most part futile, as each year violence increases in most of the world.

Violence is closely tied to, and is even the outgrowth of, territoriality, and the higher the social order of a species, the stronger is its instinct for defense of territory and the more sophisticated its means to defend it. Because humans use aggression, sometimes including violence, to acquire the territory they possess, they will use violence and aggression to defend it. And the more valuable the territory is perceived, the more violent the aggression will become.

Human beings use violence against each other for the following two major reasons: because they perceive themselves or their territory (including family, beliefs, and possessions) to be threatened or because there is an interference with those cerebral mechanisms that inhibit violence (as occurs in certain physical illnesses). Severe overcrowding will affect both these cause-effect relationships by sharpening territorial instincts and by lowering the inhibitions against violence. Overcrowding contributes to violence in other ways as well. As population increases significantly, individuality decreases, and human contact tends to become more superficial and less intimate. This is a source of enormous frustration that can lead to outbursts of violent rage. The less intimacy we experience with fellow human beings, the more alienated from each other we become, and the easier it is to commit acts of violent aggression. Alienation and loss of individuality result in a generalized lack of respect for persons, a situation we see developing in the United States today where in large cities there is much poverty and overcrowding and the rate of violent crime is higher than it is in areas where the population is less dense. This is caused in large measure by the factors already mentioned, and the trend seems to be toward increasing and spreading violence.

The smaller the space a human being has for his own personal territory, the stronger his sense of territoriality becomes. Lorenz and Leyhausen[18] described this phenomenon as they observed prisoners of war. Each time the prisoners were moved to a new camp or barracks, the first thing each man did was to stake out his territory by choosing a bed and then marking the boundaries of the bed and adjoining space with string or clothing. The same process was performed by all the prisoners, and each formally acknowledged and respected the other prisoners' territory. Lorenz and Leyhausen also observed that boundary-marking behavior can extend to other populations experiencing severe overcrowding. Individuals and families clearly mark off their own boundaries and then take active steps to protect their territory by greeting strangers with distrust or open hostility.

In the sociologic and anthropologic literature, there is an ongoing debate about whether the phenomenon of territoriality is inborn or cultural. Ardrey and others argue that territoriality in humans is genetic and unalterable, whereas Montagu and others disagree.

> Whether humans are genetically and instinctually territorial or this characteristic is a learned cultural and societal behavior does not seem to matter. What *does* matter, and what will have a profound effect on our future, is that we do not *like* to live too close together. Over and over we have seen from animal behavior studies, from observation of life in crowded cities, and from personal experience that when we are forced to live in close proximity to other human beings for long periods of time, when we do not have sufficient personal space, and when there is no opportunity to get away from it all, we grow snappish with each other, develop new neuroses and increase our old ones, are suspicious and paranoid, and lash out physically at the slightest provocation of threat. We begin to kill each other. There is little doubt that continued overpopulation will increase these behaviors and lead to a life that will be intolerable for most people.[19]

Racism and genocide

Almost without exception population planners and demographers who advocate drastic (and even not so drastic) steps to be taken to control population are members of an affluent society (generally light skinned), and those who are called on to decrease their population and to control their reproductive practices belong to poor societies and are generally darker skinned. This has provoked accusations of racism and even genocide, some of which appear fairly well founded. Some have even argued that the motivation for some population control policies is not the improvement of the quality of life on earth but rather genocide itself. This argument, while it may have some basis in fact in some quarters, is almost impossible to prove.

Genocide is, of course, the ultimate form and action of racism. Although genocide may not be a completely realistic fear, racism surely is. It exists in all areas of the world in varying forms and to different degrees. It is always pernicious, but its practice or effect can seem mild or severe depending on one's vantage point.

Since racist practices are always ethically wrong, we can accept it as a given that any population control program that has racism as its fundamental base is also ethically wrong. However, it is impossible to be certain of the motives of population planners and thus is difficult to assess which population control programs should not be supported because their theoretic base is primarily racist. For instance, it is undeniably true that India has more people than its resources can support; it is also true that Indians belong to a darker skinned race. Is it then wrong for light-skinned people in developed countries to support and encourage population control programs for India? Would it be wrong for Indians to support such programs for themselves? If the two questions are answered differently, what is the ethical distinction? A related issue is whether affluent countries should offer food and other aid to countries such as South Africa that have racist population policies. In that country public contraceptive programs are aimed almost exclusively at nonwhites. Although one might be generally in favor of contraception in principle, can a racist policy be supported by the governments of other countries or by international organizations such as the International Planned Parenthood Federation (IPPF)? Here it would seem that the principles of nonmaleficence and justice override the general beneficence of population control. On the other hand, in countries such as South Africa, nonwhites are the poorest and most disadvantaged and have the greatest trouble caring for the children they do have. In this view, a contraceptive program might seem doubly important. However, the surpassing concern would be the basic intent of the program, and in a country that has such explicitly racist government policies, there can be little doubt about the intent of those instituting contraceptive programs for nonwhites or persons with darker skins.

RELIGIOUS VIEWS

It is beyond the scope of this book to provide more than a brief overview of the perspective on population control of the world's major religions. And although in some instances it will be readily apparent that certain religious beliefs, practices, and policies have had a profound effect on population growth rates among certain populations and may even have a spillover effect on the world at large, it is not the purpose of this book to label some religious beliefs and practices more or less ethical than others in terms of population practices.

Judaism

Judaism is divided into three major branches (with a fourth newly developing) and has no central religious authority that formulates religious policy. Therefore there is differing opinion about both contraceptive practices and beliefs about population control. The major differences in the branches of Judaism arise from views about the acceptance of *halakah* (law) as binding. The more liberal branches feel bound to fewer aspects of halakah, and the bonds that do exist are less restrictive. The strictest interpretation of population control arises from two passages in Genesis, the injunction to "be fruitful and multiply" (9:7) and the prohibition against onanism (38: 9–10). Although certain exceptions are allowable (as when the life of a woman would be clearly threatened by pregnancy), Orthodox Judaism permits no contraception and thus no population control programs. This, however, is an oversimplification of the position of Judaism because both oral tradition and Talmudic interpretation of halakah make provisions for a variety of life circumstances, and rabbinic interpreters always entertain logical arguments. A major argument is whether non-Jews are required to abide by the Old Testament commandments regarding procreation and the multiplication of human beings. If non-Jews are not bound by Jewish law, then the Jewish position has little statistical significance in terms of world population. However, many Christian religions interpret these two passages in Genesis the same way as do Orthodox Jews; thus the perspective becomes more significant.

Eastern Orthodox Christianity

The threat of overpopulation has not received much attention in Eastern Orthodox Christian literature, and what there is tends to deal with the problem as it relates to individual birth control practices. The more conservative among Eastern Orthodox Christians tend to see the population crisis as a smoke screen to encourage the use of contraception, which is forbidden by the Eastern Orthodox Church. However, more liberal theologians and modern writers see birth control as a possible solution to the very real problem of overpopulation. Eastern Orthodox doctrine holds (as does Christian doctrine in general) that human beings have dominion over all other creatures on earth, and one way to achieve and assure this dominion is by steadily increasing the numbers of humans. Now that technology has taken us so far in our ability to subdue many other species, we do not need to rely on sheer numbers; thus modern Orthodox theologians are beginning to place less emphasis on this rationale. Eastern Orthodox tradition tends to focus on the family and on national cultures and heritages rather than on a global view; therefore the population problem has not captured the intensity of theologic attention that it has in other religions that have a stronger world view.

Roman Catholicism

The Roman Catholic position on contraception was discussed in some detail in Chapter 4. This firmly entrenched negative stance on individual contraception is simply enlarged to include the problem of overpopulation. The Church acknowledges the facts of hunger, famine, and death by starvation, but it does not see prevention of pregnancy as an acceptable answer to the problem. During Pope John Paul II's 1979 visit to the United States and in subsequent visits to other countries, many of which have severe population problems, he reaffirmed the Church's position on contraception. It is not likely he will change.

Protestantism

Protestant sects have focused discussions of the population problem on aspects that deal with public policy, sexuality and procreation, and contraception. Protestantism differs from Catholicism in that procreation, although it is a highly desirable goal, is not the only worthwhile and morally acceptable purpose for sexual intercourse. Companionship, nurture, and expression of marital love are also good and acceptable reasons for sex. Thus the way is open for individual contraception and positive support for population control programs. Many Protestant denominations take an active interest in population policy, a concern that has been steadily increasing since the First World War. When they issue policy statements, Protestant bodies tend to stress the effect of overpopulation on human beings and its strain on available resources, but they acknowledge that the problem is complicated by a number of other factors: advanced medical technology, uneven production and exploitation of natural resources, a gradual Westernization of material values (caused in large part by the export of American television programs), and the failure of the governments of many countries to provide adequate social welfare programs (even ones based on limited resources) for their citizens. Protestants are urged by their leaders to see the problem of overpopulation as an ethical as well as a pragmatic and social one. Because there is widespread recognition that simply decreasing the number of people on earth will not be sufficient to solve the complexities of the problem, the major thrust of Protestant theologians has been to support programs that encourage contraception and the alteration of existing social policies.

Islam

The dominant belief in Islam relative to the population problem is highly pronatalist. Allah (God) created sexuality and procreation, and it is Allah who controls fertility. The concept of *kismet* (fate) is strong in Islam, thus lending a highly fatalistic flavor to sexuality and procreation. Kismet is a force that prevents a good deal of social change, including the prevention of conception and the acceptance of modern technology, although in the Middle East, which except for Israel is almost totally Moslem, where the economy is based almost exclusively on oil, aversion to technology is changing. But kismet remains a dominant force in many areas of life, notably in sexual and family relations.

Islam does not officially prohibit contraception, although in Islamic law the only method discussed is coitus interruptus. Ironically, the law requires a woman's consent for her husband to practice coitus interruptus because she has a right not only to bear children but also the right to complete sexual fulfillment. The Koran is the definitive source on Moslem life and ethics, but it contains no mention whatever about contraception; therefore it must be considered permissible. The fact that Allah is omnipotent and the strong reliance on kismet can, in effect, override the permissibility of contraception; that is, if Allah wills it and if fate decrees it, a woman will become pregnant regardless of whether or not the penis is withdrawn before ejaculation. Modern forms of contraception can, however, add a new dimension to the issue. More than fate is involved if active steps are taken to prevent conception, and it then becomes a social and cultural as well as a religious matter. As most Moslem countries are male dominated, and as most forms of contraception are designed for use by the female, the locus of control shifts from the man to the woman. Moslem men are likely to regard this shift with disfavor. Thus if opposition to outside efforts to establish family planning clinics in Moslem countries springs up, one could regard it as the result of the historic prevalence of male dominance rather than a lack of desire to decrease population.

Another conflict is the one between the individual Muslim and his government, particularly in private matters such as family. It is perfectly permissible for a Muslim couple to practice contraception, but it is not permissible, according to Islam jurisprudence, for a national government to dictate contraceptive practices to its citizens. Many Muslims also see family planning programs as another ploy to manipulate life in Third World countries. The tendency in recent years has been a populist movement to shake off the effects of Westernization and return to some old Islamic traditions. In this regard, population programs are not likely to achieve a high degree of success.

Hinduism

Almost the entire population of India, as well as that of many surrounding countries, is Hindu. The population is growing at the staggering rate of 13% a year. Despite enormous economic growth, there are more Indians starving to death now than ever before because the ratio of population to resources is out of control. Hindu ethical ideals, or karma, are a comprehensive combination of the well-being of persons as individuals and as part of the larger society. Karma also encompasses other-worldly aspects of life, is equal to wealth and righteousness, and involves an expectation to marry (Hindu gods are married). It is the obligation of each Hindu couple to produce a son and a daughter (one of each will fulfill the obligation), but for practical purposes many more children must be born to ensure that at least one son and daughter survive.

Family planning programs cannot be considered without taking into account the entire context of karma, that is, the total personal and social welfare of Hindus. The goal of a population control program should be a "better" life, which is admittedly a nebulous goal, particularly where a program is conceived and administered by non-Hindus. In recent years the infant mortality in India has dropped significantly, as has the death rate in general, but the birth rate has remained consistently high. Therefore it would seem that factors other than ensuring the eventual survival of two children are contributing to the ongoing population growth rate in India, Pakistan, and other Hindu countries.

There is no specific opposition to contraception in Hinduism, and the religion has a tradition of sexual abstinence under a variety of circumstances (for instance, prohibition of widow remarriage or abstinence during lactation). Child marriages are common in Hinduism, ensuring a longer period of fertility in women within marriage, although in recent years the Indian government has encouraged postponement of marriage. Abortion is condemned in Hinduism and is therefore not a practical method of lowering the birth rate. There is, however, nothing in Hinduism to prevent sterilization, and that is the avenue that most population control programs have elected to take, although there are political aspects to be considered.

PUBLIC POLICY

Public policy implies that a government or other group of people will intervene in the reproductive practices of some other group of people. The purpose of the policy is most often to change conditions that affect birth and death rates and infant mortality. Interventions include various incentives to change behavior, educational programs, provision of free or low-cost contraception or sterilization, and outright coercion.

Public policy is ordinarily authored by individuals, government representatives, or spokespersons from private organizations. All are influenced not only by the conditions they are attempting to rectify, but also by personal and societal values, personal and societal aspirations and goals, and the history of other population theories and proposals. For example, an individual might write a book that is calculated to be shocking or unusual so as to increase sales, or a government might tie a population policy proposal to arms or trade agreements (for example, the unlimited purchase of some mineral resource in exchange for a significant drop in the birth rate). This does not negate the presence of altruism, a genuine concern for the ecology, or a desire to better the quality of life of future generations, but there must be a careful distinction between altruistic and egoistic intent. Most public policy has a strongly utilitarian flavor, which is difficult to avoid when dealing with an ethical problem of global ramifications.

In all instances, however, the author of a particular policy should be able to defend or justify it, and this engenders considerable public debate. Debate is always controversial, always incredibly complex, and almost always inconclusive. Factual data on which policy is based is ever changing, and its accuracy can be called into question, as can the motives of persons providing the data. Decisions or proposals based on such data can never be conclusively proved to be correct or even the most effective or appropriate from a wide range of choices.

During public debate it is generally appropriate to explore the following issues as they pertain to any proposal:

1. How will the balance among the various cultural or ethnic groups in a particular country or region be affected?
2. How will the personal lives of the people who are the targets of the policy be affected?

3. Can charges of racism or genocide be legitimately levied?
4. What methods will be used to implement the policy, and how strong will the coercion be? What forms will it take? (It must be assumed that some form of coercion, no matter how benign, will be proposed to change the status quo.)
5. What normative ethics will be used in formulating the policy?

National policies

National governments have tried, with varying degrees of success, to affect the reproductive beliefs and practices of their own citizens. Most of the programs have been aimed at reducing the population, although a few such as Israel and Australia have tried to increase population. Veatch[20] describes several factors inherent in governmental population incentives as follows:

1. Good offered as an incentive. Monetary inducements are the most commonly used, although one sometimes sees tax rebates, social security bonuses, and goods and services such as food, clothing, and jobs. This type of incentive has been widely used in India where money or other items of value were given in exchange for submission to sterilization.
2. The behavior to be induced. It makes a distinct difference to the success of a population control program whether the expected behavior is permanent or temporary, designed for men or women, physically invasive or not, or whether the person is inconvenienced by travel, physical discomfort, and other such factors. The less permanent the behavior and the less disruptive to one's life, generally the higher the rate of acceptance.
3. The timing of the incentive. The primary beneficiaries of any population control program are the offspring of the generation in existence at the time the program is put into effect. These offspring (or absence of them as the case may be) are totally innocent and passive recipients of the actions of others. Another aspect of timing is the fact that some have advocated the delayed awarding of incentives until the period of fertility has passed to ensure small family size. This delay tactic would have no bearing, of course, on incentives for sterilization.
4. Identity of the incentive recipient. Traditionally this has been the individual submitting to sterilization or agreeing to practice birth control, but another group of incentive recipients has recently come to the fore and created a new ethical dilemma, the person who "finds" or identifies a potential candidate for sterilization. Some programs even offer incen-

tives to physicians or paramedics who perform the sterilization procedures, thus placing a kind of bounty on the program. A person who is greedy or unscrupulous enough could use coercive methods to convince people to be sterilized and could make quite a profit on the endeavor.

5. The amount of the incentive. This may be a flat rate for certain categories of agreements, perhaps more for sterilization than for a promise to use contraception, or there may be different rates depending on different variables, such as age or number of children already parented.

6. The psychologic impact of the incentive. This can vary considerably, depending on the relationship of the government to its citizens, the severity of the population problem, and the kinds of incentives used.

Ethical aspects of incentive programs revolve mostly around the conflict between the general welfare and individual autonomy, and frequently the national economy plays a role in a government's decision to institute an incentive program. Cost-benefit analysis can be used, that is, balancing the value of what a child can contribute to the national economy with the cost of preventing the birth of that child. This is a strongly utilitarian view and disregards individuals' autonomy and reproductive rights. It is easy to oversimplify the matter and see it only in terms of economics or goods and benefits produced and consumed. However, classical utilitarianism requires accounting for other factors that tend to produce happiness when calculating the utility of a proposed population control program. There is still the risk of harm to innocents, which would subtract from total happiness. It is never a child's fault that his parents bore him, and the child of parents who experienced some negative incentive (an additional tax burden, for instance) or the absence of a positive one might tend to be blamed by his parents for their own choice of not participating in the incentive program.

Although a deontologic approach would provide for a better guarantee of reproductive rights and personal liberty, the eventual negative outcome of putting such a theory into practice might be so severe that it would be worse than a certain restriction of liberty. The price for maintaining traditional practices may be too high.

China is an example of a country that has encouraged coercive population control measures. China acknowledges having 975 million people,[21] and if the present birth rate continues, the population could reach a billion and a half by the end of the century. Unless the population growth rate is slowed, China's efforts at economic recovery could be thwarted. Mao Tse-tung at first believed that an ever increasing population was a good thing, mainly in terms of cultural development and defense. As the Communist regime continued, however, and as the birth rate soared precipitously, Mao gradually came to support policies to control reproduction. In the early 1970s a population control program began in earnest. Contraceptives were made available at no cost, and couples were encouraged to have no more than two children. Abortion and sterilization were also free. The program has not been as successful as Chinese officials had hoped, although they claim to have reduced the birth rate by 50% in the past decade. United States population experts, however, claim that China underreports births and has reduced its birth rate by only 10% or so. Moreover, 50% of China's population is under age 21, a fact that would ordinarily signal a huge population surge.

As a result of this failure, population control policies have become even more coercive.

> . . . Worried officials of the Provincial Revolutionary Committee ordered that all pregnant women who already had one child or more be "convinced" that they should have an abortion. And, somewhat ominously, a top official announced, "beginning next January [1980], no one in the province is allowed to have the third child."[22]

In Yunnan province various positive incentives are given to couples who marry late and who have only one child. At the same time negative sanctions are to be imposed on couples who refuse to practice planned parenthood. The programs are bound to meet with a great deal of resistance, mainly because of the agrarian nature of Chinese life. Sons are needed to work in the fields (there is a Chinese saying, "More sons, more bliss"), and those families that have daughters keep trying to have sons. If a daughter is born, the next pregnancy will try to make up for that "error." Now that China has opened its doors to cultural and economic trade with the West, the population control program is certain to be affected, but it is difficult to predict whether the birth rate will increase or decrease and which segments of the Chinese population will be affected.

International policies

Discussions of international population policy result in conflict. In theory most population planners usually acknowledge a complex of factors (grouped into questions of fertility, mortality, and migration) that affect population. But in actual practice most program proposals concentrate only on fertility. Even at the World Population Conference, held in Bucharest in 1974, delegates concentrated mostly on debating whether rapid population growth does indeed pose a problem for most governments and for the world at large. Strategies for decreasing fertility were also discussed. "Similarly, governmental population programs in the developing countries may call attention to issues of mortality and migration, but most often their operational emphasis is on fertility."[23]

There are several major concepts and schools of thought on the issue of international planning. Developmentalists maintain that the best way to lower fertility is by economic, social, and political development, which many would class as a Marxist view. The main thrust of the argument is that people are more likely to be motivated to have small families if their lives are satisfactory in terms of employment, income, nutrition, living conditions, and the like. There is no opposition to family planning programs per se, but it is believed they will be mostly ineffective if other aspects of people's lives are not improved. A somewhat opposite view is that of the family planners who hold that high fertility and birth rates impede economic and social development, and one major cause of a country's social ills is the reproductive practices of its citizens. Therefore a lowered birth rate will result in an improved economy and life-style. The survivalists maintain that human life on earth is in clear and present danger of severe catastrophe because of overpopulation. They point to the existence of widespread famine and starvation, the steady erosion of topsoil with a resultant decreased growing capacity of the land, chaos and depersonalization of human life, and increased violence. The solution, they maintain, is immediate lowering of the birth rate, using some form of coercion or strong incentives. The Bucharest conference did not acknowledge the position taken by the survivalists (the most notable of which is Garret Hardin of "lifeboat" fame), but it did discuss developmental and family-planning approaches, as well as the various values inherent in deontologic and utilitarian approaches.

One of the toughest problems in international population control programs is the matter of foreign aid. This is a complex subject in itself, and the reader is referred to the literature of international diplomacy for a general discussion, but a few things might be mentioned here about the exchange of other benefits for assistance with family planning. Very rarely, except in cases of disastrous emergencies, such as earthquakes, do countries provide foreign aid without expecting something in return. That something need not be expressed in tangibles. Aid in family planning might be tied, for example, to the expectation that the business people of the donating country will receive top priority in certain trade negotiations, or there might be an arrangement whereby certain literacy levels will be attained. Or the gift of aid might be more blatant in its request for a return agreement, for instance, a mutual defense treaty.

There are also ethical questions surrounding the priority with which one country provides aid to others. For example, between 1965 and 1975 the amount of money spent by the U.S. Agency for International Development (AID) for family-planning programs increased drastically, while the amount spent for health, education, and agricultural assistance dropped precipitously in the same period.[24] Choosing which countries are to be recipients of aid can also raise ethical questions. What if, for example, primarily African countries were found to be beneficiaries of vast amounts of foreign aid for family planning, while those Latin American countries with heavily Catholic populations suddenly found their sources of funding drying up? One could certainly be suspicious of both racial and religious factors.

There is little debate over the fact that the population problem is a global one, and that overpopulation in Bangladesh will have a definite and lasting effect on Americans or that the greed of Western corporate business can affect the daily lives of millions of Indians. The problem is how to achieve an equilibrium between production and consumption while committing the least number of ethical errors.

SUMMARY

The world is overpopulated today, and the distribution of population to land mass and to the production capacity of the land is such that vast numbers of people starve to death each year, and famine is a way of life for much of the world's population. There are only a few ways to solve the problem—limit the number of people born, increase production of food and other resources, exclude certain groups of people from sharing in the available resources, decrease each individual's allocation of resources, or some workable combination of all of these. The number of ethical dilemmas engendered by the population problem, however, is infinite.

There are a number of reasons why population tends to increase at an escalating rate in certain parts of the world; these involve religious, cultural, economic, and social factors. For example, in many places a couple finds it necessary to have many children to ensure the survival of a few because infant mortality and the death rate in general are so high. Migration also affects population size, although to a lesser extent. There are aspects of the population problem that might be termed intermediate, that is, causing severe misery and disruption of living conditions but not resulting in mass death by starvation. Some of these intermediate elements are high rates of illiteracy and entire generations of uneducated people; increasing environmental pollution from growing amounts of waste and refuse; economic inflation; a general decline in health despite the eradication of many communicable diseases; hunger and malnutrition; inadequate housing; loss of topsoil; urbanization and crowding with a resultant increase in personal violence; and a decreasing quantity and quality of health care.

There are several theories of population control, but the most controversial one is social triage. This is a variation of the medical triage concept used on the battlefield or in disasters when large numbers of people are wounded. Triage is designed to save only those individuals who will die unless immediate aid is given. Translated to the context of entire countries, only those that are not considered beyond help would receive infusions of foreign aid and would be the target of birth control programs. Social triage is strongly utilitarian in theory and has ardent proponents and detractors.

The major ethical conflict in population control in general is individual freedom of reproduction balanced against the good of (some say the ultimate survival of) an entire society. This is basically a conflict between deontologic and utilitarian theory, and reasons can be found both to support and to oppose the restriction of personal reproductive liberty.

Famine, starvation, and violence, which are already increasingly evident throughout the world, are important components of overpopulation. There seems to be little doubt that more and more people will die violently as a result of the lack of food if population growth continues unchecked.

It also seems apparent that religious beliefs, which cannot be easily separated from some cultural practices, are responsible for burgeoning population growth in some areas. Since few people would deny that the practice of one's religion is a right to be closely guarded, a conflict arises between this personal right and the ultimate survival of a population.

Public policy creates conflicts, an amalgam of all the dilemmas discussed. There may be ethical differences between the way a national government can act toward its own citizens and the way one government (or an international agency) can act toward the citizens of another. Many of these conflicts revolve around incentive programs, most of which call for some type of coercion.

Notes

1. Family planning programs. *Population Reports* (Series J.). No. 11. Washington, D.C.: Department of Medicine and Public Affairs. George Washington University Medical Center, November, 1976. p. J-178.
2. Family planning programs, p. J-183.
3. Family planning programs, p. J-184.
4. Family planning programs, p. J-188.
5. Teitelbaum, M. S. The population problem in demographic perspective. In W. T. Reich (ed.), *Encyclopedia of bioethics* (Vol. 3). New York: The Free Press, 1978. p. 1219.
6. Coale, A. J. The demographic transition reconsidered. *Proceedings of the IUSSP International Population Conference*. Liege, Belgium: International Union for the Scientific Study of Population, 1973. pp. 53–72.
7. Hinds, S. W. On the relations of medical triage to world famine: an historical survey. In G. R. Lucas, Jr., & T. W. Ogletree (Eds.), *Lifeboat ethics: the moral dilemmas of world hunger*. New York: Harper & Row, Publishers, Inc. p. 42. © Vanderbilt University and the Society for Values in Higher Education, 1976.
8. Hinds, pp. 47–48.

9. Fletcher, J. Feeding the hungry: an ethical appraisal. In *Lifeboat ethics*.
10. Fletcher, p. 54.
11. Hardin, G. Lifeboat ethics: the case against helping the poor. *Psychology Today*, 1974, pp. 38-43, 124-26; Living on a lifeboat. *Bioscience*, 1974, *24*, 561-568.
12. Shriver, D. W., Jr. Lifeboaters and mainlanders: a response. In *Lifeboat ethics*.
13. Potter, R. B. Normative aspects of population policy. In *Encyclopedia of bioethics*, pp. 1245-1248.
14. Brown, P. G. Ethical perspectives on population. In *Encyclopedia of bioethics* (Vol. 3.), pp. 1237-1238.
15. Engelhardt, H. T., Jr. Individuals and communities, present and future: towards a morality in a time of famine. In *Lifeboat ethics*, pp. 73-74.
16. Harrelson, W. Famine in the perspective of biblical judgments and promises. In *Lifeboat ethics*, p. 89.
17. Fromer, M. J. *Ethical issues in health care*. St. Louis: The C.V. Mosby Co., 1981. p. 106.
18. Lorenz, K., & Leyhausen, P. *Motivation of human and animal behavior: an ethological view*. (B. A. Tonkin, trans.) New York: Van Nostrand Rheinhold Co., 1973.
19. Fromer, p. 111.
20. Veatch, R. M. Governmental incentives. In *Encyclopedia of bioethics* (Vol. 3.), pp. 1290-1292.
21. Kramer, B. Braking births *Wall Street Journal*, October 3, 1979, p. 40.
22. Kramer.
23. Warwick, D. P. Contemporary international issues. In *Encyclopedia of bioethics* (Vol. 3.), p. 1274.
24. Warwick, p. 1276.

Bibliography

Ardrey, R. *The territorial imperative*. New York: Atheneum Publishers, 1966.
Brown, P. G. Ethical perspectives on population. In W. T. Reich (Ed.), *Encyclopedia of bioethics*. New York: The Free Press, 1978.
Coale, A. J. The demographic transition reconsidered. *Proceedings of the IUSSP International Population Conference*. Liege, Belgium: International Union for the Scientific Study of Population, 1973. pp. 53-72.
Dyck, A. J. Definition of population ethics. In *Encyclopedia of bioethics*.
Engelhardt, H. T., Jr. Individuals and communities, present and future: towards a morality in a time of famine. In *Lifeboat ethics*.
Family planning programs. *Population Reports*. (Series J.). No. 11. Washington, D.C.: Department of Medicine and Public Affairs. George Washington University Medical Center, November, 1976.
Fletcher, J. Feeding the hungry: an ethical appraisal. In *Lifeboat ethics*.
Fromer, M. J. *Ethical issues in health care*. St. Louis: The C.V. Mosby Co., 1981.
Golding, M. P., & Bayles, M. D. Population distribution. In *Encyclopedia of bioethics*.
Hadley, J. N. The demography of the American Indians. *Annals of the American Academy of Political and Social Science*, 1957, *311*, 23-30.
Hardin, G. Lifeboat ethics: the case against helping the poor *Psychology Today*, 1974, pp. 38-43, 124-126.
Hardin, G. Living on a lifeboat. *Bioscience*, 1974, *24*, 561-568.

Harrelson, W. Famine in the perspective of biblical judgments and promises. In *Lifeboat ethics*.

Hinds, S. W. On the relations of medical triage to world famine: an historical survey. In *Lifeboat ethics*.

Johnston, D. F. *An analysis of sources of information on the population of the Navajo.* Smithsonian Institution, Bureau of American Ethnology (Bull. 197.). Washington, D.C.: U.S. Government Printing Office, 1966.

Kramer, B. Braking births. *Wall Street Journal*, October 3, 1979, p. 40.

Lorenz, K. & Leyhausen, P. *Motivation of human and animal behavior: an ethological view* (B. A. Tonkin, trans.). New York: Van Nostrand Rheinhold Co., 1973.

Lucas, G. R., Jr., & Ogletree, T. W. *Lifeboat ethics: the moral dilemmas of world hunger*. New York: Harper & Row, Publishers, Inc., 1976. © Vanderbilt University and the Society for Values in Higher Education.

Montagu, A. *The nature of human aggression*. New York: Oxford University Press, Inc., 1976.

Potter, R. B. Normative aspects of population policy. In *Encyclopedia of bioethics*.

Sellers, J. Famine and interdependence: toward a new identity for america and the west. In *Lifeboat ethics*.

Shriver, D. W., Jr. Lifeboaters and mainlanders: a response. In *Lifeboat ethics*.

Spengler, J. J. History of population policies. In *Encyclopedia of bioethics*.

Teitelbaum, M. S. The population problem in demographic perspective. In *Encyclopedia of bioethics*.

Veatch, R. M. Governmental incentives. In *Encyclopedia of bioethics*.

Verghese, P. Muddled metaphors: an asian response to Garrett Hardin. In *Lifeboat ethics*.

Warwick, D. P. Bullying birth control: american infatuation with family planning for export. *Commonweal*, September 12, 1975, pp. 392–394.

Warwick, D. P. Contemporary international issues. In *Encyclopedia of bioethics*.

Warwick, D. P. Contraceptives in the Third World. *Hastings Center Report*, 1975, 5 (4), 9–12.

CHAPTER 6

ABORTION

DEFINITION

Abortion is commonly defined as the deliberate termination of a pregnancy by causing the fetus to be expelled from the uterus before the pregnancy terminates spontaneously. The fetus, in most cases, dies as a result. However, there are some exceptions to this definition of abortion. For example, abortion sometimes refers to labor artificially induced to increase the chances of the fetus being born alive and healthy, as when the pregnant woman suffers from diabetes, heart disease, and the like. But the term *abortion* usually refers to those procedures performed before the fetus reaches the age of viability, which is the arbitrary point at which the fetus has a better than even chance of surviving outside the uterus (the concept of viability will be discussed in detail later in the chapter). Deliberate termination of pregnancy after the age of viability (after 6 months' gestation) is almost always done to save the fetus from some medical disaster, and the intent of the procedure is life, not death for the fetus. Similarly all cases of termination of pregnancy before the age of viability are not regarded strictly as abortion. The most common instance is the case of ectopic pregnancy when the fetus is indeed removed, but for the primary purpose of saving the pregnant woman's life (this will be discussed in more detail in the section on double effect).

There are several methods of abortion, and descriptions can be found in any text on gynecology and obstetrics. The procedure chosen is based almost entirely on uterine size and gestational age, and postoperative risk is directly proportional to uterine size; that is, the later in the pregnancy the abortion is performed, the greater the risk to the woman. Abortion in general, however, carries a very low risk, lower even than term delivery.

A word should be said here about the vocabulary used in discussing abortion. Because it is one of the most emotionally charged of all subjects of bioethical debate, the language used in discussions of abortion can fan the flames of emotion. The problem with language is to strike a balance between unnecessarily inflammatory vocabulary and that which so neutralizes the topic that one tends to forget that it is real women and real fetuses being discussed.

One of the most important linguistic differentiations is the one between the words *kill* and *murder*. They are not precisely synonymous, although they are often used interchangably. To kill means to deliberately end a life—any life. When we cut flowers, exterminate cockroaches, or casually slap mosquitos, we are killing. To murder means to unjustifiably kill an innocent human being. The latter always has a negative connotation, whereas *kill* sometimes is a positive action as in ridding a city of rats. Admittedly the word *kill* has a mostly negative aura, although in many instances killing, even killing persons, is morally justified. Persons who are opposed to abortion usually tend to use *murder* to describe the action done to the fetus to create as negative an image as possible. Those who favor abortion try to avoid the use of either word in favor of words like *abort* or *remove* when describing the action done to the fetus. They will, however, always use *kill* in preference to *murder*.

In the abortion debate there seems to be confusion about *life*, *potential life*, and *alive*.

> Few argue whether an embryo or fetus is alive or is a potential human life. What is more arguable is that a fetus *is* a human life rather than an entity that *has* life. To say that a fetus is a life is to imply that it is a separate and unique being, already an individual, even though it is still physically attached to its mother. This is the picture painted by antiabortionists. Pro-abortionists acknowledge that a fetus has life but do not view it as a separate individual.[1]

The third confusion of terms occurs in differentiating *fetus* and *embryo*. The latter is the word appropriate early in gestational development before human form is recognizable. Some time during the latter part of the first trimester the embryo becomes a fetus. The word *fetus* is more emotionally charged than is *embryo*, which seems almost cooly clinical, and when one pictures a fetus, a babylike figure is usually imagined. Although the two words do not mean the same thing, for the purpose of readability here, *fetus* will be used exclusively to describe that which is the product of conception. Although I will make an effort to use language in this chapter that is as neutral as possible, one runs the risk of so sterilizing the language that the humanness of the dilemma as it relates to people's lives can be lost.

RELIGIOUS VIEWS

Before looking at some traditional and evolving religious views about abortion, it is appropriate first to examine what place, if any, religion should hold in the debate. Is religion relevant to the abortion issue? Newton thinks not.[2] She sees it as an ethical, legal, and political issue but not one that necessarily involves God-given moral values or ethical norms. She separates an essentially ethical issue from one that is basically religious by describing the latter as one that appeals in some way to the will of God. The average person, Newton argues, sees a difference in the two, although there is admittedly considerable overlap in many areas of human conduct. Some questions, however, can be answered by appealing to manifestations of divine commandments (such as the Ten Commandments or the Sermon on the Mount) and some can be answered only by appealing to the principles of justice, rights, duties, and obligations. Settling the abortion debate cannot be done by appealing to religious questions because nowhere in the Bible is God's will revealed on the subject.

> The belief that the fetus is a fully independent human being has evolved only slowly, in certain religious traditions, traditions (Orthodox Judaism, Anglicanism, Roman Catholicism) that otherwise have many differences. There simply is no religious root for this belief, which might be reached by anyone meditating on the implications of the available data on prenatal growth and development. . . . when the dispute about the ethical issues of abortion is joined, the appeals are to scientific evidence of fetal activity; to legal and moral conceptions of "the person"; to property rights, rights of privacy, the right to life and the right to liberty; to parental duties, duties of care and compassion; to the state's interest in future life; and even, unfortunately, to the taxpayers' interest in smaller welfare rolls.[3]

Secular issues, according to Newton, are more than sufficient (and more than complex, one might add) to debate the ethics of abortion. God is irrelevant to the debate because there are no definitive divine directives about it.

Jaffe[4] argues that because theologians have taken prominent views in the abortion debate, many have come to see it as a religious issue. This is not necessarily the case, any more than it would be a purely secular matter simply because nontheologians participate in the discussions as well. Philosophers have not been successful in differentiating religious and secular ethics, and the Supreme Court has never been able to satisfactorily define what a religion is. The legal debate, and to some extent the ethical one, has centered around the question of when human life begins, but this is as much a biologic as well as a religious question, and neither science nor the divine can be ruled out of the debate. Jaffe[5] lists the following six criteria that could distinguish a primarily religious belief from a secular one:

1. It is part of the doctrine of religious groups.
2. It is legitimated in religious and transcendental terms.
3. Its principal exponents and major adherents are associated with religious groups.
4. It is taught mainly through formal religious training.
5. Those organizations that sponsor legislation concerning the belief are primarily religious in nature and financial support.
6. Advocacy for the belief is dominated by religious references and symbols.

On the basis of these criteria, it is clear that abortion is not only, perhaps not even primarily, a religious issue, although religion plays an inescapable role. It is sometimes difficult to know whether a religious group becomes involved in the abortion debate out of a sense of social and civic responsibility, much as various religious organizations take an active part in many secular community affairs, or because the issue itself is religious in nature. There is, however, no doubt that major religions have taken positions on abortion. A summary of these views and positions follows.

Judaism

Laws governing the conduct of Jewish life derive from the Torah, the first five books of the Old Testament, and the comment on those laws that are found in the Talmud, Mishna, and other series of rabbinic interpretations of halakah (law).

The basic premise regarding abortion is that the fetus is part of its mother, not a separate entity, although there is nothing in halakah that specifically permits or prohibits abortion. The fetus has no legal rights or status, and it is specifically excluded from the laws against killing persons because it is not a person until it is outside the mother's body. However, one is not permitted to deliberately harm a fetus, although the crime of doing so is not as serious as the crime of murder and is not punishable by death (Exodus 21:22). According to the Talmud, only monetary compensation is required for harming a fetus. The concept of ensoulment will be discussed in greater detail later in the chapter, specifically in the context of Catholicism, but it is interesting to note that Judaism takes a different position on the ensoulment question as it relates to abortion. Because ensoulment is not the issue, abortion is not murder. The question of when the soul joins the body is irrelevant to the discussion of abortion "because the soul is immortal no matter when it enters or leaves the body. And, more important than being immortal it is a pure soul, free of the taint of 'original sin'."[6]

Judaism has no concept of original sin and personhood implies having an identity separate from the mother. Therefore *murder* is not the appropriate word to use in regard to abortion in the Jewish perspective. Abortion is then permitted to save the life or protect the health of the pregnant woman, and Talmudic interpretation views the fetus as an "aggressor" that can be forfeited or destroyed to save its "intended" victim. This view holds true, however, only if the woman's life or health is clearly in jeopardy; the gravity of the act of abortion should not be minimized or undertaken with less than utmost seriousness.

Since there is no absolute prohibition of abortion in halakah, the way is open for almost unlimited debate about the circumstances of its permissibility. The most conservative view is that abortion is permissible only when the pregnant woman's life is clearly threatened; more liberal views hold that jeopardy to a woman's health can be defined more broadly, for example, including her mental health, the viability of her marriage, her actual desire for motherhood, and her ability to provide both emotional and material support for the child. Judaism always looks at the issue from the maternal view, that is, how the presence of the fetus affects the pregnant woman. Fetal rights, although not nonexistent, are always secondary to those of the pregnant woman. For example, if it is possible, or even probable, that a fetus is defective, and the pregnant woman wants to abort it because she believes the child will have a less than normal life, a rabbi would probably refuse permission for the abortion. If, however, that same abortion was sought because having such a child would cause anguish to the mother, permission would be granted. "The fetus is unknown, future, potential, part of the 'secrets of God'; the mother is known, present, alive, and asking for compassion."[7]

The issue in Judaism is not the "right to life" (a currently popular political phrase that has been hackneyed out of almost all clear meaning and is reduced to a cliché), which is demonstrably clear; it is instead the right to be born, which is neither clear nor settled. The right to life is absolute*; the right to be born is relative. Life may indeed begin at the moment of conception, but it is not the life of a human person and therefore cannot claim all the legal, moral, and civil rights of a human being. Human life begins at birth, but *potential* human life exists before that. Abortion should not be undertaken casually, nor should it be done solely for economic reasons because killing of any life form is a serious act and requires moral justification. But abortion is permissible in Judaism.

---

*The right to life may not indeed be absolute (for example, as in killing the enemy in war and capital punishment), but for the purpose of comparing it to the right to be born, I shall assume that the right to life is absolute in this instance.

Protestantism

Early Protestant reformers such as Martin Luther and John Calvin were as conservative about the matter of abortion as the Catholic Church from which they broke away. Their concern arose from the doctrine of original sin, that is, that full humanity is bestowed on the fetus from the moment of conception, and the fetus is ensouled from that beginning. The Catholic Church, although opposed to abortion at all times, viewed the sin with varying degrees of gravity depending on the gestational age of the fetus (as derived from Aristotle's concept of the vegetative, animal, and rational souls that also depend on gestational age). Luther, Calvin, and other early Protestant theologians, however, made no such distinction; abortion was a sin of equal and utmost gravity regardless of gestational age.

By the seventeenth century in England the Protestant position on abortion had softened somewhat. Although both Anglicans and Puritans still opposed abortion, a distinction was made between the "unformed" and "formed" fetus. At the same time the Protestant view of marriage evolved from a strictly procreative one to a view that stressed love and companionship. Therefore contraception became permissible, and in some quarters so did abortion, but this was a minority view. In eighteenth and nineteenth century America three major theologic developments led to a shift in the Protestant view of abortion.[8] The first was a declining interest in the fetus as a full human being; that is, fetal humanity was considered a foregone conclusion. Debate instead centered on using abortion as a cover-up for sexual sins and viewing the frequency of abortion as a form of sexual promiscuity and depravity. The second development was a strongly profertility view of society. To be fulfilled as full human beings, women had to bear children, and the more children she had, the more worthwhile a woman's life was. Moreover, burgeoning population growth was crucial to the survival and development of the United States; therefore abortion was a social evil as well as a personal sin, although the former was more heavily emphasized than the latter. Third, in opposition to the first two developments, was the small but growing sense of social idealism, of class and gender equality, and of personal autonomy. This gave birth to the women's suffrage movement, which, after a long hiatus, gave rise to the feminist movement we are currently experiencing.

Twentieth century Protestantism is undergoing a certain amount of secularization and has been strongly affected by the various American social movements that have swept by.

> Under the impact of secularization, certainties that had once undergirded theological opposition to abortion became less certain. If to an earlier Protes-

tant the presence of each fetus in the womb was an expression of God's mysterious providence, to a later Protestant the fetal presence was explained by natural processes, including mistakes as well as human planning.[9]

Since midcentury there has been a growing trend toward personal autonomy, self-determination, and the obligation to exercise rational control over one's life. Coupled with legal abortion reforms, this has caused Protestant theologians to review traditional attitudes and beliefs about abortion.

There are now a variety of Protestant viewpoints regarding the ethics of abortion. In the absence of specific Biblical injunctions, many Protestant theologians seek guidelines elsewhere in the Old and New Testaments. The belief that life is considered a gift from God and that human beings are created for reasons other than fulfilling their own pleasures can be seen as reason to condemn abortion. A common Biblical theme in support of this view is that not only has God control over life and death, but that human intervention in these matters is forbidden. However, surrounding these themes are the Scriptural commands of love, justice, and mercy, which can be interpreted to mitigate the taboo against abortion, depending on the circumstances surrounding the pregnancy. The major Protestant arguments against abortion, espoused by Ramsey, Thielcke, Bonhoeffer, and others, is that ensoulment is not the important question, rather, it is, the potentiality of the fetus. That is, a fetus is on the way to becoming a full human person, it can be nothing other than a person, and therefore it deserves the protection of the sanctity of human life. There can be no relative degrees of human worth when life is conferred by God (as in the belief that abortion is a worse sin later in pregnancy than earlier); therefore all fetuses, regardless of gestational age, should be protected as though they were already full human beings.

Those Protestant theologians who favor abortion hold that only children who are fully wanted should be born and that the permissive legislation of the past decade or so is well designed because it promotes individual autonomy and minimizes social discrimination. A third Protestant view lies somewhere between the conservative and the liberal. According to this middle view, both the pregnant woman and the fetus have rights, but neither are absolute. The ascendance of some rights over others lends a moral authority to the permissibility or prohibition of abortion that does not exist in reality and tends to oversimplify the complex issues involved.[10]

Roman Catholicism

Catholic doctrine regarding abortion is almost entirely based on the status of the fetus, that is, on the belief that it is a full human being and has been since the moment of conception. Although the early Church differentiated an animate from an inanimate fetus (based on the phenomenon of quickening, which are the first fetal movements felt by the pregnant woman), there was no moral differentiation about the permissibility of abortion; it was unlawful at any time during pregnancy. However, as with any formal doctrine there was dissent. John of Naples, the fourteenth century Dominican, and others argued that it should be permissible to abort an inanimate fetus, and Thomas Sanchez, in the sixteenth century, held that if a fetus is an unwanted aggressor on the woman's body, it could be expelled (this is reminiscent of the Jewish perspective). But these were minority views, and by the thirteenth century excommunication was the usual punishment for the sin of abortion—the same punishment as for homicide.

The status of the fetus is in turn based, in the Catholic view, on the concept of ensoulment, first seen in the writings of Aristotle. He believed in a sequence of three souls: the vegetative, the animal, and the rational. The last of the three appears at birth, but the first two souls are present before birth. The vegetative soul appears at some indeterminate time after conception, but the switch to the animal soul occurs at the time when the first fetal movements are felt by the pregnant woman, a phenomenon known as quickening, meaning proof that the fetus is alive. This, Aristotle believed, occurs on the fortieth day for a male fetus and on the nintieth for a female. St. Thomas Aquinas, who formulated a great deal of modern Catholic dogma and who was very much influenced by Aristotle, termed this change from mediate to immediate animation and deemed that abortion after immediate animation (or the appearance of the animal soul described by Aristotle) was forbidden.

The shift from Aristotle and Aquinas to modern Catholic dogma occurred somewhat arbitrarily, at least as it relates to abortion. The birthday of the Blessed Virgin had been set at September 8, but the Church believed that it also needed a date for her ensoulment, which, following Aristotle and Aquinas, would have been 6 months earlier. But in 1708 Pope Clement XI chose December 8 as the date of ensoulment, thus suggesting that ensoulment occurred at the time of her conception. In 1854 Pope Pius IX proclaimed the doctrine of the Immaculate Conception and in effect removed the previous distinction between an ensouled and an unensouled fetus. Thus we have the concept of an ensouled fetus, a full human being, from the moment of conception.[11] In the Catholic view, because the presence of a soul is one of the characteristics that differentiates humans from all other animals, we have the concept of the fetus as a full human being.

The modern Catholic Church has not changed its stance on abortion since establishment of the official Immaculate Conception in the midnineteenth century. In his 1930 encyclical, *Casti Connubii*, Pope Pius XII condemned direct abortion (indirect abortion will be discussed in the section on double effect); this position has been reaffirmed by the Second Vatican Council (Vatican II) in 1965 and by every pope since.

It is most likely that official Catholic doctrine will not change, but the same cannot be said for the attitude of American Catholic laypersons, particularly women who are undergoing serious emotional conflict over abortion. On one hand, they see abortion legislation growing ever more permissive, and on the other they see high Church officials remaining adamant in their condemnation of abortion. American society is leaning more toward personal autonomy and freedom of life-style for women (this includes the freedom to be a mother only the number of times one wishes), whereas the Church remains dogmatic and conservative. The cost of bearing and raising children is escalating to unbelievable heights, yet the Church insists that no pregnancy be terminated for any reason. It is well known that Catholic women have abortions (the Executive Director of Planned Parenthood of Philadelphia claims that approximately 40% of all abortions performed are on Catholic women) for which the Church would officially demand excommunication. This creates conflict for the Church as well. Should it excommunicate all women who confess to abortion (thus forcing many women not to confess and denying themselves an important sacrament), or should the Church change its stance on punishment, thus leaving the way open for a renewed discussion of the abortion issue itself? It seems clear that the debate is far from closed. If so many members of a religion disobey one of its most important laws, a basic conflict exists between the Church and its members.

ETHICAL ISSUES
When life begins

Although fetal life exists on a developmental continuum, and it is a biologic fact that the fetus is alive and has life, controversy exists over when that life becomes human life and when the fetus becomes a human being. There are three different points at which this is commonly believed to occur: at conception, at birth, and when the fetus becomes viable.

Viability generally creates the most interesting ethical dilemmas, primarily because it is not a precisely fixed point and because its moral significance is somewhat hazy. Viability has become a legal and medical dividing line; many of the rules governing fetal research have to do with viability, and several guidelines having to do with resuscitation of premature infants are based on viability. In other words, some people have placed strong moral significance on this very shadowy concept of viability, and the ethical dilemma consists of asking whether this should indeed be so.

There are several medical and legal definitions of viability, most specifying a fetal weight (usually about 400 grams), a gestational age (most often 26 to 28 weeks), and the stipulation that the fetus have a better than even chance of surviving outside the uterus—with the use of both ordinary and extraordinary life-support systems. Fost et al.[12] claim that viability is so complex a concept that the following four different distinctions must be delineated: (1) intrinsic vs. extrinsic viability, (2) natural vs. artificial means of support, (3) short- or long-term viability, and (4) empirical vs. predictive viability. A fetus may or may not be viable, depending on the outside environment into which it is born. Thus a fetus that could survive outside the uterus with only ordinary care and feeding would necessarily be more gestationally advanced than one that could survive only with the help of sophisticated technology. Therefore viability becomes a relative term and depends, to a great extent, on the immediate world into which the fetus will be born. In addition, a fetus must have achieved a certain intrinsic developmental momentum so that if it is born before term it can continue its biologic development as well as simply surviving. Life-support systems can, in many cases, maintain vital functions, but it is questionable whether they can adequately provide for fetal development.

The distinction between natural and artificial means of support implies that the definition of viability could possibly be determined by geography (a fetus delivered in a modern American hospital as compared with one born on the Steppes of Russia or even in a rural area in this country far from health care services, for example) or circumstances of birth. Chance or fate becomes more significant to the concept of viability than do ethical components. One must also question the degree to which "artificial means of support" should be interpreted. A healthy full-term neonate needs to be artificially supported in that it cannot fend for itself and thus depends for its very existence on outside sources. This type of support, of course, is different from that required by a fetus that cannot even breathe on its own. Where is the line drawn between natural and artificial means of support?

Viability can also be measured by length of survival. A fetus that gasps once or twice and then dies is not generally considered viable, although it did breathe. On the other hand, a fetus that has survived for several weeks with intensive technologic care would generally be considered viable even though it would surely die without the support. A decade ago this fetus would not have been considered viable. Is one fetus more viable than the other, and if so, what are the distinctions?

The matter of empirical vs. predictive viability is a rather academic or statistical one, involving the chances of a fetus surviving outside the uterus at various points along its developmental continuum. It has little ethical significance.

Viability, therefore, is relative; it does not exist at a particular point in time and might even be conceptualized as a miniature continuum within the larger gestational one. Because viability is not a specific descriptive entity, value judgments become part of determinations, not only of viability itself, but also of the actions that might be taken based on those determinations. However, does viability carry any moral significance? In other words, can it be said that the fetus becomes a human being and is thus owed moral obligations when this elusive viability is attained? The answer is a typical philosopher's one: no, yes, and maybe. No, the fetus does not become a full human being at viability; that occurs only at either conception or birth, depending on one's view of ensoulment and the necessity of a soul for personhood. Yes, the fetus is owed some moral obligations because of its greatly increased potentiality, because after a certain point it deserves legal and moral protection if for no other reason than that the pregnant woman has thus far chosen not to abort and must be considered ambivalent about her desire for abortion, and because a rudimentary mother-child relationship is beginning to develop even though the fetus is by no means a social being. And maybe, because the idea of changing the status of a fetus at viability makes no purely logical sense; the fetus is no more than it was a week or two earlier, except larger and slightly more biologically sophisticated. But yet there is a progressive difference that must be taken into account.

One other aspect of viability should be considered.

> Viability might contribute to one unusual issue in the abortion debate. "Abortion" can refer to two interventions: fetal *removal* and fetal *destruction*. Before viability removal is, by definition, tantamount to destruction. After viability this need not be the case. One may envision a time when women's rights to control their bodies are recognized by granting them power of decision over fetal removal, while reserving to the state decisions on fetal destruction. If such a change in the law came about, a judgment on fetal viability might enter into a moral argument concerning abortion (qua removal) in a perfectly straightforward way.[13]

In other words, a woman would have the right to be relieved of carrying the fetus, but she would not have the right to its death. There is a significant moral difference in these two concepts, with the implication that an attempt at resuscitation should be made on all aborted fetuses if they are thought to be viable.

Ontologic status of the fetus

By ontologic status, we generally mean the moral obligation owed simply by virtue of the fact of a being's own moral existence. One can owe moral obligations to persons, animals, or societies; to religious or ethical ideals; or even to an amorphous entity such as an ecologic system. However, we will confine our discussion here to the moral obligation to a fetus. If a fetus is a person, it is certainly owed a moral obligation; if it is not a person, it is not owed the obligations that one usually thinks of being owed to persons. The question is really two questions: when does the fetus become a person, and what is a person?

Feinberg[14] discusses the following three ways of defining or describing personhood: normative, descriptive, and commonsense. A normative definition of personhood implies that moral and legal rights and/or duties are owed to the being so described. "To be a person in the normative sense is to have rights, or rights and duties, or at least be the sort of being who could have rights and duties without conceptual absurdity."[15] That is, one would never think of a rock, an abstract idea, or a tree as having rights and/or duties. To do so would be absurd. This description of personhood, however, could include animals and fetuses as the sort of beings that could have rights. Therefore, it is not sufficient for our purpose to decide whether or not a fetus is owed moral obligations.

A purely descriptive, or empirical, use of *personhood* implies a fixed set of characteristics that conveys specific information about what a person is. These characteristics are established by conventions of language that make them noncontroversial and true. For example, when the word *kitten* is used, it is commonly understood that one is referring to a young cat, and *cat* is understood to mean a fur-bearing animal of the feline species of a certain size with certain characteristics. If these linguistic conventions did not exist, we would not be able to communicate. However, the conventions are not always precisely clear, which is the case with the word *person*.

> When we use the word "person" in this wholly descriptive way we are not attributing rights, duties, eligibility for rights and duties, or any other normative characteristics to the being so described. At most we are attributing characteristics that may be a *ground* for ascribing rights and duties.[16]

Thus a descriptive definition does not suit our purposes.

A more practical and human way of defining personhood is what Feinberg refers to as "commonsense personhood," that is, examples of beings whose personhood cannot be doubted, clear examples of nonpersonhood, and examples of beings who may be persons. You and I are clearly persons. How do we know? Because we look, think, feel, and behave in ways that are common to all members of our species. We are self-conscious; we conform to certain physical characteristics; we interact with others; and we laugh, cry, eat, make love, and have fights. In other words, we look and behave like a conventionally defined person; therefore we are necessarily persons. Next there are rocks, flowers, crayfish, antelope, chairs, suitcases, and all the millions of other things that are so clearly not persons that it would never cross our minds to describe them as such. Then there are the hard cases, those beings that have many (maybe even a majority of) characteristics of personhood, in fact, so many that we do not know whether or not to call them persons—angels, dolphins, God, perhaps some extraterrestial beings, fetuses, and irreversibly comatose individuals. But are they truly persons, and if so, how do we know? To help solve the problem, Feinberg has established a set of criteria for commonsense personhood, summarized as follows (the entire set must be present for a being to be considered a person; no one or two alone is sufficient):

1. The being must be conscious of himself and of his surroundings, and he must have rationality. It is not sufficient to be merely aware without being able to reason.

2. The being must be a member of the species *Homo sapiens* to be considered a person, and only members of this species are considered, that is, all and only *Homo sapiens*.

3. All and only beings that actually or potentially possess the characteristics of commonsense personhood and who would be expected to do so in the natural course of events can be considered persons. (The difficulty with this criterion is the concept of potentiality with the attendant deduction of actual rights from potential rights.)

Given the necessity of the presence of all these criteria, it is obvious that a fetus is not a full human being, but it is equally obvious that it is a potential person having potential rights that continually and gradually increase. Therefore some moral rights are owed to the fetus at some time during its development. The only definitive right that could be logically conferred on a fetus is the right to life, but we still have not determined when this right begins to exist, if it does at all, before birth.

Those who hold extreme views about abortion based on the existence of the fetus' moral status do so either because they believe the fetus to have full human rights or to have none at all. These views are not problematic in that there is no moral conflict for the person holding them. However, the middle-of-the-road view that the fetus does have some rights at some time is fraught with moral conflict because of the dilemma of which rights exist at what time. Those who take this middle moral view claim either that there is a certain moment at which the fetus can claim rights (viability is the most frequently cited arbitrary point) or that rights evolve on a continuum so that the later the pregnancy, the greater the moral problem in abortion. There is something about a fetus that demands protection, but by the same token there is something about a fully developed woman that makes us believe that she has greater rights than a fetus and has first claim to whatever those rights are. We intuit that a fetus has rights, but we are unable to prove it logically even though

> It is clear that the unique status of the potential person has to do with its
> inherent "thrust" or predetermined tendency. A potential person is not simply
> a set of blueprints, it is an organism that itself will become the actual person
> toward which it is already developing. . . . those attracted to the potentiality
> principle do see some derivative relationship between the claims that a being
> will have in the normal course of its development and those that it has in the
> present.[17]

Although pregnancy and the status of the fetus are absolutely unique,
Langerak[18] describes an analogy between a fetus and a potential President.
A person who has been elected President, but who has not yet been inaugurated
and is therefore not the actual President, still receives many of the rights and
perquisites of office. He becomes privy to state secrets, the press hangs on his
every word, and he is listened to with more authority than the actual President
who is now a lame duck. The President-elect knows he will become Commander-
in-Chief of the armed forces; while he was running for office he knew only that
he could reach that pinnacle of power. At the moment of inauguration all the
potentialities of office will suddenly become actualities, but nothing else about
him as a person will have changed. The only change in his status is that an
arbitrarily designated time will have passed. How, then, is the President different from the President-elect except insofar as a passage of time has occurred?
And in what sense, other than in location and biologic terms of existence, is an
8-month fetus different from a 10-minute-old human infant? The distinguishing factors are difficult, if not impossible, to pinpoint.

Engelhardt[19] acknowledges that the ontologic status of a fetus cannot be
established on rational grounds alone and that the dilemma, for ease of clarifi-
cation, should be divided into two poles, the ontologic and the operational.
The ontologic refers to the meaning of a human person, of human life itself; the
operational refers to observable criteria that a person now exists where none
existed previously. The latter is based on proof of a physical body; the former is
analogous to proof of an existing soul. The distinction between the two is
difficult to draw. Although the fetus certainly has a physical body and exists in
time and space, it occupies no social role, is not referred to by gender, and is not
addressed by name except by its parents in a joking sort of way. The fetus has
whatever genetic characteristics it will have as a person, but they do not yet
matter and thus may as well not exist. Neither does the fetus have a personality
or the capacity to relate to other human beings.

> One is faced with the difficulty of distinguishing between biologic human life
> (as in a fetus or an irreversibly comatose individual) and personal human life to
> which are owed moral obligations. One could say that obligations are owed to
> the comatose individual by virtue of the person he *had been*; it is clearly more
> difficult to cease being obligated to someone than it is to begin. If an ontologic

position implies that a person is defined as such because he exists, then that existence also implies his entitlement to moral obligations owed him by others. If he is not yet a person (fetus) or has ceased to be one (a comatose individual), this principle does not apply and moral obligations are not owed.[20]

The only possible exception to this stance is the obligation of a right to life at some yet to be determined point on the continuum of fetal development. It is highly unlikely that the determination of this point will be settled to everyone's satisfaction.

The humanity of fetal life

We know that fetal life is human in the sense that it is not not human; that is, it is not a puppy, a rock, a rose, or any other entity. But is it human life as we know and recognize it? A postviable fetus looks human, but that does not mean that it is human. By the same token, a person who has just died looks human but no longer is. A dolphin, which is definitely not human, has a greater capacity for reasoning and language than does a fetus, or for that matter a neonate. Then is fetal life human life, and if not, what is it?

The only satisfactory answer, it seems, is to assign the fetus to a category of its own because it is indeed unique in the world, just as there is no other experience to compare with pregnancy (and for this reason it is difficult to draw philosophic comparisons and to make analogies). Brody[21] lists several possibilities of when one might consider fetal life human life as follows: (1) at about 6 weeks' gestation when the brain begins to have measurable electroencephalographic waves; (2) at the point in fetal development when it is more humanlike than anything else, that is, at the point at which it is recognized as a human fetus; (3) at the point at which it is capable of conscious experience, although scientists have not been able to determine just when that is; (4) at quickening, or the point at which it is perceived as an alive being by its mother and thus begins to establish some type of relationship with her; (5) at viability; (6) at the moment of birth when it breathes on its own and has established an independent existence; (7) at some point after birth when the infant interacts with other human beings, although the type and degree of interaction are not specified.

The fundamental difficulty with stating that fetal life becomes human life at any one of these seven points (or an almost infinite number of others, for that matter) is that a reasonable case can be made both for and against doing so. One might be tempted to throw up one's hands and simply set an arbitrary point for the transition (the Supreme Court came close to doing this when it permitted abortions only in the first two trimesters).

There are a variety of objections that might be raised against this view. But the most important one is that this seems to place the matter of human rights open to too many objectionable decisions. After all, there are all types of people with all types of prejudices about what is or is not required for being a living human being. And would we want to say that members of some minority group are really not living human beings just because they fail to meet the criterion of humanity established by some prejudiced majority, when the criterion in question reflects the prejudices of that majority group?[22]

Although this view seems unduly pessimistic, a political decision about when human life begins could be fraught with peril. It was, after all, not so long ago that American slaves were not thought to be full human beings. The only practical reason why one might want to arbitrarily establish such a position in the first place is for pragmatic legal purposes. And ironically, those people who seem most interested in establishing laws about abortion are those who have no doubt in their own minds about when human life begins. Most people who either have no opinion about abortion legislation or who prefer that no such laws exist doubt that such a point could be arbitrarily established.

It is society that confers rights on its own citizens, and since fetuses are closer to being human citizens than they are to being anything else, it is society that perhaps should confer rights on the fetus. It is probably not necessary to determine exactly when fetal life becomes human life but preferable to accept the fetus as a unique being with its own characteristics that is deserving of some rights but not others. What, if any, those rights ought to be will be discussed in the next section.

Fetal rights

The purest way to assign rights in any society is to have it done by those persons who are absolutely impartial, who do not now and never will have any reason to benefit directly or indirectly from the assignment of any rights. Such a person, of course, does not exist, but let us pretend for a moment that we live in a society where this impartial assignment of rights is possible. What prima facie rights could we assign to the fetus, and what rule or rationale could be given for the assignment? The one that comes immediately to mind is that it is wrong to kill a being that wants to live, and we ordinarily assume that all beings want to live unless they expressly state otherwise.* But a fetus does not know if it wants to live, although if it did know or could make a choice, we would have to assume that it would choose life.

With the exception of the right to life, which is natural and inalienable, there are generally three criteria that are imposed during the assignment of rights: the capacity for the sympathy of those assigning the rights, the vested interest of

---

*The one possible exception to this rule is the case of capital punishment.

those in assignment, and the effect of the character or moral worth of all involved. A fetus may or may not arouse the sympathy of those in a position to assign it rights, depending on one's view of its humanity. It also may be that the pregnant woman arouses even more sympathy than the fetus. A society does not have a vested interest in the survival of a fetus except in the most metaphysical way; that is, a fetus does not contribute to the good of a society insofar as the society reacts to the fetus qua fetus. The fetus, of course, has no moral character or worth to be assessed, and the moral worth of the society assigning rights has so many facets and complexities that it is impossible to determine which ones are directly applicable to fetal rights. Thus we see that no rights can be arbitrarily assigned to the fetus.

Rights should not be confused with value; they are not the same, although the two concepts are often intertwined and even sometimes conflict. To deny someone a right, or to subordinate some people's rights to others, does not mean there is no value to those whose rights were either subordinated or not granted. For example, two people might have equal value, but if one tries to kill the other, the second person has the right to kill the first in self-defense. The first may have, temporarily at least, forfeited his right to life. This does not mean that the value of either person has changed. So too in the matter of the fetus. It cannot be denied that the fetus has some value, the kind and amount depending on one's relationship to it. However, the right of a fully formed person may take precedence over fetal rights without diminishing the value of the fetus. When comparing the rights of a fetus with those of a fully formed person, the fetus' rights will almost always be the ones subordinated. "The body life of the conceptus is not of the same value as the person life of the pregnant woman, so that many considerations would justify abortion."[23]

An important concept here is the matter of whether or not the fetus' value and rights would ever override those of the pregnant woman. Even when the right to life is involved and even with the acknowledgment that the fetus, particularly in the later stages of development, does have a right to life, when the rights of the fetus and those of the pregnant woman come into direct conflict, the rights of the former are always subordinated to those of the latter, thus creating clear situations in which abortion is not only permissible but probably even mandatory in some cases (for example, when the pregnant woman's life would be clearly jeopardized if the pregnancy were to continue).

The problem of potentiality as it relates to rights is a thorny one. The analogy used previously concerning the potentiality of the President is not completely precise. When we elect a President we know pretty much how he will behave in office; he is already a person and has stated goals and intentions for his actions while President. We have no such information regarding the fetus. Aside from some possible genetic data, the fetus is a complete tabula rasa, a being of pure potentiality. There is no way of knowing what kind of person it will become; therefore no rights are owed it by virtue of what it had been or promises to be. Many believe that a fetus, although it is more personlike than it is anything else, has fewer rights than a full grown mammal because the latter already occupies a defined place and purpose in the world and thus is owed moral obligations because of the value it holds for its own sake. We see, then, that a fetus qua fetus has no rights (except the possible right to life, which can be overridden by the pregnant woman's rights), and the fetus qua potential person has no rights at all. One may believe that a fetus is a full human person and thus has all the attendant legal and moral rights, but there is no logical reason to think that this is true.

LEGAL ASPECTS

Because there are no provable rights that the fetus can claim, it might seem strange that abortion has been regulated by most modern legal systems. Legal norms vary from country to country and from time to time. Finnis[24] describes three basic legal models that are most frequently used to control or regulate abortion as follows: restriction for the sake of the child; restriction for the sake of uniform medical practice; and general availability for the sake of women's freedom.

The first model, restriction for the sake of the child (Finnis uses "child" when it is actually the fetus to which he is referring, thus placing a distinct bias on the model), was the model used in England and the United States until recently. It implied that abortion after quickening was tantamount to felonious assault, although it has never been a capital crime. All abortions are considered criminal in this model, although those that are performed after quickening carry a stiffer penalty than earlier ones. There were no antiabortion laws in the United States until Connecticut passed legislation in 1821 (antiabortionism as an American Puritan concept is thus a myth), and by 1868, 36 states had antiabortion statutes. By the next century all 50 states declared abortion illegal, although some permitted it in certain circumstances, such as when the pregnant woman's life was clearly in jeopardy or if the pregnancy was the result of rape or incest. The stated primary purpose of these antiabortion laws was to protect the fetus from wrongful attack, not to protect the pregnant woman from the risks inherent in abortion. It seems certain that such restrictive laws were designed, at least in part, to inhibit women's freedom.

The second model, restriction for the sake of uniform medical practice, was never in common use, but the earliest instance of its appearance was in Germany in 1933 shortly after the Nazis came to power. Sweden and Denmark also used this model, which required the authorization of a government official before abortion could be performed. Authorization rested on a government policy that could make certain exceptions to existing antiabortion regulations. A more informal use of this model was common practice in many American communities where hospital regulations would require the agreement of a panel of professionals (usually composed of an obstetrician, a psychiatrist, and a nonphysician such as a theologian) before the hospital would permit the abortion to take place. The usual reasons stated for permitting abortions that were otherwise forbidden were the beliefs that the fetus might be deformed or that a serious risk to the mental and emotional health of the pregnant woman existed. It is difficult to see what this model had to do with uniform medical practice, since the government officials and professional panels had nothing whatever to say about the method used to perform the abortion. Instead it seems obvious that the purpose was to keep the locus of abortion control in the hands of professionals and out of the hands of the consumers of abortion.

The third model, general availability for the sake of women's freedom, received its biggest boost from the Supreme Court decision of 1973, which will be discussed in detail later in the chapter. However, by the early 1920s in other parts of the world, notably the Soviet Union, women began to receive fairly widespread rights to abortion. The new Soviet freedom protected women from the economic hardships of an unwanted child and freed them to participate in the then burgeoning equality in education, occupation, and marriage. However, in 1936 that equality was abruptly halted when a law was passed that outlawed abortion in almost all circumstances. This repression of women coincided with the general repression of the Stalinist era. After World War II, particularly in the late 1950s in other parts of the world and in the mid-1960s in the United States, women began to look closely at how restrictive abortion laws were affecting their lives. Although avoiding the medical risks inherent in carrying a pregnancy to term was never the primary reason for a woman to seek abortion, as a result of the growing feminist movement, legislators and physicians began to compare morbidity and mortality statistics between an abortion performed by a medical professional in an adequate facility and a pregnancy carried to term. It turned out that the medical risk of completing a pregnancy was significantly higher than terminating it early. This became one of the hooks on which proabortionists could hang their argument, although it carries little moral weight.

All the abortion legislation in the United States now follows the third model, although there is a definite groundswell to return to a more restrictive era. In fact, several members of Congress (Senators Helms and Hatch and Representatives Hyde, Dornan, Ashbrook, and others) support one version or another of a Human Life Amendment (HLA) to the United States Constitution. The Helms/Dornan amendment, drawn up in early 1981, reads, "The paramount right to life is vested in each human being from the moment of fertilization without regard to age, health, or condition of dependency." If this or a similar amendment is made part of the Constitution, a woman who has an abortion, or a physician who performs one, could be liable for first-degree murder.

In anticipation of the public debate about the HLA, the United States Senate held hearings in April 1981, that attempted to gather "scientific" evidence about when human life begins. Several physicians and scientists testified, but the most forceful document in the public record was the testimony of Leon Rosenberg, a geneticist at Yale University. When asked whether there is a significant likelihood that human life begins at conception, he answered in the negative for the following three reasons: (1) there is no scientific evidence to prove such a belief; (2) the notion or concept of "actual human life" is not a scientific one; rather it is metaphysical, religious, and philosophic; and (3) the question does not belong within the purview of scientific enquiry. He concluded by saying that science and medicine should not be called on to justify a course of action that has essentially nothing to do with science and medicine. "Ask your conscience, your minister, your priest, your rabbi—or even your God—because it is in their domain that this matter resides."

Roe v. Wade

The single most dramatic and far-reaching legal action in regard to abortion (a Supreme Court decision is not a piece of legislation because the judicial branch of government does not have the power to create legislation, but its effect was tantamount to an actual law and thus is regarded by many as such) was the January 22, 1973, Supreme Court decision in the case of *Roe v. Wade*.[25] It is not inaccurate or overly dramatic to say that it changed the lives of hundreds of thousands of women. Justice Blackmun delivered the majority opinion, summarized as follows:

1. There had been three major reasons for the enactment of criminal laws regarding abortion in the United States: (a) the discouragement of illicit sexual conduct; (b) the protection of women from the medical hazards of abortion and an effort to lower mortality; and (c) the state's interest in protecting prenatal life.

2. These three reasons can no longer be considered sound because of the high degree of safety of early abortion (in fact, the mortality at illegal "abortion mills" strengthens rather than weakens the state's interest in controlling abortion) and because the states have not been able to prove conclusively that their primary reason for prohibiting abortion was the protection of fetal life.

3. Although the Constitution does not specifically guarantee a right of privacy, there has been a significant amount of case law and precedents established on the basis of those cases to make the privacy issue relevant to abortion. This implicit right to privacy can extend to matters of family, marriage, procreation, and contraception.

4. The right to privacy is broad enough to cover a woman's own decision whether or not to terminate her own pregnancy, although the Court did not agree that she has the right to terminate it at whatever time she chooses and in whatever manner suits her.

5. The word *person* as used in the Fourteenth Amendment does not include the fetus, which thus has no specific guarantee to equal protection under the law.

6. However, a point is reached at which the fetus, even though it is not a person, deserves some protection from the state. Although philosophers, theologians, and physicians have not been able to agree on when human life begins, the Court established viability as the point at which the fetus is entitled to the state's protection.

7. Therefore a state may not prohibit a woman from seeking an abortion during the first two trimesters, but it may regulate the conditions under which the abortion is performed during the second trimester. The state may establish requirements as to the qualifications of the person performing the abortion, the licensure of the institution in which it takes place, and the nature of the institution itself (hospital, clinic, etc.).

8. In the third trimester, "If the state is interested in protecting fetal life after viability, it may go so far as to proscribe abortion during that period except when it is necessary to preserve the life or health of the mother. . . . "

Two important observations should be made about the interpretation of *Roe v. Wade*. First, the right to abortion granted by the decision is a negative rather than a positive right. That is, a state may not prohibit a woman from seeking and obtaining an abortion, and it may not place any legal obstacles in her way of doing so. By the same token, however, the state is not obligated either to provide abortions or to create laws that make abortions available. A woman cannot make a claim against the state for an abortion, and no physician is required to perform one. Believing that abortion is a positive right is a common misinterpretation of *Roe v. Wade*. It grants a woman only the right not to be legally interfered with in her quest for abortion.

Second, *Roe v. Wade* did not, in and of itself, prohibit third-trimester abortions. It only granted individual states the right to prohibit them if they choose to do so. All 50 states have indeed made postviability abortions illegal, but this is a state matter, not a constitutional one, according to *Roe v. Wade*.

AFTERMATH OF ROE V. WADE. In the *Roe v. Wade* decision, the Supreme Court left several issues unresolved and even created some additional legal confusion. One was the issue of consent, that is, who is legally required to give consent for abortion and to whom does the fetus "belong." In 1976, *Danforth v. Planned Parenthood*,[26] with Justice Blackmun again writing the majority decision, stipulated a more formal legal definition of viability ("that stage of fetal development when the life of the unborn child may be continued indefinitely outside the womb by natural or artificial life-supportive systems"). *Danforth v. Planned Parenthood* allowed a state to require that a woman give her written informed consent to abortion, but the state may not require the consent of a spouse during the first trimester. Neither may the state require the consent of a minor's parents during the first trimester, nor may it proscribe a particular abortion method that is safer than continuing the pregnancy to term. The last, and perhaps most controversial and far-reaching, stipulation of *Danforth* is that the state cannot require a physician to preserve the life of a previable fetus delivered during an abortion. *Danforth* went far beyond *Roe v. Wade* in placing control in the hands of women in the matter of abortion and gave them greater freedom of choice.

The matter of spousal consent is a sticky one and has ethical as well as interpersonal overtones. Ideally both husband and wife would agree to the abortion, but in the event of a disagreement, obviously only one view can prevail; *Danforth* assured that it would be the wife's since she physically bears the child and is the one most directly affected by the pregnancy. *Danforth* was by no means a unanimous Supreme Court decision; the vote was 5 to 4, and the dissenters had strong views about spousal consent. Justice White wrote the dissenting opinion:

> A father's interest in having a child—perhaps his only child—may be unmatched by any other interest in his life. It is truly surprising that the majority finds in the United States Constitution, as it must in order to justify the result it reaches, a rule that the State must assign a greater value to a mother's decision to cut off a potential human life by abortion than to a father's decision to let it mature into a live child.[27]

Parental consent is an even more difficult matter. Parents have a legal and moral duty to protect minor children, but the dilemma is in deciding whether more harm will be caused to a young child (it is not uncommon for girls of age 11 or 12 to become pregnant) by continuing a pregnancy to term and becoming a mother or by having an abortion. Although there is a great deal to be said for the superiority of parental judgment in most cases, especially when the pregnant girl is very young and when the emotionality of an unwanted pregnancy can cloud the most mature minds, the Supreme Court maintained that Constitutional rights apply to minors as well as adults, and if women are to be permitted to seek abortion as a private decision, age should not be a factor. The matter should be between the pregnant woman and her physician, regardless of age.

There is still a great deal of controversy over this issue, and several state legislatures are now considering bills to require parental consent for abortion of a minor. If any such bills pass, there is likely to be another legal battle. Because the Court has been split over the abortion issue in general, the outcome of future cases is by no means assured. Perhaps as an indication of things to come, on March 23, 1981, the Court took a first step in the matter of parental consent. In *H.L., etc. v. Scott M. Mathieson, et al.* (79 U.S. 5903) the Court upheld as constitutional the Utah law that requires a physician to inform the parents of a minor seeking abortion. Although their consent is not yet legally required, the parents must be informed. This decision is bound to give encouragement to state legislatures that might want to require parental consent.

One of the major legal and ethical battles to arise from *Roe v. Wade* was the matter of public funding for abortion, specifically the use of Medicaid funds. The Hyde Amendment to the Social Security Act specifically denies Medicaid funds for abortion, even those that are deemed medically necessary. The constitutional issue inherent in the Hyde Amendment concerns the impingement on a fundamental right (*Roe v. Wade* created this right) of some women because of their inability to pay for the abortion. The issue was put before the Supreme Court (*Harris v. McRae*, 48 USLW 4941) in 1980 and was again a close decision, 5 to 4 in favor of the constitutionality of the Hyde Amendment. In a previous case, *Maher v. Roe*,[28] the Supreme Court had decided that it would favor childbirth over abortion by permitting public funds to be used for the former but not for the latter. *McRae* was seen by many to be a simple extension of that decision. However, the opposition charged that by denying poor women access to federally funded abortion, their rights are being impinged on solely because they cannot pay for an abortion with private funds. Dissenting Justice Stevens wrote that the state may not

> deny benefits to a financially and medically needy person simply because he is a Republican, a Catholic, or an Oriental—or because he has spoken against a program the government has a legitimate interest in furthering . . . it may not create exceptions for the sole purpose of furthering a governmental interest that is constitutionally subordinate to the individual interest that the entire program was designed to protect.[29]

Even if the interest of the state were to protect fetal life (though *Roe v. Wade* specifically states the opposite), the Hyde Amendment bears no logical relationship to that interest because the only protection granted would be to the fetuses of poor women, which is a state of affairs directly contrary to American legal principles. There seems little doubt that the Hyde Amendment is not only unfair and inhumane, it is unconstitutional as well, as two federal courts have already ruled.[30] Moreover, *McRae* overrules *Roe v. Wade*, which made no attempt to differentiate the value of fetal life based on the financial status of its mother. If the Supreme Court seemed reluctant to tell Congress how it should allocate funds (and this may have been one rationale behind *McRae*), they appear to have made a serious tactical and pragmatic error; that is, it will cost the taxpayers far more in the long run to support the children born to women who were denied abortion than it would to abort them. *McRae* represents a lost battle for all women, and it seems now that the only way to recoup those losses is by legislative action. Given the present political climate and the serious budget cut backs for health and human services, this seems unlikely.

McRae was decided on June 30, 1980, and legislative and other legal action was quick to follow. In early June the Department of Health and Human Services (HHS) notified all state Medicaid agencies that funding for abortion, except those that are "medically necessary" was to cease as of July 28, 1980. Three days before this late July deadline the American Civil Liberties Union (ACLU) petitioned the Supreme Court to reconsider *McRae*; the request was refused. On September 29, 1980, the Senate voted to allow states to decide for themselves whether to use Medicaid funding for abortion in cases of rape or incest; the House had already passed a similar but even more restrictive bill. That vote marked the ninety-sixth time the Senate had voted about some aspect of abortion, a subject many believe is not a matter for legislative debate.

Many legal and ethical questions remain unanswered after the Supreme Court has made its various decisions, and legislative action has translated the will of at least some of the people into law. Finnis[31] summarizes the major questions as follows:

1. What legal rights, other than the right not to be aborted after a certain time, does a fetus have? Can the fetus, when it becomes a person, sue its parents for "wrongful life," especially if the parents knew during pregnancy that it would be born with a deformity or genetic disease? There are strong indications to believe that the fetus will be granted these rights in certain circumstances.
2. What will be the fate of fetuses born alive as a result of abortion? Several states now require that abortion procedures be used that will be least harmful to the fetus, and California and other states have legislation requiring physicians to make every effort to save the lives of those postviable fetuses born alive.
3. Can a woman legally abort herself? It should be noted that the physician was included in the woman's right to privacy in *Roe v. Wade*, but is his presence a necessary condition for a legal abortion?
4. Can the state prevent all or some experimentation on fetuses; that is, is

the fetus a part of the mother that she can dispose of at will, or does it become a separate being after abortion even though it is not alive?

5. What forms of conscientious objection are available to hospitals, physicians, and other health workers who refuse to perform or to advise about abortion?

6. What, if any, rights does the father of the fetus have, especially during the third trimester? Can his rights ever prevail over those of the pregnant woman?

7. Can the state ever require a woman to undergo abortion, either to prevent the birth of a deformed child or to protect the interests of the state, for example, when the woman is unable to demonstrate that she can support the child she is carrying?

These questions all contain highly controversial issues; therefore it seems likely that the abortion debate will not come to rest for a good many years, if ever. It is reasonable to assume that all three branches of government will spend time and money on the issue, which will also continue to be grist for the philosophic mill.

SUMMARY: PRINCIPLE OF DOUBLE EFFECT

It is appropriate to end this chapter with a discussion of the principle of double effect as it relates to abortion, not because double effect is in such common use today, but because it embodies many of the ethical issues inherent in abortion. The reader is referred to Chapter 1 for a more thorough discussion of the principle; a short review will suffice here. The following four conditions must be present for an act that is ordinarily considered evil or impermissible to be considered permissible according to the principle of double effect: (1) the act itself must be morally good or indifferent, (2) only the good consequences of the action must be intended, (3) the good effect must not be produced by means of the evil effect, and (4) there must be some grave reason for permitting the evil.

When an abortion, which could be considered an evil act, is brought about and is justified by the principle of double effect because another, good, action must be done, the resulting abortion is termed *indirect*; that is, it occurred indirectly as a foreseen but unintended consequence of another action. If an abortion is performed for the specific purpose of ridding a woman of a fetus, the abortion is *direct*. The most common reasons for performing an indirect abortion are in the case of an ectopic pregnancy, which if not treated would result in the death of the pregnant woman, and in the case of severe and life-threatening disease or injury to the woman's reproductive organs, as for example, that sustained in a traumatic injury or in diagnosed cancer. By removing the fallopian tube or other diseased part of the reproductive tract, the fetus will necessarily be indirectly aborted, but by invoking the principle of double effect, the foreseen abortion is ethically permissible because it will meet the necessary four criteria: (1) The act of removing the diseased part is morally good because without the performance of the act, the woman would either die immediately or suffer a worsening of whatever disease is present. (2) The good consequences of the act, the surgery, are the only ones intended; the abortion and the resultant death of the fetus are foreseen but not directly intended. (3) The good effect of saving the woman's life is not brought about by the evil effect of abortion. In other words, it is the surgical procedure, not the abortion itself, that will save the woman's life. (4) The evil of abortion is permitted for the gravest possible reason—without it the woman would die.

Thus we have what many consider to be the irony of abortion. It is considered a generally evil and therefore impermissible act, but if some serious circumstances can render it permissible and those circumstances are not specifically dictated, where is the line drawn between permissible abortions and those that are not? For instance, if the primary reason to forbid abortion is the protection of fetal life, and if it is not the fetus' fault that the woman carrying it was a victim of rape or incest, why are these two circumstances, which have nothing to do with the fetus' life as an entity, almost always used as an exception to the antiabortion rule? If these exceptions are permissible, then the reasons to be opposed to abortion do not rest primarily on the value of fetal life but instead on the circumstances surrounding the pregnancy, which is an entirely different matter.

And if those people who are opposed to abortion on the grounds that all human life, from the moment of conception onward, is valuable and should be protected, then all human life should be protected, and those who are in favor of the HLA should be equally vociferous in their antiwar statements and in their strong opposition to capital punishment. One does not, however, see this moral consistency and might therefore assume that the value of human life is not the sole reason for strong antiabortion views.

More instances of inconsistency and less than total commitment to a principle when the issues are applied to abortion could be given. The point, however, is that all debate is morally legitimate because there are valid claims that can be made by those in favor of and those opposed to abortion, depending on the moral theory from which one is operating, on one's total value system, on the vested interests involved, and on religious and cultural beliefs. It is impossible to solve the dilemma, and recent legislative and judicial attempts to do so in the United States should be viewed as only temporary political decisions that are bound to change as social conditions and political power shift. Perhaps this is as it should be.

Notes

1. Fromer, M. J. *Ethical issues in health care*. St. Louis: The C.V. Mosby Co., 1981. p. 210.
2. Newton, L. The irrelevance of religion in the abortion debate. *Hastings Center Report*, 1978, *8*(4), 16–17. Reprinted with permission of the Hastings Center.© Institute of Society, Ethics and the Life Sciences, 360 Broadway, Hastings-on-Hudson, N.Y. 10706.
3. Newton, p. 17.
4. Jaffe, F. S. Enacting religious beliefs in a pluralistic society. *Hastings Center Report*, 1978, *8*(4), 14–16.
5. Jaffe, p. 15.
6. Feldman, D. Abortion: Jewish perspectives. In W. T. Reich (Ed.), *Encyclopedia of bioethics*. New York: The Free Press, 1978. pp. 6–7.
7. Feldman, pp. 7–8.
8. Nelson, J. B. Abortion: Protestant perspectives. In *Encyclopedia of bioethics*, pp. 14–15.
9. Nelson, p. 15.
10. Nelson, p. 16.
11. Fromer, p. 213.
12. Fost, N., Chudwin, D., & Wikler, D. The limited moral significance of 'fetal viability'. *Hastings Center Report*, 1980, *10*(6), 10–13. Reprinted with permission of The Hastings Center.© Institute of Society, Ethics and the Life Sciences, 360 Broadway, Hastings-on-Hudson, N.Y. 10706.
13. Fost, et al., p. 13.
14. Feinberg, J. Abortion. In T. Regan (Ed.), *Matters of life and death: new introductory essays in moral philosophy*. New York: Random House, Inc., 1980. pp. 186–198.
15. Feinberg, p. 186.
16. Feinberg, p. 187.
17. Langerak, E. A. Abortion: listening to the middle. *Hastings Center Report*, 1979, *9*(5), 24–28. Reprinted with permission of The Hastings Center.© Institute of Society, Ethics and the Life Sciences, 360 Broadway, Hastings-on-Hudson, N.Y. 10706.
18. Langerak, p. 25.
19. Engelhardt, H. T., Jr. The ontology of abortion. *Ethics*, 1974, *84*, 217–234.
20. Fromer, pp. 213–214.
21. Brody, B. On the humanity of the feotus. In R. L. Perkins (Ed.), *Abortion pro and con*. Cambridge, Mass.: Schenkman Publishing Co., Inc., 1974.
22. Brody.
23. Curran, C. E. Contemporary debate in philosophical and religious ethics. In *Encyclopedia of bioethics*, pp. 22–23.
24. Finnis, J. M. Abortion: legal aspects. In *Encyclopedia of bioethics*, pp. 27–32.
25. *Roe v. Wade*, 410 US 113 (1973).
26. *Danforth v. Planned Parenthood of Missouri*, 44 USLW 5199 (1976).
27. *Danforth v. Planned Parenthood of Missouri*.
28. *Maher v. Roe*, 432 US 464 (1977).
29. *Harris v. McRae*, 48 USLW 4941 (1980).
30. Annas, G. J. The Supreme Court and abortion: the irrelevance of medical judgment. *Hastings Center Report*, 1980, *10*(5), 23–24.
31. Finnis, pp. 30–31.

Bibliography

Annas, G. J. Abortion and the Supreme Court: round two. *Hastings Center Report*, 1976, 6(5), 15–17.

Annas, G. J. The Supreme Court and abortion: the irrelevance of medical judgment. *Hastings Center Report*, 1980, 10(5), 23–24.

Bleich, D. Abortion in Halakhic literature. *Tradition*, 1968, 10, 72–120.

Brody, B. On the humanity of the foetus. In R. L. Perkins (Ed.), *Abortion pro and con*, Cambridge, Mass.: Schenkman Publishing Co., Inc., 1974.

Brody, B. Religious, moral, and sociological issues: some basic distinctions. *Hastings Center Report*, 1978, 8(4), 13.

Connery, J. R. Abortion: Roman Catholic perspectives. In W. T. Reich (Ed.), *Encyclopedia of bioethics*, New York: The Free Press, 1978.

Curran, C. E. Contemporary debate in philosophical and religious ethics. In *Encyclopedia of bioeth...*

Engelhardt, H. T., Jr. The ontology of abortion. *Ethics*, 1974, 84, 217–234.

Feinberg, J. Abortion. In T. Regan (Ed.), *Matters of life and death: new introductory essays in moral philosophy*, New York: Random House, Inc., 1980.

Feldman, D. M. Abortion: Jewish perspectives. In *Encyclopedia of bioethics*.

Finnis, J. M. Abortion: legal aspects. In *Encyclopedia of bioethics*.

Fost, N., Chudwin, D., & Wikler, D. The limited moral significance of 'fetal viability'. *Hastings Center Report*, 1980, 10(6), 10–13.

Fromer, M. J. *Ethical issues in health care*, St. Louis: The C.V. Mosby Co., 1981.

Grisez, G. G. *Abortion: the myths, the realities and the arguments*. New York: Corpus Books, 1970.

Gustavson, J. M. A Protestant ethical approach. In J. T. Noonan (Ed.), *The morality of abortion: legal and historical perspectives*, Cambridge, Mass.: Harvard University Press, 1970. pp. 101–122.

Hellegers, A. E. Abortion: medical aspects. In *Encyclopedia of bioethics*.

Huser, R. J. *The crime of abortion in Canon Law: an historical synopsis and commentary*. Catholic University of America, Canon Law Studies. No. 162. Washington, D.C.: Catholic University Press, 1942.

Jaffe, F. S. Enacting religious beliefs in a pluralistic society. *Hastings Center Report*, 1978, 8(4); 14–16.

Klein, I. Abortion (1959). *Responsa and Halakhic Studies* (Chap. 4). New York: Ktav Publishing House, Inc., 1975. pp. 27–33.

Langerak, E. A. Abortion: listening to the middle. *Hastings Center Report*, 1979, 9(5), 24–28.

Mechanic, D. The Supreme Court and abortion: sidestepping social realities. *Hastings Center Report*, 1980, 10(6), 17–19.

Moore, H. F. Acting and refraining. In *Encyclopedia of bioethics*.

Nelson, J. B. Abortion: Protestant perspectives. In *Encyclopedia of bioethics*.

Newton, L. The irrelevance of religion in the abortion debate. *Hastings Center Report*, 1978, 8(4), 16–17.

Noonan, J. T., Jr. The Supreme Court and abortion: upholding Constitutional principles. *Hastings Center Report*, 1980, 10(6), 14–16.

Spitzer, W. O., & Saylor, C. L. (Eds.). *Birth control and the Christian: a Protestant symposium on the control of human reproduction*. Wheaton, Ill.: Tyndale House Publishers, 1969.

Warren, M. A. On the moral and legal status of abortion. *The Monist*, 1973, 57(1).

CHAPTER 7

GENETICS

James Watson and Francis Crick's discovery in 1953 of the double helix structure of DNA was undoubtedly the greatest scientific achievement since the dawn of the atomic age several decades before. Knowledge of structure leads to research about function, which is followed by an irresistible impulse to tinker with or manipulate that structure and function. This is the essence of genetic engineering (some refer to it as genetic manipulation), the alteration of genetic and cellular structure and function for the ultimate purpose of altering life itself. It is one of the most interesting, awesome, and frightening areas of research ever attempted and will have profound effects on the nature of all life. Because of the depth and range of the research possibilities, the attendant ethical issues are particularly complex.

Genetic determinism has played an important role in the history of humanity. Genetic traits have been and still are endowed with moral values; social position is frequently assigned by conditions of birth and family, and entire populations have been enslaved and slaughtered on the sole basis of their genetic configuration. These situations have existed for thousands of years. To attempt to change them is to cause a furor, although a reexamination of the assignment of human values and worth on the basis of genetics might be beneficial.

This chapter will examine some of the ethical dilemmas inherent in genetic engineering. Veatch[1] suggests that the following eight essential questions ought to be asked in regard to the ethics of genetic engineering:

1. What is meant by genetic health? Health is a value-laden concept, and all conditions of health or the lack of it are assigned a set of values by the health-care system and by society in general. Since one cannot be held morally responsible for one's genetic makeup, should a value be placed on it? Some

genetic configurations, such as retinoblastoma, are unhealthy, and others, such as hair or eye color, are not. The assignment of values by a society decides which genetic conditions are described as unhealthy and which ought to be changed.

2. Who should decide about genetic intervention? This question has special implications for genetic counseling and will be discussed later in the chapter. Suffice it to say here that there are a variety of actions that can be taken once the likelihood of bearing children with genetic defects is determined. This variety leads to conflicts concerning reproductive liberty, public policy, and genetic research.

3. How should conflict between the interests of clients and those of society be resolved? These are classic bioethical dilemmas, compounded in genetics by sometimes not knowing who the client is (the pregnant woman, the married couple, the fetus, or even a fetus yet to be conceived). Rights are also at issue here; that is, does society have rights in this regard that can be superimposed on individuals, or is it the other way around?

4. Is the most beneficial course of action always the right or just course? This question reflects in part the conflicts between the individual and society and between right and good. It is also the conflict between utilitarianism and deontology, that is, between general societal happiness and obedience to certain ethical principles.

5. Must genetic information and prenatal or preconceptual interventions be kept confidential? The principle of confidentiality is the medical application of promise- and contract-keeping, but relatives of persons with genetic anomalies or potential genetic defects and diseases surely have a vested interest in having such information. Whose rights take precedence in these instances?

6. Does the genetic counselor have a duty always to tell the truth or only if it will be beneficial? Does the principle of truth telling always hold, even if the truth will be profoundly psychologically disturbing or even if nothing can be done to intervene in an unfortunate chain of events?

7. What is the relation of abortion to genetic problems? Although abortion is a separate moral issue, it is closely associated with the ethics of genetic engineering. If, for example, we assume that abortion is the correct action when a fetus is discovered to be genetically imperfect, we have made a statement (pro or con) about the value of human life and about the hierarchy of rights.

8. What is the nature of human life and how should human beings use technology to change that nature? This is probably the most fundamental question regarding ethical issues in genetic engineering, and answers to it depend heavily on one's interpretation of human nature.

In addition to ethical principles, there are some basic physical principles inherent in genetic engineering. Davis[2] believes that two major ones should be considered: (1) the interaction of polygenic traits with behavioral genetics and (2) the interaction of heredity and environment. Polygenic traits depend on multiple genes; thus their characteristics vary continuously from generation to generation (in contrast to a monogenic trait, such as eye color or certain diseases like hemophilia, which depend on only one gene and therefore can be specifically traced in succeeding generations). Moreover, each gene can vary by mutation and thus can exist in several different forms. The traits of human nature that are most interesting to study genetically—temperament, intelligence, and physical structure—are highly polygenic; therefore research on their nature is an imprecise and inexact science at best.

> The study of polygenic inheritance has received little public attention. Education on the distinction between monogenic and polygenic inheritance is clearly important if the public is to distinguish between realistic and wild projections for future developments in genetic intervention in man.[3]

The second principle, the interaction of heredity and environment, is important to understand because genes contribute only to a range of potential for any given human trait, while environment contributes much to a person's actual state within that range. Genetic structure is now known to determine protein structure, but the regulatory mechanisms within that genetic structure (the pattern or blueprint, as it were) determine how much protein is produced. Since protein is essential for the development and adequate maintenance of all body cells, including those in the brain, genetic structure may have more to do with human behavior than had been previously thought. Behaviors that had been believed to be a function of culture, interpersonal relationships, and the like might indeed be a function of genetic endowment.

PRESENT AND FUTURE GENETIC TECHNOLOGIES
Enzyme replacement

Genetic disease is usually caused by the mutation of a gene that translates to a defect in the enzyme molecule that is enclosed by that particular gene. Thus the enzyme functions poorly or not at all. Enzymes are the catalysts that control all chemical reactions in the body; therefore the loss or defect in function of any one enzyme can set off a potentially devastating chain of biochemical events. An enzyme must be supplied to counteract this effect. Those enzymes that normally function within a body fluid can be replaced; those that function within cells cannot, except in very few instances. Lysosomes are one of those exceptions, and the process by which this is done is extremely complex, involving a fairly great risk of harm to the person as a result of inadvertent introduction of microorganisms and other impurities. The chance of untoward side effects is high, and treatment must be instituted slowly and cautiously. The therapeutic value of this treatment is still unknown, the cost is astronomic, and major ethical questions exist as to the relative benefit to be gained at such high cost.

Transformation of DNA molecules

Isolated fragments of purified human DNA containing functional genetic information can be introduced into human cells with the intent of treating genetic disorders. Mammalian (including human) cells can be grown in vitro and exposed to various pieces of foreign DNA to determine whether they can permanently alter the cell's characteristics. Some successful results have been achieved with this method, but so far none of them have been reproduced after further investigation. Permanently modifying human cells by adding DNA would involve the following complex process: the added DNA would have to be taken up by the cells and transported to the nucleus; the new DNA would have to become permanently associated with the original chromosomal DNA in the cells; and the newly introduced genetic information encoded in the DNA must be correctly transcribed into another molecule and the message translated into a functional protein to express the new genetic information. Technical problems, such as destruction of DNA by intra- and extra-cellular enzymes and the low density of any specific DNA segment (frequently one part in ten million), have so far prevented the successful genetic alteration of mammalian cells. However, much research is currently being done to overcome these problems, and there is reason to believe that it will be accomplished within the foreseeable future. Side effects and untoward reactions as a result of transformation of DNA molecules and other genetic engineering research could be disastrous. Chromosome damage might be permanent in the individual treated and might then be passed on to future generations. Interfering with natural processes in cell nuclei could damage them sufficiently to cause a malignancy or a carcinogenic tendency in offspring. These and other ramifications of research will be discussed in detail later in the chapter.

Transduction of DNA molecules

Transduction is the process by which something is received from one place and is carried or transferred to another place. Transduction as a form of genetic engineering research will use viruses or viral DNA as carriers of specific foreign DNA sequences into cells. It has already been accomplished with a monkey virus which, when added to cultures of human cells grown in vitro, was integrated into the chromosomal DNA of the human cells. Foreign pieces of DNA could be attached to the monkey virus, which would then act as a carrier to link the foreign DNA with the cell that was its destination. One serious problem with this technique is that the DNA in the virus may become integrated with that of the recipient cell with deleterious effects. For example, infection of human cells with certain kinds of DNA may cause them to resemble cancer cells, even though they may not be cancerous. Moreover, new genetic material (that is, new to the cell to which it was transferred) may not act in an expected manner and may thus establish an entire chain of untoward and unanticipated events.

A variation of transduction of DNA molecules is germ cell alteration in which a synthesized gene would be introduced into a cell in vitro.

> This would result in directed mutagenesis; that is, specific agents could bring about a specific alteration in the DNA. It could be used to reverse a current gene mutation or to create a new one. This process is incredibly complex and has not yet been accomplished. To date, all known mutagenic agents occur randomly and their effects are generally negative. For a particular gene to be directed toward a specific place on the DNA strand, it would have to be attached to a molecule that could selectively recognize the distination. Without this tracking device germ cell alteration would be like telling an Amtrak train to find its way from Boston to Washington without providing an engineer, tracks, and signals. It would likely wander off into the Atlantic or end up in Cleveland.[4]

Cell fusion and hybridization

Cell fusion to create a hybrid nucleus seems like a relatively simple matter, rather like grafting different varieties of rose bushes, but the resistance of cells to being fused in vitro makes it difficult to accomplish. In theory, different cells are fused so that the combination of their genetic material will form a single new nucleus. This has been accomplished in isolated instances with both human and animal cells, the results of which have been inconclusive at best. Some nuclei have been capable of fusing, but cells in general do not have the capability for recognition of compatible DNA strands.

However, one successful use for cell fusion has been the development of the human genome, that is, the assignment of specific genes to individual chromosomes and the analysis of the linear order of genes on single chromosomes. This provides a relatively simple, accurate, and fast way to accomplish a generational analysis of genetic pedigree. Hybridization will also provide a system whereby the general organization of cells and factors relating to their function can be studied.

To date all work with cell fusion has been done in vitro, but there is no reason to believe that it will not eventually be carried out in animals and humans. There are several possibilities inherent in these future uses.

1. New genetic information can be introduced into the cells of any given species, thereby changing the genetic nature of that species, although admittedly this would be extraordinarily difficult to accomplish.
2. New nuclei could be introduced into newly fertilized eggs from which the nucleus had been removed. These transferred nuclei could then be used to create embryos of specifically defined genetic constitution. The embryo would then have a genetic makeup identical to that of the individual that donated the transplanted nucleus, that is, it would be a clone.
3. Cell fusion could result in increased knowledge of genetic defects by introducing genes from persons with known genetic disorders to see if the genes could somehow correct themselves when fused with a similar but normal gene.

Four-parent individuals

The rather startling genetic engineering feat of four-parent individuals is accomplished by removing embryos while the cells are still undifferentiated and placing them in a culture medium. The cells of two genetically unrelated embryos are made to adhere to each other to form an artificial composite. Each embryo had its own two parents, and the composite now has four. The new unified embryo maintains cells of disparate genetic composition that do not fuse until late in embryonic development (the bone and muscle formation stage). The composite is then transferred to the uterus of a surrogate mother. This has already been done successfully in experimental animals, who are then born as a sort of genetic mosaic, that is, with different tissues having different genetic makeup. Four-parent experimental animals can be of benefit to researchers in that the original tissue site of various diseases can be accurately pinpointed.

This procedure has not yet been done in humans because so far it has not been feasible to remove embryos in a sufficiently undifferentiated state. Moreover, the legal and ethical ramifications of a child with four parents would be mind boggling. For instance, what would happen to the conventional concepts of self, family, heritage, race, and personal identity? What would be the fate of ordinarily recessive deleterious genes when they are mixed with either normal or deleterious genes of the other embryo; would the normal cancel out the abnormal, or would the latter somehow be stimulated by the presence of other genes? And what about the sex of the embryo? Would we have supermales and superfemales, or a person who is a little of both? That issue alone might be enough to deter the most enthusiastic research geneticist.

Cloning

The word *clone* is the part of the genetic engineering lexicon that is most familiar to most people, although they only vaguely understand that it somehow involves asexual reproduction. Cloning is indeed asexual reproduction and in theory is a relatively simple procedure. In practice it becomes quite difficult. The theory behind cloning, which is called the theory of nuclear equivalence, is that all cells in the body contain the same genetic information that made the body's original fertilized cell able to form the entire being. As the fertilized cell develops and increases in size and complexity, it becomes differentiated in form and function and somehow loses this ability to reproduce. Or perhaps the ability is temporarily switched off but is still there. To turn this regenerative capability back on, a technique known as nuclear transplantation is used, which was briefly described. The idea is that placing the nucleus in a new environment (another cell) will somehow stimulate it to begin mitosis and eventually to develop into a completely new being. The technique is extremely precise and difficult to accomplish without destroying either the cell nucleus or the surrounding cytoplasm. However, cloning was first accomplished in 1951 and is now quite routine in certain species of vegetables and animals. Human cloning has not yet been done, although technologic barriers will undoubtedly be broken.

Cloning has been an enormous step forward in genetic engineering and has led to increased knowledge about cell function. The most important piece of information derived from cloning is that any cell of the body can be made to reproduce, a function that was thought to belong only to sex cells. Asexual reproduction is vastly different from sexual reproduction in that all offspring will be genetically identical to the parent, whereas natural reproduction provides almost infinite genetic variety.

Eisenberg[5] believes that those who oppose human cloning for ethical or social reasons do not understand its implications.

> Were human cloning to be accomplished, it has been assumed that the result would be psychological as well as physical identity between the originator of the clone and his or her cloned offspring. This unwarranted assumption reveals the persistence of the concept of predestination as a causal force in development, despite its incompatibility with biological evidence. The basic problems with the fiction of human cloning are not ethical or political but scientific. Pseudo-science serves to distract attention from fundamental social and moral questions.[6]

Eisenberg holds that wide use of human cloning would invite biologic disaster because it would lead to a significant decrease in the size of the gene pool (persons who are to be "parents" of clones would likely be chosen in the selecting scientists' image—intelligent and of certain social and psychologic characteristics). This would reduce humanity's chances of surviving major evolutionary changes, and the risk of extinction would increase significantly. Nature has been arranged so that there is a tremendous biologic investment in sexual reproduction, and Eisenberg believes this arrangement indicates its importance to species evolution.

> The benefit of sexual reproduction is the enhancement of diversity (by cross-over between homologous chromosomes during meiosis and by combining the haploid gametes of a male and a female parent). The new genetic combinations so produced enable the species to respond as a population to changing environmental conditions by selective survival of adaptable genotypes. The deliberate imposition of a restriction on human genetic diversity would violate the very biological principles basic to the evolution of our species.[7]

The process of selecting donors to be cloned would be insurmountable unless society in general would be willing to leave such decisions to a tiny minority—scientists who specialize in genetic engineering. This possibility is highly unlikely.

Cloning as a method of perpetuating the species is one thing; using the technique as an aid in the solution of health problems of individual human beings is something entirely different, and the ethical issues are not the same. Individual infertile couples might benefit from cloning, although there would surely be psychologic difficulties as well as ethical dilemmas. Cloning a variety of cells to produce certain enzymes, hormones, and other substances used in the treatment of human disease is a distinct possibility for the future and in some instances is currently available technology. The ethical issues inherent in these forms of technology will be discussed with those of genetic engineering in general.

Recombinant DNA

Of all the forms of genetic engineering presently available or possible within the foreseeable future, none has had the dramatic impact of recombinant DNA. This process was pioneered by Paul Berg and Stanley Cohen of Stanford University and again is deceptively simple in theory and incredibly difficult in practice. In essence, recombinant DNA is the insertion of foreign genes into a cell, splicing the foreign and host genes to each other, and then allowing cell division to take place naturally. A bacterium such as *Escherichia coli*, which contains a single chromosome and several plasmids (small rings of genetic material), is broken open by exposing it to a detergent to remove its outer protective covering. The plasmids are removed by centrifugal force and then immersed in an enzyme solution. This causes the plasmid to open at a specific place on the ring (the exact place is determined by the nature of the enzyme solution). Meanwhile, by the same process, a gene from a completely different cell is removed from a segment of DNA and is spliced into the opening in the bacterial plasmid. Thus recombinant DNA is formed, that is, DNA made up of two different organisms. These hybrid plasmids are then reinserted in a bacterial cell, which divides and replicates all the genes, including the new DNA.

The uses to which recombinant DNA can be put are almost limitless, a few of which include the manufacture of interferon, hormones, enzymes, and other naturally occurring substances; the manufacture of new life forms; gene therapy to correct certain hereditary defects such as thalassemia and other blood diseases; the ability of certain agricultural crops to draw their own nitrogen from the atmosphere, thus eliminating the need for fertilizers; and the creation of bacteria that will be able to leach metals directly out of the earth. Without doubt recombinant DNA could radically alter many of the ways in which we live.

There has been a great deal of publicity in the past 5 years or so about recombinant DNA, much of it sensational, that is, horror stories of new and bizarre life forms escaping research scientists and wreaking all kinds of biologic havoc. These stories make exciting science fiction, but the facts are less dramatic. Cohen,[8] one of the developers of recombinant DNA, points out some basic information that is essential to have if one is to rationally discuss the ethical issues involved.

1. Recombinant DNA, which is a group of techniques rather than a single one, is neither good nor bad in itself and as a piece of technology holds no moral value per se. Certain recombinant DNA experiments are hazardous and should not be done, as are many types of research that have nothing to do with genetic engineering.

2. Regarding the possibility that some particular DNA molecule that has thus far shown no evidence of being hazardous could suddenly become so, Cohen says that this view is correct, but by the same token no one is able to say for certain that other seemingly safe procedures will not suddenly turn dangerous. For example, a vaccine that has been used for years could produce contagious cancer some years from now, or some traveler from afar could bring a virulent virus into the United States at any time. Moreover, hybrid plants that are now so much a part of agricultural research could suddenly turn into weeds that will overcome major crops and contribute to worldwide famine.[9]

3. Experiments involving genes that could eventually produce toxic substances or are now known to do so are prohibited.

4. Cohen believes that scientists are, for the most part, responsible enough

not only to bring to the public's attention possible hazards inherent in recombinant DNA research but also to voluntarily call a moratorium on such hazardous experiments. Not everyone believes that scientists are capable of such self-regulation, but in a free society government regulation of scientific endeavor is not regarded with great favor.

5. The anticipation of benefits is well worth whatever minor risk exists, and these benefits will be both theoretic, in that they will advance fundamental medical and scientific knowledge, and practical, in that they will alleviate some human misfortunes.

Although it is impossible to completely eliminate risk from any scientific research (if outcomes of experiments were predictable, the activity would not be research), there are certain actions that can be taken to significantly decrease risk. The National Institutes of Health (NIH) has established guidelines for research carried out at its own establishment to increase the chances that recombinant DNA research will be done safely. Although the NIH does not have the authority to impose these guidelines on other research institutions, the prestige of the NIH is such that some of the guidelines have been voluntarily adopted elsewhere. These guidelines are as follows:

1. Experiments in which there is some scientific basis for anticipating a hazard are prohibited. In addition, if an experiment involves a speculative hazard, that is, a hazard that is believed to exist rather than known to exist because the same or similar experiments have never been done before, and if the NIH considers it to be potentially serious, the experiment is prohibited.

2. NIH requires that a large class of experiments be carried out only in high-level containment facilities, known as type P4, designed for work with the most hazardous viruses. These laboratories are specially built and designed with air locks, autoclaves, safety cabinets for personnel, and the like. They are the safest possible environment for research; the only thing safer would be not to do it at all.

3. As the level of potential risk decreases, restrictions on research loosen, but in no instance of recombinant DNA research are regulations absent. All work areas must be decontaminated daily, and laboratory personnel are required to obey strict rules about clothing and bathing.

4. Recombinant DNA research uses molecules from cells that have been designed not to propagate outside of specific environments, that is, to self-destruct if they should somehow escape from the laboratory. By contrast, work is done at NIH with *Lassa* fever virus (also in P4 containment laboratories), but no such effort to destroy the virus outside the laboratory is possible. If the *Lassa* fever virus were to escape, there would be no natural barrier to prevent it from propagating. *Lassa* fever is

particularly virulent, it has a 100% mortality, and there is no known cure. All current recombinant DNA research is tame by comparison.

Ethical issues inherent in genetic engineering research will be discussed in more detail in the next section, but it is important to point out here that one must look at the hazards in a rational way. Genetic engineering research is not necessarily any more hazardous than nuclear research, space exploration, and a wide variety of general medical research. It is true that there may be some danger to the environment and the creatures in it as a result of genetic research, but this does not mean that such research should be halted. Without genetic research, a good many forms of human healing would be impossible. If we as a society want certain benefits, then we must be willing to pay the price in possible environmental damage.

ETHICAL ISSUES

Ethical issues in genetic engineering, although they cover a wide range of territory, are usually based on one essential and fundamental question: Do human beings have the right to experiment with natural life forms? This question is important to consider, but from a pragmatic view, it is beside the point because there is no doubt that genetic engineering research will continue. According to Callahan there are two basic reasons why genetic research cannot be stopped.[10] The first is that both the public and the scientific community are prepared to go ahead with it. Whatever opposition exists has not been strong enough to prevent the research from proceeding.

> Moreover, whenever there has been a scientific breakthrough, the general reaction has been one of wondrous excitement, in the scientific no less than in the public media. Whatever ethical reservations or objections may have been voiced prior to the breakthrough have been swept away with astonishing rapidity once the actual events have taken place.[11]

The second reason is that those opposed to genetic engineering have not been able to argue persuasively enough against it. To be persuasive, Callahan believes, the argument must have sufficient emotional impact as well as logical consistency.

There are various reasons why people argue for and against genetic engineering. First, individual liberty is a strong compelling force that encompasses the right to seek new knowledge as long as it is not likely to harm others. Second, people tend to weigh good against evil, that is, the degree to which theoretic knowledge can be applied to the alleviation of human suffering as opposed to the potential (or real) hazards to our present quality of life. Third, there is a strong belief that one has a moral obligation to do good, that is, translate the principle of nonmaleficence (the duty to do no harm) into the principle of beneficence.

Among the many problems in discussing the ethical issues in genetic engineering is the fact that the endeavor is so new that no codes of ethics or rules of behavior exist (as they do in medical research, for example), and general ethical principles must be adapted to a field of study that barely existed a decade ago and that will change drastically in form and function a decade from now. One could begin the debate from the principle that doing good is indeed good, that is, that using genetic engineering to learn about and eradicate certain diseases will benefit humankind. That is true, of course, but what if in the course of doing good an equal or greater harm is brought about? What if, for example, a disease exists for a biologic purpose that we have yet to understand; what if its presence prevents another disease from being released from its even more recessive genetic trait? What will have been accomplished if disease Y replaces disease X, especially if it is even more harmful? Most people do not find this to be a persuasive reason not to do genetic engineering for the same reason that Columbus was not disuaded from setting out for India because he might fall off the edge of the earth. But the lack of a firm groundwork of experience in genetic engineering, while not a reason to halt it altogether, does create problems in solving the ethical dilemmas.

Another philosophic argument concerning the "ought" and "is" of genetic engineering is that expressed by G. E. Moore and other intuitionists. Moore believed that a demonstration of an empirical truth about nature (an "is") permits no inferences to be drawn about appropriate standards of behavior concerning those truths (an "ought"). In other words, it is illogical to move from a set of *descriptive* empirical facts about some aspect of nature, for example, the fact that certain nuclei can be snipped apart gene by gene and attached to the nucleus of another cell, to a set of *prescriptive* or normative conclusions about those facts of nature, for example, that recombinant DNA is or is not morally acceptable. A scientist who attempts to build an ethical position on an empirical fact of nature is committing a logistical fallacy. It is important to be able to separate an "ought" from an "is."

Sinsheimer,[12] who tends to be less than totally optimistic about the outcomes of genetic engineering, asks a series of troubling questions about the uses to which this research will be put. How far will we eventually want to go; will we want to assume basic responsibility for life on earth, or only certain forms of life? Do we want to create new life forms, and if so, what will they be like? Shall we control evolution? Sinsheimer doubts that the consequences of genetic engineering can be fully forecast, especially as they relate to social structure, personality, culture, and other important aspects of human operations. Although he does not call for a moratorium on all such research, he urges scientists to look more closely at the consequences of seriously interfering in the course of nature and human evolution.

Individualism and liberty

In 1974 a committee of molecular biologists, chaired by Paul Berg, one of the discoverers of recombinant DNA, wrote a letter to *Science* magazine (July 26, 1974, p. 303) expressing concern about the possible hazards resulting from the artificial molecules used in recombinant DNA research. The letter requested that "scientists throughout the world join with members of this committee in voluntarily deferring [certain] experiments." The letter was followed by a conference at Asilomar, California, which will be described later in the chapter, and it sparked heated, sometimes acrimonious debate among scientists (the public press was curiously silent about the matter) as to whether or not there are some forms of research that simply should not be done and some types of knowledge that human beings should not have. At issue here is the individual scientist's liberty to seek knowledge both for its own sake as an intrinsic good and for the ultimate use to which it can be put. It should be noted here that the Berg letter and the debate that followed did not concern research of which the consequences or outcomes are known to be harmful or even evil. It is a given that these types of research ought not to be done.

One reason for the Berg letter was to alert the public about the possible hazardous effects of DNA research. This proved to be an irony, not only because the general media did not pick up on the issue, but also because within a few years the members of the committee realized that they had overestimated the seriousness of the risks, and this particular letter turned out to be a tempest in a teapot. But the problem of the conflict between the individual scientist's freedom to do research and laypersons' natural fear of arcane goings-on in the laboratory still exists. Some of the public's trepidation is perfectly well founded, but most is not. Safety standards in research must be established; no reasonable person disagrees with that. But the problem with research in genetics is the fact that almost the entire endeavor is an uncharted course, and the nature of the hazards is potential in two senses of the word; that is, are there indeed hazards, and if so, what form will they take? Even space exploration, with which genetic engineering is often compared in terms of its magnitude and ultimate effect on human life, contains hazards that are more familiar to the explorers than to those in genetic research. Therefore what precautions should be taken? Those that are too stringent will hamper the course of research, and those that are too lax could be the cause of an accident. Then, too, establishment of precautions implies the existence of a hazard that may or may not even exist.

The political and social mood of a country, or at least a particular segment of the population, has a great deal to do with the extent to which people are willing to tolerate potential political hazards. Scientists are viewed as members of the Establishment, particularly if they work for such institutions as the government, universities, and large corporations. If the social mood is strongly anti-Establishment, as it was during the latter years of the Vietnam war or during the great depression of the 1930s, the amount of potential risk (real or fancied) that people are willing to subject themselves to is significantly less than they are willing to tolerate when the mood of the country is relatively complacent and sluggish, as it was during most of the 1950s, for example.

The Berg letter caused a great deal of controversy and even trouble for some of the scientists involved. Was it a necessary or even appropriate action for the committee to take, and should scientists in the future encourage the public to involve itself in genetic engineering laboratories? On balance, the answer must be affirmative. When asked to comment on it several years later, Nobel laureate David Baltimore, one of the signers of the Berg letter, said,

> I think the Berg letter was certainly necessary and possibly good. It was necessary because it represented a reasonable response to a request from the scientific community to consider the potential hazards in recombinant DNA. I think the letter may have been good because I think the initial statement was right—there was an unthought-out potential for hazard—and because we cannot shy away from actions that are right even if they are inconvenient.[13]

Because the letter was written by responsible scientists who were familiar with the process of recombinant DNA, it carried a tone of both scientific and moral authority that would not have been the case if it had been written by unknowledgeable laypersons. The fact that the scientists themselves were able to question their own actions is an encouraging sign, although serious conflict about liberty still exists.

What is the meaning of genetic disease?

Which is a personal and social liability, blue eyes or brown? Tawny skin or fair? Left-handedness or right? Down's syndrome or normal intelligence? The first two are easy to answer; the personal worth of a person has no correlation whatever to eye color or skin tone, nor do these factors matter to the way one lives. Left- or right-handedness is also irrelevant to moral worth, although because only about 10% of the population is left-handed, most instruments and other mechanical accoutrements of daily life are designed for the right-handed. It probably would be more convenient to be right-handed, but in general it does not matter.

However, the last distinction, that between a person with Down's syndrome (characterized chiefly by mental retardation) and one of normal intelligence is significant. It is safe to say that not only is Down's syndrome a tragedy for all concerned, it is an enormous social, ethical, and economic problem. No one wants to bear a child with Down's syndrome, and many women, when they discover that the fetus they are carrying is afflicted with the condition, choose to abort it. People with less than normal intelligence are scorned, neglected, abused, and even isolated from the general society all because of an accidental genetic configuration over which they and their parents have no control. Eye color, skin tone, and handedness are also genetically caused and are equally beyond human control. Why, then, is there such a significant difference between some genetic traits and others? What is a genetic liability, and what are simply differences among people? The answer must surely lie in social and cultural values. Some differences are labeled *genetic illness* because of the way society chooses to define illness. Shinn says that the meaning of the language used to discuss illness is as much social as medical. This is particularly true in the case of mental health and illness where societies can define a person as *mentally ill* and hospitalize him involuntarily if it so chooses. "If we broaden the concept of genetic illness to include genetic liabilities, it becomes still more obvious that some definitions may be arbitrary, socially conditioned, and prejudiced."[14]

In addition to human prejudice, a cultural life-style can determine whether or not a genetic factor is regarded as an illness. For example, a genetic predisposition toward being exceptionally thin is looked on as a quirk of body build by most of Western society (and regarded with considerable envy by those who must count every calorie). However, among the Eskimo and other people who live in the far North, thinness can be a dangerous and possibly life-threatening trait. It is also costly to the community because thin people must consume more food to manufacture enough fat to keep them from freezing to death (or alternatively, they must wear more clothing, which is also costly to the community). Hence excessive thinness would be a social and cultural liability.

Sometimes genetic liabilities are linked to genetic assets. For example, Shinn[15] notes that it appears that the sickle-cell anemia trait is linked to a capacity to resist malaria, which provides for a combination of qualities that has been advantageous for survival among some people in certain situations. In some cultures the ability to resist malaria may far outweigh the deleterious effect of the sickle-cell trait, whereas in places where malaria is almost unknown, it may be desirable to attempt to eliminate sickle-cell anemia. The ethical dilemmas become quite apparent in cases such as these. In other words, should manipulation of genetic structure be considered in view of geographic area? If, for example, the sickle-cell trait is bred out of a certain group of people, those people will be constrained from going to a place where malaria is endemic. By the same token, what if malaria suddenly increases in incidence and virulence? Those people who no longer are subject to sickle-cell disease will also be easy prey for malaria, and the intended beneficence of the geneticists will backfire. Should the genetic restructuring have been done in the first place in view of the always uncertain future?

One famous example of the value components of genetic traits is the Boston XYY case.[16] It provides an excellent illustration of what can happen when a particular genetic configuration is believed to contain moral characteristics. During the 1960s several studies revealed that about 2% of the inmates of mental-penal institutions had the XYY chromosome type (XY is normal in males, that is, one female and one male chromosome). Chromosome studies done on newborn infants revealed that about 0.11% of all male neonates had XYY. It was hypothesized that the extra Y chromosome was the cause of aggressive or sexual psychopathology. The reports received wide attention in the public media and raised the serious possibility of social stigmatization of male infants born with XYY, although statistically the vast majority of XYYs do not end up in institutions. There was no logical reason to predict that males born with XYY would be likely to engage in aggressive antisocial behavior.

Despite the lack of a workable hypothesis, some scientists elected to study behavioral development in males with XYY. One study was conducted by Dr. Stanley Walzer and Dr. Park Gerald in Boston. The study involved both genetic screening and a detailed psychologic and behavioral study of these children. Newborn infants were subjected to chromosomal study and distinguished as one of the three following types: those with an extra X chromosome (Klinefelter's syndrome), those with an extra Y, and those with balanced chromosomes. A 20-year follow-up study was planned that involved interviews with the parents of children with abnormal chromosomal configuration by a scientist who knew that the children were affected and behavioral observations and testing by a scientist who did not know which children were affected and which were not. School and home behavior were observed. "An unusual component of this program has been its willingness to intervene therapeutically in the event that some specific treatable disabilities are detected."[17] Therein lies the ethical dilemma. If only a small minority of XYY children (statistically predicted to be 3%) will engage in aggressive antisocial behavior, two problems immediately become evident: which are the 3%, and should the remaining 97% also be treated? There are other issues as well. The study assumes that future antisocial behavior can be predicted and that causes of the behavior will be genetic, but no proof exists for either assumption. If proof existed, what treatment modality would be used, and would benefits of any treatment chosen be worth the risks? What kind of information should be given to parents? Considering the sketchiness of information available to scientists, why would parents consent to participation in such research?

The study was eventually halted but not before great controversy had arisen. The question of whether the study should continue was taken up first by the Harvard Medical School committee on medical research, then by the human studies committee, and finally by the entire medical school faculty. These three bodies voted in favor of continuing the study, but several lay groups (Science for the People and Children's Defense Fund, for example) were bitterly opposed to it and continued to fight to have it terminated. Finally Walzer stopped the screening portion of the study because of the emotionally exhausting atmosphere caused by the controversy.

It seems that the only benefits of the Boston XYY study, if any can be found, are purely observational, and even this aspect is fraught with danger. If parents know why their child is being so assiduously observed (to give informed consent, they would have to be aware of the scientists' hypotheses), would not their behavior toward their child be affected? If they knew the hypothesized correlation between the XYY chromosomal type and antisocial behavior, would their mode of raising their child affect this behavior and thus negate the study results? Would the parents misinterpret every childhood aggressive act and punish it severely, possibly increasing future aggression by significantly altering the parent-child relationship? They could, on the other hand, adopt a dangerously laissez-faire attitude and remove all discipline and controls from the child's upbringing, thinking that whatever they did would have no effect because the child's behavior was genetically determined. Early diagnosis and screening might prove to be of some benefit if there were a definite treatment or known way to prevent the antisocial behavior that might occur in 3% of XYY children. Giving parents this information necessary for informed consent would automatically skew results of the study, but not telling parents why their children are being observed would violate a number of ethical principles. It seems that in this instance the possible benefits are not worth the risk; in fact, it is almost impossible to isolate and identify any benefits at all.

DO GENETIC DIFFERENCES HAVE MORAL VALUE? Why are we as concerned as we are about genetic disease, and why do we feel differently about genetic diseases than we do about nongenetic ones? In terms of human tragedy one might say that a child who dies of Tay-Sachs disease causes its parents about as much grief as one who dies of leukemia after having been ill for several years. But somehow, in a way that we cannot quite explain, the emotional component of the grief is different.

The history of the way we regard genetic disease (and to some extent congenital defects that are not known to be genetically caused) provides some indication of the moral value attached to them. Until recently persons who were born defective were regarded as mysterious, awe-inspiring, and terrifying creatures who, in many cultures, were isolated from the rest of society and untouchable by "untainted" persons. Sometimes the phenomenon of genetic difference, which was of course not recognized as such, was endowed with religious or mystic qualities, and many times it was thought to be the work of the devil. Fear that still lingers today was a predominant emotion surrounding genetic disease. Callahan expresses it well:

> But it would be a mistake to think that the old sense of mystery, awe, and terror does not live on. Surely the pervasive prenatal fear of bearing a defective child is not just because of the troubles of raising such a child, though that is a most serious matter. The fear seems much deeper than that, as if a defective child would represent a supreme undoing of the parents' image of themselves and reality. I am reminded of the conviction of many philosophers of antiquity that there is an irrational, irreducible, surd element in the universe, which constantly breaks through our visions and structures of ordered rationality. Genetic disease, long before it was labeled as that, was a case in point. One might in the instance of a hunting accident be able to discern a causal logic; the accident, however unacceptable, at least made sense. Genetic disease made no sense whatever; a defective child just arrived, out of some primeval darkness. A terror before the darkness still endures.[18]

We are now beginning to understand what happens in genetic disease, we can in some cases diagnose its presence or potential, and in rare cases we can cure it. But we still do not know why genetic disease and nondisease traits exist and what the causative factors are. One belief of those who do genetic research is that some genetic configurations should not exist and that human beings, via science and technology, can and should change those configurations. Callahan[19] indicates that this philosophy has some aspects that are not altogether positive. First, if genetic counseling continues to advance at its current pace, it will soon be possible to predict an even greater number of statistically significant chances of bearing a genetically defective child. From there it is only a small step to labeling parents socially irresponsible who choose to bear a child that they know will likely be defective. It is easy to see how genetic counselors could apply subtle or not so subtle pressure on parents, thus labeling their choice morally wrong and indeed lessening the value of the affected child. Society could then wash its hands of all responsibility toward these parents and children and provide them no financial or social support.

Second, cost-benefit analysis has become a popular exercise attached to all bioethical dilemmas. Its application to genetic matters could conceivably permit every child to be born with a price on its head. Again, Callahan sums it up beautifully:

> But let us observe a curiosity. It was counted a great advance of the modern mind when a bookkeeping God, with his minutely maintained ledger of good and bad deeds, was noisily rejected. Yet here we are, beginning to keep our own books, and using them increasingly as a determinant in deciding whether or not defectives should be allowed the privilege of birth, and their parents the privilege of parenthood. Moreover, we seem to have forgotten the reason why the bookkeeping God was rejected—because it seemed eminently unjust, insensitive, and outrageous that a scorecard be kept on

human lives. Indeed, we are even worse than the old God; for at least in his ledger everything was supposedly recorded. But our cost-benefit analysis totes up one item only— what the financial liability of the defective will be, what he will cost us in terms of taxes, institutional facilities, the time of medical personnel, and so on. Needless to say, this kind of reckoning is prone to be weak in comparing the costs of the defective against the cost of other patently foolish public and private expenditures which are accepted with barely a word of protest.[20]

Third, the concept of genetic disease, deformity, or difference must be compared with something, probably an image of a perfect human being. There have been various movements throughout history to achieve this ideal, but for the most part it was thought too expensive, technologically impractical, and socially undesirable. However, now that genetic engineering is a reality and developing rapidly, this ideal form again becomes possible. Callahan believes that there are already indications that the desire for perfection is increasing among prospective parents and that anxiety about producing a defective child is increasing, that is, that everyone must be able to measure up to some vague societal standard of perfection and achievement.

Fourth, the idea of social democracy where everyone has an inherent right to the opportunity for equality would be seriously jeopardized if the present trend toward desiring genetic perfection continues. In the past 50 years or so American society has made tremendous strides toward the humane care and treatment of "defectives," although this care is by no means completely adequate. All that could change if society decreased its commitment to the care of defectives.

There is no reason to believe that these rather unpleasant possibilities should be used as justifications to halt genetic engineering research, for genetic disease is surely a tragedy and determined steps should be taken to eliminate it. But these observations should give us pause to examine our social and philosophic attitudes about genetic disease; that is, how can we adapt to its existence while still striving to eradicate it? This involves a serious examination of the moral meaning of genetic disease and a determination of which, if any, moral values should be assigned to various genetic traits. From what we now understand about the nature of human genetics, it seems that all genetic traits are morally neutral and equal (that is, an XYY genotype has the same moral value as the trait for blue eyes or the one for Down's syndrome); the phenomenon that assigns moral value is the way in which we react to those traits and what we choose to do about them.

Advantages and disadvantages of genetic engineering

As stated earlier, there is no doubt that genetic engineering will continue despite whatever philosophic and scientific dangers lurk (an analogy can be made to current research in developing nuclear energy, which has sparked much public debate). There is also no doubt that genetic engineering will prove to have both beneficial and adverse effects on society. For example, although human cloning is not now possible, it is surely within the realm of probability. How will human life be affected when the genetic configuration of future offspring can be totally predictable? Creating "people to order" may not be only a bizarre fantasy if human cloning becomes commonplace—and legal. Part of the joy and tragedy of human uniqueness is its element of surprise, a characteristic that might be lost in cloned individuals. There might be decreased incentive to strive for achievement because a certain sense of potentiality might be lost, and we could be faced with a life much like Aldous Huxley's *Brave New World*: calm, ordered—and stultifyingly boring.

On the other hand, certain negative antisocial qualities could be gradually bred out of the human race. With the advent of cloning we would be less and less likely to read about the senseless, unprovoked, and random murder that has become a part of daily life, for persons who exhibit violent behavior simply would not be considered candidates for clonal parenthood. However, by making such a decision, members of society will find themselves at the top of that ethically dangerous slippery slope—determining which human behaviors are too negative to be allowed. How will differences be drawn between "too negative," "questionably negative," and merely unlikeable but morally neutral behavior? Should the human race become so homogenized, bland, and "good" that it might slowly grind to a halt from sheer inertia?

In the future, when asexual reproduction is a viable choice, what will happen to the always tenuous relationship between men and women? If each person has the ability to reproduce without the physical presence of a person of the opposite sex, how will the feelings that men and women have toward each other change? Will whatever natural animosities that exist now increase in scope and depth because there is no longer a reason to need each other for reproductive purposes? Or will that lack of need relieve some of the other tensions that exist between the sexes and improve the relationship? Natural reproduction will still continue in the present manner unless geneticists so drastically change human nature that the ability to reproduce sexually is "engineered out." Since this is a remote possibility, will men and women take advantage of this reproductive choice and begin to see each other as persons to be enjoyed for themselves sexually, emotionally, and intellectually without the tension of regarding each other as marriage partners and parents? Will homosexuality increase or decrease? And what of the institution of marriage itself; if one wishes to be a clonal parent, will one still want to participate in a formal marriage, or can the form and legality of marriage change? Infertile men and women will surely find asexual reproduction beneficial if the presence of another person's traits is not important to the goal of parenthood.

And what of the asexually produced child; what kind of bond will it have with its parents? One could imagine that a married couple with a child who is the genetic duplicate of one parent and not at all genetically related to the other may develop some interpersonal problems, both in terms of their marriage and in raising the child. What could be expected in the way of individual development on the part of a child who is the genetic duplicate of one parent? If he is fully aware of that part of his future that is genetically determined, he might grow up with a lessened sense of excitement about or anticipation of the future. A way to counteract this problem is to rear children in an environment completely removed from their parents to provide them with a sense of individuality and purpose. But as the Israeli social experiment of raising children on a communal basis with greatly decreased parental input has shown, this method of childrearing is a mixed blessing. Asexual reproduction will be problematic for parents and possibly devastating for children.

Genetic engineering could prove to be an irony; that is, certain techniques may turn out to be beneficial to individuals but may be detrimental to society as a whole. Or the opposite may be true in that the process of natural selection will be disrupted—to either a positive or a negative end.

Physicians, scientists, and genetic counselors will find themselves faced with increasingly difficult dilemmas about the conflict between the individual and societal good. For example, a woman carrying a child with a known and severe genetic defect will have to decide whether to abort or to bear the child, or perhaps submit to an in utero surgical technique. It will be the physician or the genetic counselor who will stress the advantages and disadvantages of each choice. They can also withhold certain information, thereby applying coercive factors to the woman's decision-making process. Bearing the child might be a desirable individual choice for the woman, but if societal resources for the care of defective children have been reduced, her choice will be limited by circumstances. The woman then may experience strong societal pressure to abort, which might have a strong adverse personal effect.

Again genetic engineering might ultimately be highly successful in eradicating certain genetic defects or diseases, but in the process the gene pool will be significantly altered, a change that undoubtedly will mean a narrowing, rather than a widening, of available genetic configurations. Although some might believe this to be intellectually and socially desirable, it would surely be an evolutionary disaster in that human adaptability, which has always been one of the species' greatest strengths, would be severely curtailed, and environmental changes of significant magnitude could leave the species defenseless and faced with eventual extinction. It is, however, endlessly fascinating to speculate how and in what manner these changes would take place, and it opens up possibilities for debate about the question of how much, if any, responsibility the present generation and the ones to come in the immediate future have toward generations of the distant future.

Genetics and human behavior

All human behavior springs from traits that Gottesman[21] holds are defined, explained, or described in the following three ways: (1) people differ in the way they behave, and those behaviors have commonalities or similarities that are called traits, such as aggression, kindness, and recklessness; (2) a quality or trait is ascribed to an actor instead of simply existing in the abstract; and (3) traits are named and grouped according to some kind of societal judgment.

The range and diversity of behavioral traits is almost infinite, and it is difficult, if not impossible, to determine which are genetic in origin, which are environmental, and which are a combination of both. This makes research in genetic aspects of behavior difficult to accomplish and highly questionable in its conclusions, as the example of the Boston XYY case showed. The field of behavioral genetics is extremely complex and uncertain because the cause and effect relationship between genetics and behavior is weak, that is, the biology of behavior remains unknown. Since these ambiguities exist, consumers of health-care services should be aware of the fact that hard data are almost impossible to obtain.[22]

The foundation for modern behavioral genetics was established by Francis Galton, an English scholar who was greatly influenced by Charles Darwin. In 1859 Galton's book, *Hereditary Genius*, was published (only a decade after Darwin's *Origin of Species*) in which he applied Darwin's theories of natural selection to the transmission of mental, especially intellectual, traits. However, Social Darwinism (the application of the principle of natural selection to social and economic institutions, a theory that is still hotly debated by sociologists) can be attributed to Herbert Spencer, an English philosopher who believed that certain behavioral traits could be used for perfecting the species. This formed part of the eugenics movement (about which more will be said later), which Spencer evolved into both a religion and a social policy. The combination of Mendelian laws, Darwin's theory of evolution, science's belief that the study of most sciences can help to solve many of humanity's problems, and the growing psychologic and sociologic knowledge of class stratification created a kind of conglomeration of data (and a good many unproved hypotheses) that formed the basis for behavioral genetics.

Scientists eagerly embraced, applied, and misapplied these ideas to such ills of society as feeblemindedness, insanity, pauperism, and alcoholism; contemporary research on the same problems (in modern clothing) must struggle with both the stigma of past distortions and the complexities of the issues involved in making advances.[23]

Variations in genetically determined behavior are assumed to arise from the simultaneous occurrence of many small polygenic effects that produce variations in phenotype (the observable, measurable characteristics of a person) rather than genotype, which underlies the demonstration of observable traits.

> A useful way to conceptualize the contribution of heredity to a trait is in terms of heredity's determining a reaction range.... It helps to remember that different phenotypes may have the same genotype, and different genotypes may have the same phenotype.[24]

However, it is impossible to assign genetic causative factors to particular behavioral traits as well as to predict future patterns of behavior based on either phenotype or genotype.

But what if some time in the future geneticists can isolate genetic behavioral traits, as opposed to environmental ones? And what if these traits could be transferred from cell to cell via the recombinant DNA process? It would not be difficult to envision parents who desire offspring with certain character or behavioral traits requesting a "nuclear plasmid transplant treatment," that is, having particular genes spliced into an oocyte and then either reimplanted in the woman's body or submitted for in vitro fertilization with the sperm of either her husband or an anonymous donor. It would thus be possible to create unique genetic sequences that do not now exist in nature or exist in so random a pattern that the chances of any particular offspring exhibiting that particular genetic sequence would be, for all intents and purposes, nil.

Racial and genetic differences

Most racial differences are obviously genetic. The typical eye shape of Orientals, skin color of Negroes, hair texture of Caucasians, and skin texture of American Indians are genetically determined. But what of other differences between races that may or may not be genetically determined, and if they are, may or may not be the basis for certain characteristics on which moral judgments are made? For example, what if race X is shown to have a genetic characteristic that, when developed and nurtured, will produce highly undesirable traits? Let us also suppose that although environment can have an effect on these traits, they are definitely genetic. Assuming that the behavior produced by these traits is not desired by society, what should be done about it? Should all embryos of race X be subjected to genetic surgery in utero to remove the trait? Should members of race X be prohibited from reproducing unless they are willing to submit to this procedure? Should all infants of race X be submitted to behavior modification techniques that will "erase" this trait before it has a chance to develop? Would it ever be justified to single out members of race X for special societal consideration because of a genetic trait over which they have no control and the existence of which is, in and of itself, morally neutral?

Examples of comparisons between social and genetic differences in regard to race can be seen in the history of blacks in their relation to whites in the United States. Although there are no racially pure boundaries between blacks and whites because of much cross breeding, for practical purposes blacks and whites can be identified as biologically and socially different from each other in many ways; and in many ways there are no differences. The differences that do exist, however, can be traced not only to genetic/racial ones but to historic background, educational levels, social variables, and present social and economic conditions. The question that is most ethically and genetically interesting is if whites and blacks differ in some behavioral characteristics, are the differences associated primarily with biologic ancestry (genetics) or with differences in social and cultural history (environment)? The question is difficult to answer on a purely empiric level, and it is complicated by sociopolitical factors. However, according to Loehlin,[25] there has been a good deal of evidence amassed over the past several decades about why such differences should exist. He describes some of the postulated reasons as follows:

1. Random samples of blacks and whites who are given standardized intelligence tests can be expected to differ in that whites score 10 to 20 points higher than blacks, although because intrarace differences can also be significant, there is no empirical reason to believe that IQ tests are an accurate predictor of intellectual performance.

2. The test score differences exist before school entry and "ordinary educational manipulations have not been notably successful in changing them. . . . " These differences have been fairly constant over the past 50 years, and attempts to match blacks and whites on the basis of socioeconomic criteria tends to reduce but not altogether eliminate the differences.

3. A wide variety of environmental conditions such as nutrition, general health, educational background, and even sleep patterns can affect IQ test scores to some degree. Therefore it is reasonable to conclude that some of the IQ score differences are environmental in origin, but it is impossible to know to what extent this is true.

4. There have been questions about the nature of the tests themselves; that is, do they measure only intelligence, or is there a hidden factor having to do with conformity to certain social norms? Can individual results on test scores be compared with group results; that is, how strong are environmental factors on test scores?

Although the argument about these observable differences in test scores can be expected to go on indefinitely, let us assume for the moment that there is indeed a genetic difference between blacks and whites as a group. Should this have ethical significance; that is, should blacks and whites be treated differently on the basis of differences in intelligence among large, randomly selected groups of people?

The answer, using either of the two major ethical theories, must be no. Intelligence, by itself, does not create happiness; happiness is created in part by what is done with intelligence. Therefore the utilitarian, in an effort to choose the action that would result in the greatest amount of total happiness, would not only not discriminate on the basis of intelligence, he would take those actions that would tend to make the most of intellectual capacity, thereby increasing total happiness. The deontologist would choose among any of several principles (justice and nonmaleficence, for example) and apply it to the act of discrimination based solely on genetic configuration and find it to be morally incorrect.

Are there, though, any instances in which it is permissible to take racial differences into account? One might, in the interest of social policy, wish to equalize certain opportunities, as occurs in the handicapping system of certain sports such as golf, in which the better player has to achieve a better than usual score in each individual game to give the poorer player an equal chance at winning. This handicapping system does not operate in all sports; in tennis, for example, no scoring advantage is given to the poorer player. In social policy as well, advantages are not given in all aspects of life, and there are those who believe that no advantage should be given on the basis of race alone.

It is important to increase the fund of general human knowledge by learning about genetic differences, but it is equally if not more important that the research be reported not only accurately but in a light in which it is least likely to be misinterpreted. With the exception of identical twins, individuals are completely genetically unique, but social, cultural, and racial groups have characteristics that can be identified as genetic in origin and that can be environmentally influenced. Some groups wish to preserve and capitalize on certain aspects of their uniqueness even though a particular characteristic may have been the source of tragedy in the past. And to preserve uniqueness is to learn more about it. The danger in paying a great deal of attention to certain genetic characteristics is that the knowledge gained can be used for social evil as well as either social good or simply a neutral acquisition of knowledge. Dubos[26] believes that knowledge about genetic differences is not as important as understanding the social context of those differences and that genetic structure is so dependent on the social structure in which it operates that any alteration in genetic configuration could have disastrous social consequences.

The question of justice frequently comes up in regard to the matter of race and genetics. A utilitarian would argue that the only just basis for the distribution of a certain societal good or benefit would be the performance of a particular action in regard to that good or benefit. For example, only those persons with a "sufficient" amount of intelligence should benefit from certain educational opportunities for the greatest amount of good or happiness to result. Deontologists, in particular a social contract theorest such as Rawls, would argue that just bases for the distribution of societal goods or benefits must take into account social position and arrangements, capacities and aspirations, past inequities, and human attitudes. Although it is now possible in some cases to prove empirically that some human differences are indeed genetic, arguments concerning justice raise the question of whether these genetic differences should be socially relevant. Rational theories of justice can be devised to prove different points. If one holds the theory that benefits or goods should be distributed on the basis of merit or societal contribution, then genetic attributes would make no difference one way or another. If one holds the theory that goods or benefits should be distributed on the basis of need or overall equality, then genetic attributes may indeed make a significant difference if a particular group has a greater need because of the results of a certain genetic configuration. Recent court cases involving reverse discrimination show what a complex dilemma this is.

Although the matter of retributive justice, which is based on retribution or punishment, is far too complex an issue to be discussed here, a few observations can be made. The central issue in regard to race concerns genetic determinism, that is, whether a person or group of people can be either expected to exhibit or excused from exhibiting certain forms of behavior because of genetic inheritance, such as the XYY chromosomal configuration discussed previously. Another issue is whether certain biologic groups differ markedly in behavior from other groups specifically because of genetics. A third and related issue is whether certain forms of antisocial behavior can be either excused or justified because of race. Although there has been some research in the area of behavioral determinism, it is far from conclusive and surely no social policy should yet be based on it.

Many argue that retributive justice should take racial contexts into consideration, not only for genetic reasons but also for environmental ones that are based on race. For, example, if a person from race X were to be caught stealing, and if he stole because he was poor as a result only of racial discrimination, should he be punished less harshly because of this, or should his race be irrelevant? The answer to this question, if there is one, may lie in one's views of ethical relativism as compared with ethical absolutism. Some philosophers have argued that behavioral determinism is not compatible with the development of moral responsibility, and some have claimed that social irresponsibility may have been an indirect cause of behavioral determinism.

GENETIC RESEARCH

Ethical issues in genetic research can be best understood in the context of ethical issues in scientific research in general. The basic issue here is freedom of scientific inquiry, that is, the liberty of scientists to pursue whatever research path they choose with little or no control over the nature of the research. Should scientists have this total freedom, and if not, where and how should controls be instituted? Those who favor scientific research with no controls hold that the acquisition of all knowledge is intrinsically good, that there is nothing that human beings should not know, and that scientists have no responsibility for the use to which the knowledge they discover is put. Knowledge is, they claim, in essence nothing more than ideas, which in and of themselves cause no harm.

Those who are opposed to total freedom of scientific research believe that although knowledge itself may not be harmful, its potential for evil will always exist in the uses to which it can (and probably will) be put; therefore science simply should not enter into certain realms of knowledge.

Both views must be taken seriously, especially since the emphasis and purpose of science has shifted from pure theory to practical benefits in the past few decades. This trend began with the Industrial Revolution and has gained momentum ever since; hardly any scientific research is now done only for the sake of increasing theoretical knowledge (the one notable exception is the science of astronomy). Given the fact that all scientific knowledge in some way affects human lives, all scientific research then has ethical overtones. And if knowledge is indeed power, then scientists with their incredibly arcane knowledge that is barely comprehensible to most of us could be the truly powerful of the earth.

It is too simplistic to say that scientists have no control over the uses to which their discoveries will be put; in many cases they can and surely should. The Manhattan Project was a good case in point. Scientists in the 1940s who worked on atomic fission knew that the ultimate purpose of their research would be a bomb that could kill hundreds of thousands instantly and have life-long effect on hundreds of thousands of others. I am not stating that dropping the bomb on Hiroshima and Nagasaki was morally right or wrong; what I am saying is that the scientists who developed nuclear fission knew that their research results would be capable of such devastation.

What, then, is the relationship between science and the rest of society? Jonas[27] sees the following four essential ingredients in this relationship: (1) much of science lives on the intellectual feedback from its technologic application;

that is, science creates technology, which in turn makes more science possible; (2) science receives assignments from the rest of society, especially corporate business; (3) science uses the most advanced technology and thus creates for itself more need for research; that is, science convinces society that it is indeed essential; and (4) the cost of science and technology is underwritten by the rest of society.

> In sum, it has come to be that the tasks of science are increasingly defined by extraneous interests rather than its own internal logic or the free curiosity of the investigator. This is not to disparage those extraneous interests nor the fact that science has become their servant, that is, part of the social enterprise. But it is to say that the acceptance of this functional role (without which there would be no science of the advanced type we have, but also not the type of society living by its fruits) has destroyed the alibi of pure, disinterested theory and put science squarely in the realm of social action where every agent is accountable for his deeds.[28]

The fact that science will end up in the marketplace creates a moral obligation on the part of scientists. The morality of scientists and the nature of their work can no longer be separate entities. It is also almost impossible to separate pure scientific theory from actual scientific experimentation because the development of theory causes a natural inclination (indeed, an irresistible urge) to empirically test the theory. And in the testing lies the danger. No reasonable person would question the right of scientists, or any other member of society, to have absolute freedom of thought. By the same token, however, no member of society has absolute freedom of action, and controls must be placed on scientists as well as laypersons. The dilemma comes in deciding where and how those controls should be instituted.

Present dangers and future benefits

It is most appropriate to use the recombinant DNA paradigm when discussing controls and regulation of genetic research because not only is it a present technology, but it has the greatest potential of any known genetic technology for both good and evil. It can be used to work almost miraculous wonders to benefit humankind, and it could be used for monstrous evil.

Partly because of the Berg letter, mentioned previously, and partly because of general debate over recombinant DNA and other forms of genetic engineering, the idea of government regulation began to be discussed in the mid-1970s. This debate involved (and continues to do so) the attitudes of scientists toward risk taking and exposing others to the risk of possible harm; scientists' attitude toward outside regulation (not generally a positive one); and the purpose of regulatory agencies and their past successes and failures. Underlying all this is the central issue of the comparison of risk to benefit, including the separation of facts from value judgments and an attempt to exclude emotionality from the entire issue. Scientists are naturally inclined to minimize risk, and nonscientists lean toward emphasizing it, often to the point of hysteria. Because one can never isolate the absolute probability of the nature and incidence of accident in genetic engineering, whatever policies and regulations are instituted must be based on estimates, educated guesses. Inherent in this regulatory process is the willingness to accept risk (for example, to go ahead with a manned lunar landing knowing that, despite all evidence to the contrary, some pathogen may exist on the moon that could prove ultimately harmful to humans on earth).

The risks we are willing to take are predicated on the benefits that are expected to be gained. But the "catch-22" of genetic research, because it is so new an endeavor, is that one cannot predict these risks and benefits. For this reason Dismukes[29] proposes several principles as follows for research when the risks and benefits are hazy at best:

1. The potential benefit to society of such research should be proportional to the scientific importance of the fundamental discovery. In other words, whatever benefits are gained should be practically applicable and not useful only in theory.
2. Because scientists and the general public differ so markedly in what is considered acceptable risk, there should be vigorous public debate to explore the advantages and disadvantages of genetic research.
3. Because, with the exception of medical experimentation involving human subjects, scientific research has not been regulated, and the only constraints placed on its conduct have been put there by scientists themselves in the name of "good" science, more emphasis should be placed on the consequences to human life of the research rather than simply on the process of "doing" science.

The point, however, to any assignment of risk and benefit is determining the value to society of those risks and benefits. In the absence of hard facts about outcomes, society must remain neutral about whether the consequences of the research will be ultimately beneficial or detrimental. That is, if one has no way of knowing what will happen as a consequence of an action, it seems only smart to adopt a wait-and-see attitude, not to form opinions before there are facts on which to base opinions. When making normative decisions one cannot necessarily appeal to consequentialist theories because consequences may not be predictable, but using a deontologic base also poses problems. It is not always possible to know which principles apply, although one can make estimates of right-making and wrong-making characteristics of particular research on the basis of certain similarities to past actions. But decisions must be made even when complete facts are unavailable, and sometimes this must be done on the basis of an educated guess or calculated gamble, which is essentially what research is all about.

> What is the best policy for society to pursue? One that proceeds cautiously, fearing the worst when the outcomes of frontier research are largely unknown? One that is willing to take considerable risks—even as described in the "worstcase scenarios"? The ultimate practical decision would seem to depend on what sort of society we want to live in. There is surely some disutility attached to an outcome that fails to benefit people who might otherwise have been helped by research. But unless we subscribe to a research imperative that places freedom of scientific inquiry above all other values when potential danger lurks, we need to examine closely the value dimensions of each instance of decision making under uncertainty.[30]

At the crux of this issue, however, is the power that human beings have over their own nature and that outside their immediate selves. Each generation succeeds in controlling nature a bit more than the preceding one, but in each generation exists only a tiny fraction of all the people who are yet to be. Should a few thousand existing persons and a few thousand still to be born be given power to control the nature of billions? Each measure of power that human beings win or exert over nature is also power over others because human beings and nature are inextricably bound to each other. Therefore how much power do we want to give ourselves over our present and future selves? How much liberty and autonomy are we willing to sacrifice for future generations? Should we let future generations worry about themselves, or should we take steps now to protect them? Shall we research, experiment, and satisfy our own intellectual curiosity because tomorrow we will not have to live in the disaster we may create today? Or should we take the attitude that today's research will lead to advances in solving problems that will surely be with us tomorrow and forever, for example, genetic malformation and hereditary disease, pain and aging, viral infections that decimate large segments of the population, and starvation? All these problems of human existence have some chance of being solved or at least partially alleviated by genetic engineering, and all involve considerable risk that we may or may not be correct in taking.

Public policy

In 1975 a conference at Asilomar was called by a group of prominent scientists who had pioneered research in recombinant DNA.[31] The purpose of the conference was to review scientific progress and to discuss appropriate ways to deal with actual and potential hazards. Although the scientists convened at Asilomar were not members of a government regulatory agency, the recommendations and principles of the conference had all the earmarks of public policy. Two major principles were that (1) containment (of potentially hazard-ous research material) is to be made an essential consideration of research design and (2) the effectiveness of the containment procedures should match as closely as possible the estimated risk. The conferees also discussed possible technologic means to accomplish this containment and decided that experi-ments were to be graded according to degrees of anticipated risk from minimal (which was not defined) to high, which was defined as carrying a serious potential for ecologic disruption or the pathogenicity of a modified organism that could create a serious biohazard. The conferees also distinguished specific types of experiments that would be likely to result in particular risks.

Although the specific scientific recommendations resulting from Asilomar were important, the essential aspect of the conference was the willingness of scientists to publicly acknowledge the potential seriousness of research risks and to voluntarily place some controls on the manner in which experiments are conducted. There is, however, an irony involved. Since so little is known about the potential hazards of DNA research, it is necessary to conduct experiments to find out what hazards do indeed exist. There is risk in determining risk.

Asilomar marked the beginning of active public debate about recombinant DNA research; since then several states have held public hearings, and in the most dramatic public outcry, citizens in Cambridge, Massachusetts, sought to block the building of a recombinant DNA laboratory at Harvard University. The building went ahead only after a citizens' commission approved construc-tion plans. Several environmental groups have also become involved in the issue. Now that the public is firmly and irrevocably involved in the issue of genetic engineering, Callahan[32] believes public concern should concentrate on the following key questions:

1. Why did it take the public so long to get involved in the issues? Scientists did not deliberately keep the public out; in fact, the press was invited to conferences from the beginning. There is always a lag between a major scien-tific discovery and public interest in it, but the issue of recombinant DNA research took longer than usual to pique public interest. Callahan notes that the public did not take a real interest until some noted scientists spoke out on the side of the opponents. It seems that people needed these scientists to lead them into the fray. Although Callahan does not speculate about this, it almost seems that the public, at least in this instance, was waiting for a group of scientists to tell them how to think. The implications of the public's apathy about genetic engineering are frightening.

2. Now that the public is involved, what options are open, and how can issues be evaluated? The first option is to turn NIH guidelines (summarized previously) into law; this would apply only to federal grantees, not to private industries that do not receive public funds. Another option is to ignore the

present guidelines and begin debate all over again. A third is to call a full moratorium on all recombinant DNA research until public policy guidelines can be developed using the democratic process. Yet another choice is to appoint a presidential or congressional commission to study the ethical and social issues. Callahan favors turning the present NIH guidelines into law and at the same time establishing a commission to further study the issues.

3. What ethical and social criteria should the public use in judging and deciding the future of recombinant DNA research? Callahan points out that there has yet to be a public discussion of the issues that addresses both content and criteria. The public needs to think about scientific progress in general and about the ethical issues of genetic engineering in particular.

The development of public policy is a difficult issue to confront because the public, who will be the most affected by decisions, is not in a position to have sufficient knowledge on which to base a workable and fair policy. There are several levels to be considered in the formulation of that policy.

1. The agency responsible for creating and administering policy must also be responsible for clarifying and responding to issues brought to its attention by the public. This implies knowledge of the nature of the research and might therefore eliminate nonscientific bodies such as Congress or state legislatures.

2. Public policy must be evaluated on two levels, the technical and the social. Dilemmas arise in deciding which specific questions (such as how much should be spent on containment procedures to reduce risk) should be decided on which levels.

3. Public policy implies that rules and regulations will be established by law, which in turn implies that an agency will be established to authorize and administer that law. Both control (of scientific experiments) and accountability (to scientists and to the public) are inherent in authority and regulation.

> Any agency deciding policy affecting public welfare must be responsive to public values and attitudes. This is not guaranteed simply by accountability through Congress, as illustrated by the number of government agencies which have been co-opted by the industries they regulate. Several years of public interest activism demonstrate that responsiveness to public concerns is greatly improved when business is conducted in public view and discussion and comment are invited at each stage of policy making.[33]

The primary pragmatic purpose for research in genetic engineering is the cure or alleviation of human genetic disease; thus formulating public policy creates an emotional tone to the ethical dilemmas. This is compounded by the fact that many of the diseases for which cures are being sought affect only a small portion of the total population, and although it could probably be agreed that eradication of any disease is in general a good thing for society, there are still racial and cultural overtones to be considered. In view of this, Lappé[34] suggests three approaches to the formulation of public policy: the fatalist approach, the individualistic approach, and the social-welfare activism approach.

The fatalistic approach simply recognizes the existence of vulnerabilities in certain population groups for which society as a whole cannot be held responsible, for example, Tay-Sachs disease in Ashkenazic Jews or sickle-cell anemia in blacks. This approach, although it might satisfy those with a utilitarian bent, tends to be problematic in that the acceptance of the inevitability of genetic disease (although this inevitability, according to Lappé, has not been proved conclusively) would tend to create resentment on the part of those who suffer from the disease or who belong to minority groups in which the disease is prevalent. It also clearly violates the principle of beneficence and perhaps nonmaleficence if one interprets halting research in a specific disease as tantamount to causing an increase in the number of cases of that disease.

The individualistic approach provides for assistance to individuals by social institutions to better understand the genetic problem and to provide a variety of ways to deal with it. This approach recognizes the fact that genetic disease affects people's lives in a variety of ways and attempts to alter life-style and/or environment to help the sufferer. The individualistic approach suggests that public and private health-care agencies provide both direct care and education; it provides for laws that ensure equal access for the handicapped and research funds to study genetic disease.

The social-welfare activism approach uses principles of justice and equity that also apply to other aspects of society; that is, there is a collective obligation to correct genetic inequities, for example, to try to cure genetic disease. Rawls' social contract theory is one of the principles that is applied to this approach. The "difference principle" in his theory states that when conditions are found to be socially unequal, those factors that contribute to the inequality should be rectified. Society should be willing to devote resources to cure genetic disease (social contract theory can be interpreted to include a societal effort to cure other diseases as well because itself creates social inequities).

Even before one settles on one or a combination of these public policy approaches, it is important to understand how a society as a whole reacts to individual genetic differences. Blatant or subtle social stigmatization is probably the most common reaction, regardless of its basic motivation. There are, however, ways in which this stigmatization can be minimized. First, labeling a person handicapped or at a disadvantage in some other way because of a particular genetic configuration should be done as seldom as possible. The fewer detrimental labels that are attached to genetically "different" people, the more likely they are to think of themselves as normal and thus to lead relatively normal lives. Second, society should recognize that all three approaches (or a combination of any of them) in the formulation of public policy might be an appropriate course of action in any given situation. Of primary importance, however, is individual assessment of problems to best benefit human life. Third, it is important to know when and to whom to provide information. This may appear to be a particularly paternalistic statement, but in the example of the Boston XYY case, justifiable arguments could be made not to inform parents of the hypotheses made by some scientists.

GENETIC SCREENING AND COUNSELING

Genetic counseling is the discussion, usually with parents or prospective parents, of the probabilities of bearing a child with a particular genetic disease or trait. Counseling implies the existence of a problem (I shall assume as a given that the presence of genetic disease is indeed a problem); it also implies the imparting of information and sometimes advice, although the giving of advice should be held to a minimum if people are to be as autonomous as possible.

Genetic counseling is predicated on genetic screening programs begun in Baltimore in 1971 with a community-wide program to detect the existence of Tay-Sachs carriers.[35] Mass genetic screening programs tend to fall more under the rubric of public health than do genetic counseling services, which are classified as an individual health service. Sometimes the screening programs do not include counseling services, and clients are provided with raw data but no means to interpret them and no one with whom to discuss them. Although such programs could be said to benefit society as a whole, at least in theory, they often cause serious harm to clients.

Some screening programs are government mandated, usually by a state, sometimes by a municipal agency. Although the government's intent was probably beneficent, the result is frequently highly paternalistic and unethical. Some of the screening programs are actually compulsory, such as ones for phenylketonuria (PKU), which can detect the propensity for certain kinds of mental retardation that are largely preventable in many cases if detected in time. Mandatory and compulsory* state screening programs for sickle-cell anemia and Tay-Sachs disease have also received widespread attention, and there is considerable debate about the ethical permissibility of these programs. Veatch[36] presents one such dilemma in regard to sickle-cell disease in which an American accused the state of genocide. Wilbur Johnson and May Sanford, both black, decided to marry and have a family. When they appeared for the premarital venereal disease blood test, they learned that their state also required black applicants for a marriage license to be tested for sickle-cell disease.

---

*In this context *mandatory* means that the program itself is mandated by state law, and *compulsory* means that certain classes of persons are required to participate in the program.

Sickle-cell disease is autosomal recessive, that is, both parents must be carriers before there is a risk of producing a child with the disease. When both parents are carriers, each child has a risk of 25% of having the disease. Mr. Johnson had a younger brother who died of the disease; therefore both his parents were carriers, and the chances were 50% that he was also. About one black in 12 is a carrier of the trait. Two prospective parents who are both carriers have only the three following options: (1) risk a 25% chance for each child to have sickle-cell disease; (2) resort to artificial insemination with sperm of a noncarrier donor; or (3) refrain from childbearing altogether. Mr. Johnson found all these choices unacceptable and argued that mandatory testing for sickle-cell disease in blacks is an attempt by a white-dominated society to control the reproductive capacity of blacks and thus is tantamount to genocide. The government's beneficence in providing free information to blacks is merely a guise for frightening them and discouraging them from bearing children. He refused to be tested, as did his fiancée.

Mr. Johnson's point is well taken, although his rationale is not entirely accurate. Since there is no treatment for sickle-cell disease except for a degree of palliation, there is no point in making screening compulsory. Even if there were treatment, compulsory screening for one particular minority group does raise one's suspicions about racism. Tay-Sachs disease is also autosomal recessive, but Ashkenazic Jews are not required by law to be tested before marriage. PKU testing is compulsory, however, and is based on a specific rationale. It is also possible that if a parent refused to have a newborn infant tested for PKU, that refusal would be upheld in court. Syphilis screening before marriage and during pregnancy is required by law (mandatory) in most states, but syphilis is a contagious disease that affects public health and safety. Sickle-cell testing should surely be encouraged among blacks, and educational programs about the disease should be increased. However, one must question the state's right to interfere with an individual's right to bodily privacy and autonomy by making sickle-cell testing compulsory. "The responsibility to make informed parental decisions does not necessarily justify a compulsory information supplying program."[37]

Diagnostic methods

Murray[38] defines a gene carrier as a clinically healthy person who is heterozygous for a mutant gene that determines an autosomal or X-linked recessive trait. The carrier has two genes at the same place on a specific pair of chromosomes, and both genes carry the same genetic code for the function in question but differ slightly in structure. One gene is normal, and one is not. If two of the abnormal or mutant genes must be present to produce a clinical manifestation of the disease in question, it is termed recessive; if only one gene is required for a clinical effect, it is termed dominant. Carriers can be identified for some traits or diseases by taking an electromicroscopic picture of their chromosomes and then matching and pairing the chromosomes and arranging them in numerical order (this technique is known as a karyotype). Because some genetic diseases or traits do not become evident until later in life,

> the definition of the heterozygous gene carrier can be justifiably broadened to include any persons who carry in their genes or genetic material a genetic abnormality that may possibly produce disease in them at some time during their lives and can be inherited by their offspring in whom it may or may not produce a disorder of clinical significance.[39]

In theory it is possible to identify all heterozygous carriers of autosomal dominant traits before parenting and to prevent them from having offspring. This could, in one generation, significantly reduce the number of offspring born with a particular trait, and if a childbearing prevention program were carried out assiduously, the only offspring born with that trait or disease could be attributed to mutation. As the technology for genetic detection becomes more sophisticated, these programs could be carried to the point where all known genetic diseases could be eliminated. Obviously these kinds of programs are ethically insupportable, but since the control of genetic disease depends to a great extent on accurate diagnosis, we are left with the dilemma of when to institute genetic screening programs. Murray[40] identifies four instances in which this would be acceptable as follows: (1) when a defined high-risk subgroup exists in a population, that is, a group that runs a significant risk of genetic disease, such as Tay-Sachs disease in Ashkenazic Jews; (2) when a relatively simple and reliable detection test exists; (3) when couples who are both heterozygous for an autosomal recessive trait are willing to abort defective fetuses detected through amniocentesis or other prenatal diagnosis; and (4) when effective medical treatment is available for the affected individuals.

Although diagnosis of genetic diseases or traits may be highly desirable on an individual basis, mass diagnostic programs, especially when they are government sponsored (as they frequently are), present certain ethical dilemmas. Screening programs are usually conducted with a great deal of publicity, and if they are to be considered cost effective, as many people as possible must participate. At issue, then, is the concept of individual freedom. Although no programs are specifically designed to instruct people as to what course of action to follow, coercion always lurks behind the screen of "social responsibility" or "environmental genetics," two euphemisms that tend to create pressure not to reproduce in the event that an abnormal trait is discovered. The value of individual human life must be weighed against whatever social responsibility is perceived.

Abortion is also a major ethical issue because many genetic diseases are not diagnosed until a fetus actually exists. If there is no effective therapy for a particular disease and if the couple does not consider abortion an acceptable action (or if the disease cannot be detected in utero), there seems little reason to participate in a diagnostic evaluation, and the establishment of a screening program then has the earmarks more of research than therapy. Thus those persons participating in the research program become human subjects rather than clients. This can change the ethical focus.

Another dilemma occurs in the detection of X-linked recessive disorders in which the female is the carrier and the male develops the clinical disease. There are two major choices in this case: (1) male fetuses who are diagnosed as having the disease can be aborted and (2) female fetuses that are offspring of affected males can be aborted in an attempt to reduce the number of carriers, thus destroying an otherwise healthy fetus. Of course, one could take no action at all. In the first choice the decision is between a genetically defective child and no child, and in the second the choice is between a healthy child, who may later pass the disease on to other offspring, and no child. In a family that already has one or more affected children, the ability to make an ethical decision based on logical moral reasoning may be seriously clouded by emotional stress and a severe drain on financial resources.

Prenatal diagnosis carries even more serious ethical overtones than does karyotyping because of the existence of the fetus. Even if one is absolutely unopposed to abortion, the presence of the fetus changes the emotional tone of the problem, which can cloud the ethical issue even if it does not change it. Well over 200 diseases can be detected in utero, and there has been a significant amount of debate recently about doing too many amniocenteses, that is, performing the procedure when it is not necessary. But when is it necessary? When is the risk to the pregnant woman and the fetus (which is minimal but not nonexistent) outweighed by the need to know the condition of the fetus? Should it be routine for all pregnant women on the slight chance that the fetus is genetically or congenitally damaged? This proposal is both impractical and unnecessary for reasons of cost and risk. Should amniocentesis be performed on all women who have, or whose husbands have, a family history of genetic disease? The obvious answer would be yes, of course. But should these persons not be counseled to undergo karyotyping before pregnancy to avoid the risk of amniocentesis? Again yes, but they cannot be denied amniocentesis because they did not participate in genetic screening. One might wish to include all those women who, for a variety of reasons, run a higher than normal risk for bearing a child with a genetic or congenital disease, such as older women, who are statistically more likely to bear a mentally retarded child. Those women who have previously borne a child with genetic disease should surely have the option of amniocentesis, as should those whose husbands' previous wives have born such a child. However, making amniocentesis available might create yet another ethical dilemma. What rules, if any, should be made about the results of the amniocentesis? That is, if it is found that a woman is carrying a defective fetus, should she be required to abort it? Or should she be required beforehand to promise to abort it if disease is identified as a result of amniocentesis? The second requirement is not as hard hearted as it might first appear because if a woman would not consent to abortion even if the fetus is shown to be defective, one could question the purpose of exposing both herself and the fetus to risk and in using scarce financial resources for the procedure. The only possible reason to gain this piece of information about the fetus is to prepare psychologically and financially for the burden of caring for such a child, but this does not seem to be a sufficiently strong justification for amniocentesis when abortion would be unequivocably refused.

Screening techniques and programs

Genetic screening programs are either voluntary or nonvoluntary (for instance the PKU testing and syphilis screening described previously) and involve three different kinds of testing: detection of carriers, detection of affected individuals (both newborns and adults), and prenatal diagnosis. The Research Group on Ethical, Social and Legal Issues in Genetic Counseling and Genetic Engineering[41] (hereinafter referred to as the Research Group) of the Institute of Society, Ethics, and the Life Sciences described some principles it believes to be essential to the operation of genetic screening programs. The following is a summary:

1. The screening program should be based on one or more clearly defined goals that should be identified before screening begins. The Research Group believes that the most important goals are those that contribute to improving the health of persons who suffer from genetic disorders, that allow carriers of a variant gene to make informed choices about reproduction, or that move toward the alleviation of anxiety of families faced with the prospect of serious genetic disease.

2. The screening program should be able to demonstrate benefits to persons or couples who receive services such as genetic counseling, detecting asymptomatic persons at birth, and detecting carriers of variant genes.

3. The screening program should also contribute to knowledge about genetic disease by determining the frequency of rare diseases and the incidence and prevalence of all genetic diseases.

4. The operation of a screening program should not begin until pilot

projects have demonstrated that its goals are attainable and flexible enough to update procedures and objectives as new knowledge becomes available.

5. Committees should be involved in planning and operating the screening program, and mechanisms must be established to assure equal availability to all members of the community.

6. Testing should be accurate. The screening program must ensure the reliability of laboratory services, whether its own or an outside contractor's.

7. Compulsion of any kind must not exist in either the screening policies or in the childbearing practices of affected couples. Voluntarism must be assured. Screening must be done only with informed consent.

8. The Research Group believed that even though there is minimal physical risk in genetic screening, psychologic or social injury could be great because the programs are relatively new. Therefore genetic screening ought to be considered a form of human experimentation and subjects protected according to DHHS guidelines.

9. All policies and procedures for screening should be disclosed to individuals being tested and to the community in which the program is located. Results of all diagnostic tests should be made available to the individual or couple.

10. Well-trained genetic counselors should be available for interpreting diagnostic tests and for explaining options open as a result of the tests. Counseling should be nondirective; that is, the counselor should inform clients but should not make choices for them. There is an urgent need to define and establish appropriate qualifications for genetic counselors, but the quality and effectiveness of the work done by the screening program remains the responsibility of the program director.

11. Information about available therapy and its cost, the facilities for maintaining afflicted offspring, and the risks and benefits involved should be given to all clients. Decisions about whether to participate in the program are not possible without this information. Clients' privacy must be protected at all times.

The Research Group concluded, "Even if the above guidelines are followed, some risk will remain that the information derived from genetic screening will be misused. Such misuse or misinterpretation must be seen as one of the principal deleterious consequences of screening programs."[42] The most serious kind of misinterpretation involves labeling and stigmatizing people. For example, people who have sickle-cell trait are erroneously believed to be handicapped and unable to function. This can result in job discrimination and social isolation. Physical activities of schoolchildren with the trait have been restricted, and adult carriers have been denied life insurance coverage. None of these opinions is medically warranted; all are the result of public misinterpretation of fact. The Research Group believes that screening programs have a definite educational function to prevent or minimize such occurrences.

There are reasons to favor and to oppose genetic screening programs. A utilitarian view based on cost-benefit analysis would likely be in favor of mandatory genetic screening, at least for certain diseases that can be easily and positively identified such as Tay-Sachs disease or Down's syndrome. Not only would families be spared the emotional agony and financial disaster of a defective child, but society, which bears much of the financial burden, would be relieved of one aspect of health-care cost. The cost of a defective child can be reasonably calculated in terms of money and resources. Emotional costs can be acknowledged but not calculated. What of the benefit side of cost-benefit analysis? Are there personal or societal benefits to be gained by the birth of deformed children? The matter is entirely subjective and completely unanswerable. One sometimes hears of parental pleasure from the frequently sunny disposition of children with Down's syndrome, and coping with the crisis of a defective child can reveal strengths people did not know they had. But are these benefits? Other children have equally loving personalities, and there are more than enough family crises to test anyone's strength. Would a person honestly prefer to have a defective child than a normal one? If the answer is no, then finding a benefit becomes more difficult. However, even if no benefits exist and personal and societal costs become astronomic, it does not necessarily follow that genetic screening should be mandatory.

A deontologist would look at the right or wrong nature of the act itself and seek ethical principles in a given situation, regardless of consequences. The obvious moral principle in genetic screening is the liberty of individuals to reproduce as they please, or autonomy. Paternalistic arguments might center on the purity or determination of the genetic pool, societal cost, and even the unnecessary grief families might experience. All these arguments are pragmatic and all have merit, but they all eventually crash headlong into the fundamental concept of personal freedom and liberty. There is no way to get around this barrier unless one is willing to change many of the principles by which we live.

There are physical reasons as well to oppose genetic screening. Motulsky of the University of Washington and Neel of the University of Michigan have found that large-scale prenatal abortion could affect the diversity and quality of the gene pool.[43] Such programs could result in an inadvertent increase in genes for certain genetic diseases. For example, detection of affected males with an X-linked disease such as hemophilia cannot yet be accomplished in utero, although carrier mothers can be detected and the gender of a fetus determined. If all male fetuses of carrier mothers were aborted, the gene frequency would increase by 50% with each generation. There are, of course, diseases that could be eliminated by selective abortion, but the ultimate long-term effects cannot be determined. It is possible that by eliminating one disease by genetic engineering or selective abortion, a new and far worse mutation could occur with an even greater incidence. Perhaps some diseases hold others at bay.

Why do we want to rid ourselves of genetic disease? What do we instinctively dislike or fear about people who are born different? Is it that they are sometimes misshapen and ugly? Not all are. Is it that they will die soon and cause us grief? Some live normal life spans. Is it that we are forced to do something to help them? We could simply throw them into pits the way lepers and other outcasts were in Biblical times. Is it that they remind us of our own mortality and lack of perfection? Not everyone is forced to think about persons with genetic disease. Do they represent an intellectual challenge to cleanse or purify the human race? We are obviously not satisfied with ourselves the way we are.

Most of the fear of these different people and the desire to eliminate genetic disease is linked to a horror of what we are capable of producing and the guilt or shame that a freak or defective person could have sprung from a perfectly normal body. The ancients cast their defectives out of society so that they would not have to acknowledge or deal with them (Aristotle recommended that they simply be eliminated). Moderns retreat to their laboratories to devise ways to prevent them from coming into existence.

What actually is wrong with being different, or retarded, or deformed? Why are we so anxious that everyone be similar, smart, and physically perfect? There is, of course, nothing intrinsically wrong with being born with below-average intelligence, but society values intelligence. There is nothing immoral about ugliness or imperfection, but society values beauty and physical wholeness. Differences can be unique and interesting, but society values similarity and homogenization. These statements seem to imply that society is at fault for wanting to decrease or eliminate genetic disease. Disease or defect, if it causes suffering to the individual and to those who love him, should be fought and eliminated. Differences that are not intrinsically painful or dangerous to the individual are another matter. Being unable to cope with individual or psychologic differences is a grave societal problem, and it is then society, not fate or chance, that inflicts pain on the different person.

One must wonder why society values sameness so much, why intelligence is prized, and why we all strive to be as beautiful as possible. Parents often are blamed for bringing defective children into the world, especially if the defect could have been predicted by genetic screening or even by the couple's decision not to bear children together. Do we "then share with our ancestors the view that a defective child is a curse but then unlike them, provide no comfort whatever, other than the aescetic reward of praise or blame for socially acceptable behavior in the face of the curse?"[44] With the advent of the use of cost-benefit ratios in health care, society can find even greater justification for blaming parents and for encouraging people to do everything in their power to prevent the birth of a defective child. Even the language we use indicates societal values. *Defective, abnormal, diseased*, and so on are negative words when used in this context, and striving for physical perfection rivals religious zeal in some quarters. This is not meant to imply that diseases or defects in and of themselves are good and are to be encouraged; what is implied, however, is that society needs to reexamine its values about those people who are born different from the average. Can we continue to discriminate against or reward people on the basis of physical or mental characteristics over which they have no control?

Genetic counseling

Genetic counseling differs from the usual physician-client relationship in that there may be no overt disease to be treated, or if disease is present, it may not be treatable in the usual sense. The focus of treatment is usually on the future rather than on the present, the client is ordinarily a couple or a family instead of an individual, and the therapist is not necessarily a physician.

The American Society of Human Genetics defines genetic counseling[45] as an attempt to communicate to a counselee (individual, couple, or family) the diagnosis, genetic mechanism, prognosis, and alternative courses of action available to manage a genetically determined disorder. The counselor then guides the counselee through the decision-making process that should be consistent with the latter's psychologic, economic, and social function. Immediate and long-range goals are considered, as are religious values and ethical dilemmas. This rather concise definition covers a wide range of activities and possibilities, including, but not limited to, decisions about abortion, sterilization, divorce and remarriage, placement of affected children in institutions, coping with the knowledge of future disease in presently unaffected individuals, and grief and mourning. The presence of a genetic disease or trait affects an individual and his family on all levels of existence; therefore a genetic counselor must be able to function on a wide range of professional levels.

Most people who seek genetic counseling do so because they have in some way become aware of the existence of a trait or disease, usually as a result of a medical diagnosis. Most have been referred to genetic counseling by a health professional or by a layperson who has some knowledge of a community program. Many couples enter counseling when a genetically diseased or deformed child is born, either to the couple in question or to a close relative. Another common beginning is knowledge of a family history of a genetic disease or membership in a group known to have an increased incidence of a genetic disease. These persons frequently decide to have a "genetic check-up" before marriage or childbearing.

The counseling process involves obtaining a detailed medical history, a thorough physical examination, and a variety of laboratory tests including tissue typing and karyotyping. All information should be given to the client along with the statistical probability of bearing children with a particular disease or trait. Murray[46] divides the counseling process into four distinct parts as follows: (1) client characterization in which the intellectual, psychologic, and socioeconomic characteristics of the client are determined; (2) the educational aspect in which the counselor provides information, tries to teach the client about genetic laws and how genetic diseases and traits are inherited, and explains what reproductive options are available and what the consequences of each are; (3) evaluation of the explanation in which the counselor must be certain that the client has understood the facts and concepts and determined if the explanation has made an impact on reproductive decision making; and (4) immediate and long-term follow-up to determine the effects of counseling. These four aspects of genetic counseling occur to some extent simultaneously, and all four parts are equally important.

Genetic counseling requires both scientific knowledge and excellent communication skills, a combination that is difficult to find in a single person. Most counselors are physicians, a few are geneticists with doctoral degrees, and a small but growing number are nurses, social workers, and other nonmedical health professionals. Since each professional group brings specific sets of skills to the counseling situation, it makes sense to establish a counseling team. The physician has knowledge of specific disease entities, their clinical course and prognosis, including the likelihood of mental and physical handicap. The geneticist brings highly specialized training in the physiology and future history of genetic traits and diseases. The nurse or social worker brings experience in dealing with the way in which this physical crisis will affect the lives of the individual and family. This last is especially important because of the considerable social and psychologic impact of genetic disease. Because of the societal attitudes discussed previously, the person affected with a genetic disease (usually a child) almost always experiences a negative self-image and periods of severe depression. Parents frequently have strong feelings of guilt, shame, and anger that can be almost crippling in their intensity. They may not know what to do with the affected child, that is, whether or not to institutionalize him if that is an option, how to raise him within the confines of his mental or physical limitations, and even how to pay for the increasingly expensive care. All these aspects of genetic disease require counseling that is both knowledgeable and sensitive.

ETHICAL ISSUES. There are, of course, ethical problems in genetic counseling.

Perhaps the thorniest is the matter of confidentiality, that is, to whom does genetic information belong? This issue can be best examined by looking at a case presented by Veatch.[47] Mr. and Mrs. Edwall heard about the Tay-Sachs screening program at their synagogue. They decided to be tested because they were both Ashkenazic Jews and were planning to start a family soon. Mr. Edwall was found to be a carrier. The genetic counselor assured the couple that they would never have a Tay-Sachs baby, but she questioned Mr. Edwall about the rest of his family. He had two younger brothers who were both married and who presumably planned to have children. The counselor suggested that Mr. Edwall contact his brothers so that they too could be tested. He thought about it and came to believe that he was "not quite a man" since he carried this sickness in his cells. He felt ashamed and refused to inform his brothers. The counselor tried in every way she could to convince Mr. Edwall to notify his brothers, but he was adamant. If both brothers and their wives were carriers, the chances were one in 60 of producing a baby with Tay-Sachs disease (the rate in the non-Jewish population is about one in 600, which is very high considering the tragic course and end result of the disease). The counselor argued and pleaded with Mr. Edwall, but he still refused. Finally she wrote a discreet letter to both brothers.

In addition to confidentiality, several other ethical conflicts appear in this case. Does the counselor owe absolute confidentiality to Mr. Edwall, or are his brothers in sufficient jeopardy to warrant breaking the confidence? Does the fact that the counselor never asked for Mr. Edwall's permission to contact his brothers (she only requested that he do it) place the breach of confidentiality in a different ethical perspective, or would that be using a technicality to get around the spirit of the principle involved? How will the policies and ongoing practices of the genetic screening program be affected by the two letters? If the public found out what the counselor did, its confidence could decrease; is this risk worthwhile compared to the necessity of giving the brothers the information? To whom does Mr. Edwall owe primary responsibility—to himself in keeping private information private or to his brothers who might avoid major tragedy were it not for Mr. Edwall's personal shame based on unrealistic perceptions. How much responsibility do Mr. Edwall and the counselor have toward the brothers? They are aware of their ethnic background and presumably would be tested if they so chose. Does the counselor have a further obligation to suggest that Mr. Edwall receive some kind of psychologic help to deal with his feelings?

Perhaps the crux of the confidentiality issue is whether or not genetic information should be treated as the same as other medical information, or because it directly and indirectly affects the health of other persons, it should be made available to more people than usual. If it is considered as confidential as other information, then the person identified as having a trait or disease must give permission for release of the information, perhaps then preventing other persons from receiving vital information about their future health. If genetic information is considered "publicly owned," tragedy might be averted, but some individual privacy must be sacrificed. To justify this abrogation of privacy, one might consider genetic disease in some way analogous to communicable disease. Although one does not catch a genetic disease, it is transmitted from one person to another and in that respect might be considered public health information and reportable to a government agency in the same way that the law now requires certain diseases to be reported to the Center for Disease Control of the United States Public Health Service.

Another major ethical issue is the conflict between total freedom of reproduction and the responsibility not to perpetuate genetic disease. Genetic counseling should be nondirective, but there may be instances in which it is permissible to guide a client into one decision or another. If, for example, the risk of disease is 25% or higher or if the burden of the disease is especially severe, as it is in Tay-Sachs disease, the counselor may wish to be more directive than usual. If the family has poor resources to deal with genetic disease, such as lack of intellectual or emotional ability to cope, a history of being unable to deal with another affected child, or an attitude that demonstrates that the child will not fare well, the counselor may even go so far as to suggest that the couple not reproduce. This would indeed be a rather controversial position, but if one assumes that the right to reproduce at will is not absolute, the position can then be defended, particularly from a utilitarian point of view.

Another critical issue is truth telling. A physician or genetic counselor has a prima facie obligation to tell the truth to clients, but in the instance of genetic counseling there may be cases in which the truth would cause more harm than good, although this is most difficult to predict. For example, if it could be proved that the father of a fetus is not the husband of the pregnant woman, should the couple receive this information? The woman obviously knows that there is at least a chance of this being revealed, and she may choose not to tell her husband. The counselor may not know the nature of the marital relationship, and if this information is provided to the husband havoc may be created in the marriage. Another example is more uncommon but creates an equal or greater conflict. Sometimes a female is born with XY chromosomes. She looks and acts like a female but has undeveloped testes instead of ovaries. The woman can be sexually attractive and active as a woman, but she is sterile. Many counselors believe that these women can handle the fact of sterility but not the fact of being chromosomally a man; therefore the troubling facts should not be revealed. In these or any other instances of withholding the truth, the burden of proof *must* be on the counselor who is required to justify withholding all or some of the truth.

The matter of resource allocation is an important issue in genetic counseling and screening. For example, certain genetic diseases affect only a tiny minority of any given population, yet screening and counseling programs are enormously expensive and therefore not particularly cost-effective based solely on the number of people who will use them. On the other hand, we are morally obligated to alleviate pain and suffering wherever it occurs; thus cost-effectiveness might not be an appropriate criterion to apply to this ethical dilemma. The political clout of a minority group may have a definite effect on the amount of money spent on a screening or counseling program, although one would hope that this phenomenon plays a minor role in decisions of this sort.

LEGAL ASPECTS

The most dramatic legal decision regarding genetic engineering was *Chakrabarty*,[48] in which the Supreme Court decided that a human-made micro-organism is patentable and is considered a manufactured product. The product in this particular case was a genetically engineered bacterium capable of breaking down crude oil, a property that is not naturally possessed by any known life form. The United States Patent Office had rejected the application for a patent by claiming that life forms are not patentable. Lower courts agreed and stated that "micro-organisms are alive and . . . without legal significance for purposes of the patent law."[48] Chakrabarty and his then employer General Electric disagreed and took the case to the Supreme Court, which overturned the lower court ruling. In addition to recognizing the commercial and ecologic qualities of Chakrabarty's invention, the Supreme Court did not limit the kinds of life forms that could be patented. This opens the door not only to the invention of all types of commercially useful and profitable new life forms but also to the eventual development of new life forms far more complex than the unicellular animals now possible. Although it is not likely to happen in our lifetime, it is possible that someone in a generation to come will patent a new form of "human" life and thus might be able to exert a frightening amount of political, social, and economic control. One can only hope that the Supreme Court would then rethink its position.

As can be expected, not everyone is satisfied with the Court's decision in *Chakrabarty*. One of the major reasons to oppose the decision is that no prolonged public debate took place, although listening to public debate is a legislative rather than a judicial function. There is also the claim that Chakrabarty "did not create a new form of life; he merely intervened in the normal processes by which strains of bacteria exchange genetic information, to produce a new strain with an altered metabolic pattern."[49] This point is arguable; it may not be necessary to prove that a particular life form is completely new because if its metabolic function is significantly altered, then its life function is also altered, and it may as well be a new life form.

Opponents of *Chakrabarty* have a point, however, in that the absence of reasoned public policy could lead to both immediate and long-range ethical dilemmas. This policy can affect the openness or secrecy with which genetic research is carried out; that is, if the bulk of the research is done by private commercial firms with an eye toward an eventual patent, the flow of published research papers, which is the life blood of science, could be drastically inhibited. Scrutiny by scientists of work done by other scientists has always been an incentive to do better and better science; secrecy is not an appropriate atmosphere for the intellectual development of scientific research.

There is also the matter of scientists personally profiting from an invention or discovery. Although at first blush one might view the profit motive as acceptable in a capitalist society, on closer inspection this might present problems in terms of seeking the truth about natural occurrences, admitting to and correcting errors or wrong hypotheses, and the complete objectivity that good scientists strive for.

> Traditionally the primary rewards for scientists have been the process of discovery itself and the recognition of the validity of their discoveries by their peers. It might seem unfair to restrict the business enterprise of scientists—since such restrictions are not placed on other professions—but I worry about the effect of the profit motive on the quality of science and on the public's perception of our commitment to objectivity.[50]

Others believe that *Chakrabarty* will have little, if any, effect on the quality of the scientific process, although few deny that the decision will have a profound economic effect. Chakrabarty's oil-eating bacterium is simply another patentable scientific invention, nothing more, nothing less, and it should have no lasting effect on the future of genetic engineering, which will continue regardless of patentability. The granting of a patent may be no stronger an incentive to continue genetic engineering research than other incentives such as satisfaction of the intellect or the desire to cure genetic disease. The fact that granting a patent for a new life form will provide exclusivity to a particular scientist or group of scientists is probably no more damaging to the scientific process than is granting a patent for computers, xerographic equipment, a totally implantable artificial heart, or even a better mousetrap.

Patentability is by no means the only legal aspect of genetic engineering; there are several others that are equally pressing and that in fact probably affect greater numbers of people. The matter of reproductive privacy has already been established by Supreme Court precedents (*Griswold v. Connecticut* and *Roe v. Wade*), although it is of course difficult to know if the Court will continue to protect individual reproductive privacy. These interpretations of the right to privacy mean that a genetic counselor is required to be nondirective when providing information about alternative courses of action, and it means that a client has a legal right not to be coerced into a particular course of reproductive action by a health professional.

Of increasing interest, because of the increasing number of cases, are laws regarding genetic screening. Almost all states have some form of compulsory genetic screening, the most common of which is PKU testing. Many programs are aimed at racial and ethnic minorities, such as ones regarding sickle-cell disease. It seems reasonable to believe that the primary motivation of the state in conducting these screening tests is beneficence, but it is easy for legislatures to turn beneficence into paternalism—with no real evil intent. Therefore the essential ethical issue in regard to genetic screening is to determine if and when the state's paternalistic impulses have gone too far and have abrogated the individual's right to refuse those tests—and to receive sufficient information to do so intelligently.

No state now requires that genetic counselors be licensed, although several state genetic screening laws require some type of quality control in the education and employment of genetic counselors. However, there is considerable debate over the exact nature of a genetic counselor's function; therefore state legislatures seem to be undecided about how to examine and license them. It should be noted, however, that other occupational groups in the health-care field, such as nursing, social work, and physician assistants suffer from a similar "identity crisis" about the parameters of practice, yet they are examined and licensed by states.

A new and quite unusual legal issue in regard to genetic engineering, or more specifically to prenatal diagnosis, is the matter of "wrongful life." Although this is an incredibly complex issue, the essential ingredient is the claim by either parent(s) or a fetus/child against a physician who either knew of the existence of a genetic disease and chose not to mention it to the parents or who did an inadequate genetic and/or prenatal diagnosis so that the existence of the disease was not detected when it could and should have been. It is also possible for a child who is born with a serious genetic disease or defect to sue his parents for having given birth to him. In other words, the child is claiming that it would have been preferable not to have been born at all in view of his present and future suffering. These kinds of cases are unusual, even bizarre, and some would be tempted to say that they are totally absurd. The root of these tort actions can be seen as an extension of prenatal tort law, that is, that it is unlawful to harm a postviable fetus. To date there have been several tort cases regarding wrongful life. They will be discussed in more detail in the chapter on reproductive technology.

The last important legal issue in genetics is so pervasive that a full discussion would require at least several books. This is the matter of genetic hazards in the environment. Many are believed to exist, some have a proven causal relationship with genetic disease, and all are frightening to contemplate. The most common origin of an environmentally caused genetic disease is mutation, that is, a change of some type in a gene that then becomes a permanent part of that gene, which is in turn inherited by succeeding generations. Genetic hazards in the environment are divided into several classes as follows: x-rays emanating from a variety of sources; radiation in the form of the by-products of nuclear energy; and chemicals that enter the body in the form of food additives and polluted air and water. Environmental hazards, in addition to being genetically destructive to future generations, can be carcinogenic or teratogenic (causing birth defects in an existing fetus). There has been some legislative activity in the last decade or so, as well as a proliferation of government regulatory agencies to control environmental hazards. It is undoubtedly true that laws and the agencies to enforce them have decreased the amount of genetic hazards in the environment. But by the same token it is almost impossible to know what laws must be passed to protect future persons if research is not done now to determine which environmental conditions are indeed hazardous, in what way, and to what extent. Research about these conditions on humans presents a series of almost impossibly complex ethical dilemmas, and research on animals is only partially applicable to human physiology. There is also the matter of the dilemma of resource allocation; that is, how much should be spent on research that will affect only future generations when people now existing are suffering (or soon will be) from diseases that require vast amounts of money to cure or alleviate. How much of a moral claim do future persons have, and how can their claims be compared with those of present persons?

EUGENICS

Eugenics, or good breeding, is designed to improve the condition and capacity of a species. Stock breeding of animals is an example of eugenics. Dogs are bred to ensure more perfect physical composition and to achieve species perfection. Cattle are bred to perfect the ratio of edible flesh to fat and bone, and an effort is made to improve the quality of the flesh itself, to make it tastier and more tender. Horses are bred to run faster, and cows are bred to give more milk of higher quality. Although there are ethical dilemmas involved in animal eugenics (for example, is it justified to increase the possibility of negative or hurtful genetic characteristics in animals simply to improve the positive ones?), unfortunately we tend to ignore them because a social utility is served by perfecting species; we want plumper chickens and more milk in relation to feed consumed.

Human eugenics, however, is a different story. Although the idea of genetically improving the human race has been around since Plato (he presented several interesting eugenic ideas in the *Republic*), it has been only since the nineteenth century that social scientists and politicians have seriously proposed eugenic population policies. Most eugenic theories spring from a belief in what is known as either "naturalism" or "Social Darwinism," that is, that there is an analogy between biologic organisms and social systems. In other words, only the best social systems composed of the best people will survive. A person's genetic inheritance tends to be equated with his social position and general social "fitness." Social Darwinism also holds that the human race is capable of perfection, although the criteria for perfection were never fully delineated. Certain races or groups of people are considered genetically unfit for a perfect social system. The goal of eugenics, therefore, is to use appropriate breeding techniques to improve human genetic quality and thus to attain the perfection of human social systems.

The human eugenics movement gained momentum in the United States and elsewhere around the turn of the century when people began to understand the physical laws of heredity. In the United States the eugenic movement, coordinated by the Eugenic Record Office on Long Island, was divided into negative and positive eugenic programs. The goal of the former was to improve the heredity level of the American people by discouraging "unworthy parenthood," that is, by placing restrictions on marriage, encouraging sterilization of certain classes of people, and taking state custody of defective children.[51] Various state laws were passed that prohibited certain people (the mentally retarded, alcoholics, prostitutes, paupers, the insane, and the like) from reproducing. Many of those laws are still in effect. Positive eugenics was a program that encouraged people with certain traits and characteristics, such as intelligence, good social position, and higher education, to marry and bear children.

These programs, although seemingly elitist and unfair when looked at in the light of today's social system, were designed with beneficent intent. Social science and social psychology were, for the most part, nonexistent, and the United States was a young and more naive country that had yet to realize the horrendous social problems that modern life would create. These eugenic programs, however, almost completely disregarded many of the individual rights and liberties we now take for granted and flagrantly ignored some basic civil rights. Moreover, the racism implicit in any eugenics program cannot be disregarded, and one would hope that the Nazi experience taught a permanent lesson.

Davis[52] describes three basic patterns that could be used in a modern human eugenics program as follows:

1. Selection against monogenic defects. This approach has in the past depended almost entirely on estimates of probability, for example, statistics can predict that a certain percentage of children born to carriers of a genetic disease will be born with the disease. It is now possible to detect the presence of certain genetic diseases in utero while a decision for abortion can still be made. This eugenic method, although significant to the individuals involved, has an almost miniscule effect on the general population. Even if every fetus known to have a genetic defect were aborted, the eugenic effect would still not be statistically significant on a worldwide basis. Most hereditary diseases are genetically recessive and appear only when both parents have the same rare defective gene; therefore for each such "double" mating, there will be thousands of carriers who do not marry each other.

2. Selection of especially desirable germ cells. This approach involves the establishment of sperm banks (in the future when the entire course of pregnancy may take place in vitro, egg banks may also be established) to choose whatever human characteristics are deemed ideal or desirable by society. One might assume that parental pride would increase as superchildren become superachievers, but Davis thinks the voluntary aspect of this type of program would soon disappear, and all couples would be subjected to eugenic selection.

3. Differential reproduction of large groups. This is a rather euphemistic designation for the encouragement of certain groups of people to reproduce and the discouragement of certain other groups. Those people who have demonstrated superior achievements would be encouraged to bear more children than those who are considered less socially desirable. This eugenic method has strong racist overtones and would not be acceptable to a society that sees itself as egalitarian. It also would not result in a statistically significant change unless the eugenic program were made nonvoluntary and coercive. Davis proposes a compromise solution:

> Another eugenic approach, essentially ignored in the past, may be more likely to prove acceptable: one with the humanitarian goal of increasing human satisfaction, and decreasing misery, by minimizing the production of individuals whose genetic endowment would seriously limit their capacity to find a sense of usefulness and fulfillment in a complex world. In this approach an improved endowment would not be an alternative to an improved environment, but the two would be complementary approaches to the solution of persistent social problems.[53]

This is an extremely value-laden view that essentially advocates preventing the birth of all individuals who cannot accommodate to the present social and physical environment. It would be practical if one could positively identify and define all those factors that increase satisfaction and decrease misery. It also depends on knowing what capacities lead to a sense of "usefullness and fulfillment in a complex world." If this theory were to be put into practice, we would require total agreement on all subjective components of life and the means to achieve these desired goals. If everyone were to agree on what promotes happiness and decreases misery, individual differences might disappear, and we would be a truly homogenized society. At that point it might not seem terribly outrageous to make cloning a routine part of life.

Davis finds several trends and advantages in the development of a eugenic program as follows:

1. Since population needs to be controlled anyway, it might make sense to restrict the growth of certain population segments by various licensing or incentive procedures. The gene pool would surely be unalterably affected.

2. Knowledge about genetics would increase and would become more important in the study of psychology, sociology, education, and even economics. A firm genetic base might be used to measure and predict all sorts of human endeavors.

3. Those sections of the country where biology is taught without mention of evolutionary principles would be forced to acknowledge the enormous role of genetics in human development.

4. Increased knowledge could be expected to equalize the sharing of societal goods and opportunities. If it can be definitely proved that people of certain genetic makeup have more difficulty coping with the world or succeeding in it, would it not be kinder to prevent them from being born at all? This could apply to people with mental as well as physical defects. Indeed society could define *defect* in any way it chose and could impose a genetic program that conformed to the definition and shifted with changing societal values.

Whatever eugenic or genetic technology is developed will surely be put to some use. We are too pragmatic a society to ignore or prohibit a new technologic tool without first investigating its use.

Ethical issues

These observations about what could be done with a eugenic program are at the same time fascinating and terrifying. The potential for both good and evil is limitless. Racial prejudice could be either eliminated totally by eventually having only one race or drastically increased by restricting or encouraging the population growth of certain races. We could make human beings supremely adaptable to changing environments, or we could breed out our present remarkable ability to adapt. In creating breeds of superpeople of pure genetic makeup, however, we might wish we had not eliminated the mongrelization that adds to our hardiness and adaptability. Presumably a eugenic program would encourage breeding of intelligent people with the hope that the species would grow smarter. Society, which now depends on people with average or low intelligence to carry out some of the routine tasks of keeping the wheels in motion, would perhaps be unable to maintain itself. Automation can take us only so far. If no one wanted to be assembly line workers, keypunch operators, telephone operators, and bus drivers, the fabric of life would change. Consider what happens now in England or Italy during a general strike; life is changed for the duration of the strike because essential services are halted. Multiply that times forever if the entire world were composed of geniuses.

Evolution would be unalterably affected by eugenics, and it is impossible to know whether it would be for good or ill. Eugenics is as fascinating as it is frightening, and the desire to experiment with human genes just to see what would happen is incredibly strong. To tell a scientist that intellectual curiosity must be stifled because the future of humanity is on his and his colleagues' shoulders is to place an unreasonable burden on the scientific community. Society supports the idea of creative science, and to prohibit some of it would be to deny the intellectual curiosity that is an integral part of human nature.

In a eugenics program there are, however, some specific ethical issues—even dangers—that should be briefly enumerated. The first is the objective of the program, which has already been discussed. It is the foundation for other ethical issues. The danger of beneficence turning to paternalism or outright evil is all too real, as recent history has shown. The second issue is the matter of values, that is, which human characteristics are valued by society and which are devalued. And when these questions are answered, if ever they can be, what should a society choose to do about the answers? In other words, should a eugenics program exist at all? If the answer is affirmative, then the third issue comes into play: which principles should be used as a basis for the program? Should the theory supporting those principles be utilitarian or deontologic? Considering what we know about the fundamentals of both theories, it is clear that supporting a eugenics program would be relatively easy for a utilitarian and quite difficult for a deontologist. In fact, it would be difficult if not impossible for a deontologist to support a eugenics program. The fourth issue is decision making. It is one thing for a society to define which human characteristics it finds desirable and which it does not; it is quite another thing to make hard and fast decisions about actual genetic engineering, that is, which genes to chemically obliterate in which people.

SUMMARY

Although it is a frightening and awe-inspiring prospect, it is now possible to manipulate the genetic structure of vegetables and some lower forms of animals to alter their life forms. The ability to do the same in humans is simply a matter of time and developing technology. The technologies currently in use and those being rapidly developed even as these words are written include enzyme replacement, transformation of DNA molecules from one individual to another, transduction of DNA molecules from viral carriers to humans, cell fusion for the purpose of hybridization, four-parent individuals, cloning, and recombinant DNA. The latter has the greatest and most practical possibilities for use in humans.

While the technology of genetic engineering is fascinating in itself, it is the ethical issues that present the most complex questions; that is, even though we can do certain things with genes, should we indeed do them? The issues have implications both for individual human lives and for the human race itself. Ethical questions are concerned mainly with the value of genetic health (and what we mean by genetic disease), who should decide about matters of genetic engineering, and how the conflicts that arise between individual reproductive freedom and the good of society should be resolved. Also important are matters of consequences; that is, even if a course of action would be ultimately beneficial to society, should it indeed be taken; matters of confidentiality, or to whom does genetic information rightfully belong; and matters of abortion and/or enforced sterilization. Moreover, one might want to ask what the ultimate nature of human life is, how we can be certain of the answer, and if we find it, what we should do about it. One might also ask whether genetic traits or diseases should be assigned moral value, and if so, how this should be done. For example, are green eyes better than brown, and does a person with Down's syndrome have a greater or lesser moral value than one who does not? On what basis is this value judgment made?

Other ethical issues to be taken into consideration when thinking about and undertaking genetic engineering are the differences between racial and genetic characteristics; the separation of genetic factors from sociocultural ones; the distribution of justice when allocating research funds for studying genetic disease; deciding which ethical principles ought to be the foundation for public policy in genetic engineering; and whether or not humans should indeed interfere in the natural course of evolution. Should we take evolutionary risks with the human race?

Genetic screening and counseling present separate but related issues that involve matters of personal reproductive liberty and the right to privacy in reproductive matters; the relationship of genetic counselors to clients; matters of confidentiality of information; when, if ever, the state should make certain screening programs mandatory and/or compulsory; and how social and psychologic issues can be separated from ethical ones.

Eugenics is the attempt to improve the condition or capacity of a species by means of breeding techniques. Eugenics programs began in earnest around the turn of the century when sufficient scientific knowledge about heredity became available. The programs began in a more or less beneficent way, but they quickly turned paternalistic and even downright evil. Eugenics programs seriously undermine individual liberty in regard to reproduction and disregard other civil and legal rights as well.

Notes

1. Veatch, R. M. *Case studies in medical ethics*. Cambridge, Mass.: Harvard University Press, 1977. pp. 194–197.
2. Davis, B. D. Prospects for genetic intervention in man. *Science*, 1970, *170*, 1279.
3. Davis, p. 1279.
4. Fromer, M. J. *Ethical issues in health care*. St. Louis: The C.V. Mosby Co., 1981. p. 67.
5. Eisenberg, L. The outcome as cause: predestination and human cloning. *The Journal of Medicine and Philosophy*, 1979, *1*(4), 318–331.
6. Eisenberg, pp. 318–331.
7. Eisenberg, p. 322.
8. Cohen, S. N. Recombinant DNA: fact and fiction. *Science*, 1977, *195*(4279), 654–657. © 1977 by the American Academy for the Advancement of Science.
9. Cohen, p. 654.
10. Callahan, D. The moral career of genetic engineering. *Hastings Center Report*, 1979, *9*(2), 9.
11. Callahan, p. 9.
12. Sinsheimer, R. Troubled dawn for genetic engineering. *New Scientist: The Weekly Review of Science and Technology* (London), October 16, 1975.
13. Baltimore, D. The Berg letter: certainly necessary, possibly good. *Hastings Center Report*, 1980, *10*(5), 15. Reprinted with permission of The Hastings Center.© Institute of Society, Ethics and the Life Sciences, 360 Broadway, Hastings-on-Hudson, N.Y. 10706.
14. Shinn, R. L. Gene therapy: ethical issues. In W. T. Reich (Ed.), *Encyclopedia of bioethics*. New York: The Free Press, 1978. p. 521.
15. Shinn, p. 522.
16. Roblin, R. The Boston XYY case. *Hastings Center Report*, 1975, *5*(4), 5–8.
17. Roblin, p. 6.
18. Callahan, D. The meaning and significance of genetic disease: philosophical perspectives. In Hilton, B., et al. (Eds.), *Ethical issues in human genetics: genetic counseling and the use of genetic knowledge*. New York: Plenum Publishing Corp., 1973. p. 84.
19. Callahan, p. 84.
20. Callahan, p. 86.

21. Gottesman, I. I. Genetic aspects of human behavior: state of the art. In *Encyclopedia of bioethics*, p. 528.
22. Gottesman, p. 528.
23. Gottesman, p. 529.
24. Gottesman, p. 530.
25. Loehlin, J. C. Genetic aspects of human behavior: race differences in intelligence. In *Encyclopedia of bioethics*.
26. Dubos, R. Genetic constitution and environmental conditioning. In *Encyclopedia of bioethics*, p. 549.
27. Jonas, H. Freedom of scientific inquiry and the public interest. *Hastings Center Report*, 1976, 6(4), 16. Reprinted with permission of The Hastings Center:© Institute of Society, Ethics, and the Life Sciences, 360 Broadway, Hastings-on-Hudson, N.Y. 10706.
28. Jonas, p. 16.
29. Dismukes, K. Recombinant DNA: a proposal for regulation. *Hastings Center Report*, 1977, 7(6), 13. Reprinted with permission of The Hastings Center:© Institute of Society, Ethics, and the Life Sciences, 360 Broadway, Hastings-on-Hudson, N.Y. 10706.
30. Macklin, R. On the ethics of *not* doing scientific research. *Hastings Center Report*, 1977, 7(6), 13. Reprinted with permission of The Hastings Center:© Institute of Society, Ethics, and the Life Sciences, 360 Broadway, Hastings-on-Hudson, N.Y. 10706.
31. Berg, P., et al. Asilomar conference on recombinant DNA molecules. *Science*, 1975, *188*(4192), 991–994.
32. Callahan, D. Recombinant DNA: science and the public. *Hastings Center Report*, 1977, 7(2), 20.
33. Dismukes, p. 28.
34. Lappé, M. Humanizing the genetic enterprise. *Hastings Center Report*, 1979, 9(6), 10–14.
35. Veatch, p. 201.
36. Veatch, pp. 202–205.
37. Veatch, p. 205.
38. Murray, R. F. Genetic diagnosis. In *Encyclopedia of bioethics*, p. 555.
39. Murray, p. 555
40. Murray, p. 556.
41. The Research Group on Ethical, Social, and Legal Issues in Genetic Counseling and Genetic Engineering of the Institute of Society, Ethics, and the Life Sciences. Ethical and social issues in screening for genetic disease. *New England Journal of Medicine*, 1972, *286*, 1129–1132.
42. Research Group, pp. 1129–1132.
43. Friedmann, T. Prenatal diagnosis of genetic disease. *Scientific American*, 1971, *255* (5), 34–342.
44. Callahan (The meaning and significance), p. 84.
45. Murray, R. F. Genetic counseling. In *Encyclopedia of bioethics*, pp. 559–560.
46. Murray (Genetic counseling), p. 561.
47. Veatch, p. 205.
48. *Diamond, Commissioner of Patents and Trademarks v. Chakrabarty*, 79 U.S. 136 (June 16, 1980).

49. Dismukes, K. Life is patently not human-made. *Hastings Center Report*, 1980, *10*(5), 11. Reprinted with permission of The Hastings Center:© Institute of Society, Ethics and the Life Sciences, 360 Broadway, Hastings-on-Hudson, N.Y. 10706.
50. Dismukes, p. 12.
51. Ludmerer, K. M. Eugenics: history. In *Encyclopedia of bioethics*, p. 458.
52. Davis, B. D. Threat and promise in genetic engineering. In P. N. Williams (Ed.), *Ethical issues in biology and medicine: proceedings of a symposium on the identity and dignity of man*. Cambridge, Mass.: Schenkman Publishing Co., Inc., 1972.
53. Davis, p. 27.

Bibliography

Abrams, M. Frogs, asparagus, and you—the real meaning of cloning. *Today* (Philadelphia Inquirer), October 29, 1978, pp. 14–38.

Anderson, W. F. Genetic therapy. In M. P. Hamilton (Ed.), *The new genetics and the future of man*. Grand Rapids, Mich.: Wm. B. Eerdmans Publishing Co., 1972. pp. 109–124.

Annas, G. J. Righting the wrong of 'wrongful life'. *Hastings Center Report*, 1981, *11*(1), 8–9.

Baltimore, D. The Berg letter: certainly necessary, possibly good. *Hastings Center Report*, 1980, *10*(5), 15.

Beauchamp, T. L. & Walters, L. *Contemporary issues in bioethics*. Belmont, Calif.: Wadsworth Publishing Co., 1978.

Berg, P., et al. Asilomar conference on recombinant DNA molecules. *Science*, 1975, *188*(4192), 991–994.

Callahan, D. Recombinant DNA: science and the public. *Hastings Center Report*, 1977, *7*(2), 20–22.

Callahan, D. The meaning and significance of genetic disease: philosophical perspectives. In Hilton, B., et al. (Eds.), *Ethical issues in human genetics: genetic counseling and the use of genetic knowledge*. New York: Plenum Publishing Corp., 1973. pp. 83–90.

Callahan, D. The moral career of genetic engineering. *Hastings Center Report*, 1979, *9*(2), 9, 21.

Cohen, S. N. Recombinant DNA: fact and fiction. *Science*, 1977, *195*(4279), 654–657.© American Association for the Advancement of Science.

Davis, B. D. Prospects for genetic intervention in man. *Science*, 1970, *170*, 1279–1283.

Davis, B. D. Threat and promise in genetic engineering. In P. N. Williams (Ed.), *Ethical issues in biology and medicine: proceedings of a symposium on the identity and dignity of man*. Cambridge, Mass.: Schenkman Publishing Co., Inc., 1972.

Dismukes, K. Life is patently not human-made. *Hastings Center Report*, 1980, *10*(5), 11–12.

Dismukes, K. Recombinant DNA: a proposal for regulation. *Hastings Center Report*, 1977, *7*(2), 25–30.

Dubos, R. Genetic constitution and environmental conditioning. In W. T. Reich (Ed.), *Encyclopedia of bioethics*. New York: The Free Press, 1978.

Ehrman, L., & Grossfield, J. What is natural, what is not? *Hastings Center Report*, 1980, *10*(5), 10–11.

Eisenberg, L. The outcome as cause: predestination and human cloning. *The Journal of Medicine and Philosophy,* 1979, *1*(4), 318–331.

Ephrussi, B. *Hybridization of somatic cells.* Princeton, N.J.: Princeton University Press, 1972.

Friedmann, T. Gene therapy for human genetic disease? *Science,* 1972, *175,* 949–955.

Friedmann, T. Prenatal diagnosis of genetic disease. *Scientific American,* 1971, *255*(5), 34–42.

Fromer, M. J. *Ethical issues in health care.* St. Louis: The C.V. Mosby Co., 1981.

Golden, F. Shaping life in the laboratory. *Time,* March 9, 1981, pp. 50–60.

Gottesman, I. I. Genetic aspects of human behavior: state of the art. In *Encyclopedia of bioethics.*

Green, H. P. Chakrabarty: tempest in a test tube. *Hastings Center Report,* 1980, *10*(5), 12–13.

Harris, H. *Cell fusion.* Oxford: Clarendon Press, 1970.

Hotchkiss, R. D., & Gabor, M. Bacterial transformation—special reference to recombination process. *Annual Review of Genetics,* 1970, *4,* 193–224.

Isaacs, L. The once and future clone. *Hastings Center Report,* 1978, *8*(3), 44–46.

Jonas, H. Freedom of scientific inquiry and the public interest. *Hastings Center Report,* 1976, *6*(4), 15–17.

Lappé, M. Eugenics: ethical issues. In *Encyclopedia of bioethics.*

Lappé, M. Humanizing the genetic enterprise. *Hastings Center Report,* 1979, *9*(6), 10–14.

Loehlin, J. C. Genetic aspects of human behavior: race differences in intelligence. In *Encyclopedia of bioethics.*

Ludmerer, K. M. Eugenics: history. In *Encyclopedia of bioethics.*

Macklin, R. On the ethics of *not* doing scientific research. *Hastings Center Report,* 1977, *7*(6), 11–13.

Murray, R. F. Genetic counseling. In *Encyclopedia of bioethics.*

Murray, R. F. Genetic diagnosis. In *Encyclopedia of bioethics.*

Powledge, T. M. Recombinant DNA: backing off on legislation. *Hastings Center Report,* 1977, *7*(6), 8–10.

Roblin, R. The Boston XYY case. *Hastings Center Report,* 1975, *5*(4), 5–8.

Shinn, R. L. Gene therapy: ethical issues. In *Encyclopedia of bioethics.*

Sinsheimer, R. Troubled dawn for genetic engineering. *New Scientist: The Weekly Review of Science and Technology* (London), October 16, 1975.

Veatch, R. M. *Case studies in medical ethics.* Cambridge, Mass.: Harvard University Press, 1977.

Watson, J. D. The future of asexual reproduction. *Intellectual Digest,* 1971, *2*(2), 115–125.

Zinder, N. D. The Berg letter: a statement of conscience, not of conviction. *Hastings Center Report,* 1980, *10*(5), 14–15.

CHAPTER 8

REPRODUCTIVE TECHNOLOGY

PREDETERMINATION OF GENDER

The gender of a fetus need no longer be a mystery until the moment of birth. Amniocentesis (the withdrawal of a small amount of amniotic fluid for microscopic examination via a needle inserted through the abdominal cavity) will reveal fetal gender. Although amniocentesis is almost never done for the sole purpose of determining gender, this information is available when the procedure is done for other diagnostic purposes, but it cannot be done before the second trimester. When the gender is revealed to the pregnant woman, it can be used in a variety of ways. Most often the information has only an emotional value, that is, the woman has a fact about the fetus and begins thinking of it as "him" or "her," rather than "it." Grandparents may change the color of their knitting yarn, and siblings can envision the new family member in a more concrete way. Beyond this, for most people, information about gender has little practical value, and some women even request not to be told, preferring the surprise at birth.

However, for others fetal gender makes a great deal of difference, and some women have even aborted a fetus of the "wrong" gender. These "gender abortions" take place both for matters of purely personal preference and for reasons of controlling sex-linked genetic diseases. The latter reason is discussed in some detail in the chapter on genetics; it is with the former (gender abortions) that we will be largely concerned with here. Fletcher[1] discusses several areas of argument concerning the question of amniocentesis (and subsequent abortion) for the purpose of gender selection. He poses the following series of ethical dilemmas:

1. Is gender determination alone a morally acceptable reason for performing amniocentesis, and should women or couples have the right to request it? By the same token, is it morally permissible to abort a fetus only because it is the "wrong" gender?

2. Amniocentesis is considered high technology and thus falls under the general rubric of a medical procedure for which financial resources are scarce. Because of this should amniocentesis be permitted for reasons other than saving fetal life or improving fetal health? Is amniocentesis for gender determination frivolous and thus to be discouraged or even outlawed?

3. If amniocentesis for this reason alone is considered trivial, and the literature indicates that most bioethicists believe this to be so, how can this position be reconciled with the Supreme Court's decision to allow abortion in the first two trimesters for any reason a woman chooses?

The Prenatal Diagnostic Clinic at the Johns Hopkins Hospital in Baltimore has conducted staff discussions about this problem and has evolved a workable policy.[2] All clients who request amniocentesis for gender determination are informed of the maternal and fetal risks entailed in the procedure, what a second trimester abortion is like, and how scarce the medical resources are for this procedure. If the couple still wants the amniocentesis, the clinic will comply if the couple would have terminated the pregnancy even without the amniocentesis and when the delivery of a child of unwanted sex will greatly affect the emotional health of the parents or child. The staff admits that their judgment in this last criterion is, of necessity, subjective and surely not foolproof. The clinic had not, at the time of the writing of the report, seen an increase in the number of requests for amniocentesis for gender determination, and the administrators believe that the number of American women or couples who would abort a fetus solely for reasons of gender is very small. This, however, may have to do with the fact that gender determination by amniocentesis cannot be done until the second trimester, and if a reliable test could be done early in pregnancy, the number of abortions would quite likely increase. If this were to be the case, female fetuses would be aborted almost exclusively. Fletcher states that after a thorough review of current research he concludes that

> wives are much more likely to prefer a son than a daughter and more likely to prefer either one than to have a positive underlying desire for an equal number of boys and girls. The exception to this finding were wives of Hispanic heritage, who preferred girls. These findings suggest that if a safe, inexpensive method of sex selection were available, firstborns would increasingly be male.[3]

Predetermination of gender by aborting fetuses of unwanted gender would have strong and definite effects on American society and on the functioning of both individuals and families. Gender might become increasingly important and might change the present societal trend of blurring previously stereotyped gender roles and functions. Up until the past decade or so, people had fixed ideas of what masculine and feminine behaviors were or should be. There were certain separate things that men and women did, and that was all there was to it. Recently, however, we have come to realize that men's and women's natures are not so separate, and there are many roles, functions, behaviors, and feelings that are naturally common to both men and women. This trend, while causing some adjustment problems for both sexes, has been generally healthy and positive, and it would be detrimental to American society to see it destroyed by widespread use of predetermination of gender.

There would surely be strong political backlash in reaction to the current rights of reproductive privacy; that is, if some women began to abort fetuses for reasons considered "too frivolous," it is possible that the Supreme Court could reverse itself in the matter of *Roe v. Wade* and similar cases, or Congress and state legislatures would enact restrictive abortion legislation. There is also the extremely serious matter of unbalancing the natural human sex ratio, the consequence of which will be discussed in more detail later in the chapter. Sex-linked genetic diseases could be affected, although the effect would not necessarily always be positive. Although the following example is farfetched, it is useful as an illustration. If all male fetuses who were discovered in utero to have hemophilia were aborted, and if each woman became pregnant again and again until she conceived a female and allowed it to be born, the number of female carriers of hemophilia would surely increase, and the problem of the disease of hemophilia would not only not be eliminated, it might worsen.

Individual self-perception would surely be altered, and the changes would undoubtedly be more beneficial to males than to females who would be firmly entrenched in a second-class citizen status. Some hypothesize that gender selection would reduce the total birth rate because parents would not have to bear additional children to have some or more of a particular sex. In other words, a family would not need to keep trying to have a girl when they already have a houseful of boys.

Although many will argue that gender determination is indeed a technology to be desired, surely it is more desirable to use a preconception means to that goal than to abort a fetus after its gender has been determined (in the second trimester). Preconception methods are not yet foolproof, although they are likely to be in the near future because it is known that the gender of an offspring depends on the type of sperm that fertilizes the egg.[4] Some sperm are androsperm (Y-bearing) and some are gynosperm (X-bearing). Therefore the goal of preconception gender selection is to make certain that an androsperm fertilizes the egg if a male is desired or that a gynosperm fertilizes it if a female is desired. Avenues of research in this area are proceeding along several lines,[5] for example, discovery of an antigen that will block a particular kind of sperm; knowledge about the biochemistry of spermatogenesis and how various factors affect the development of androsperm and gynosperm; study of conditions relating to the movement of sperm along both the male and female reproductive tracts, that is, what conditions affect the strength and motility of sperm; and study of the relative size of various spermatozoa and how this affects fertilization. Various treatment techniques could be initiated once the mechanism of gender determination is known, and preselection of gender would then be almost foolproof. But would this be a good idea?

Effect on society and culture

Since a good deal of the research currently being done in gender determination is funded by the federal government and large private foundations, it is reasonable to assume that the government, by granting or withholding funds, will play a major role in the essentially private matter of gender selection. Is this as it should be?

Largey[6] thinks that in terms of the social context of this issue, we might compare sex selection methods with birth control methods. Governmental regulations would probably be similar in both instances. Those sex selection methods requiring a drug, abortion, or artificial insemination would probably be more closely regulated than those that were less invasive. Largey also believes that birth control has a far greater impact on the public than will sex selection, but that remains to be seen. Birth control has undoubtedly had an enormous impact on society and culture; it is safe to say that it has affected the lives, not only of those persons who have chosen to use it, but also the character of Western culture simply because of its existence. Predetermination of gender would also tremendously affect society but in different ways about which we can only speculate.

The social effect of gender predetermination would be enormous and without precedent. In the available literature about the subject, no source reported that a majority of those surveyed would prefer female children. Campbell[7] reported that at Tietung Hospital of the Anshan Iron and Steel Company in China a technique was developed to determine the gender of a fetus as early as 47 days after conception by withdrawing a small amount of amniotic fluid via the cervix. The technique was developed ostensibly for family planning, and for the same purpose women were offered abortions after gender had been determined. Of the 100 women having experimental gender determination tests, 30 opted for abortion, and 29 of the aborted fetuses were female. Of course not all societies value men over women to the same extent, but it is safe to say that most give men an edge in terms of opportunity, value, and access to whatever a particular society believes is good and beneficial. In the history of the world in the vast majority of cultures men are more highly valued than women, and there is little reason to believe that this state of affairs will change significantly in the foreseeable future.

Consider what would happen in a country in which the ratio of males to females is increased by even a small percentage. Because many men would not be able to marry, cultural values would change. Perhaps marriage and the family would decrease in importance, leading to a more generalized bachelor existence with, as Etzioni puts it, a kind of frontier town mentality, causing an increase in aggression and violence. Men would have fewer women with whom to engage in sexual activity, a situation that could lead to a rise in homosexuality and prostitution. On the other hand, marriage and the family could increase in importance and desirability simply because opportunities would become rarer for men. Shopping for spouses, the payment of male dowries, and polyandry (one woman having more than one husband) could become prevalent and result in all kinds of legal and ethical questions: which husband would be father to which children, who would be responsible for supporting whom, how would sexuality be affected, and how would the traditional qualities of marital fidelity, intimacy, and loyalty be affected?

The entire character of society in general could change. Presently in our society men tend to be more aggressive and violent than women and are more often convicted of violent crimes. There would likely be an increase in physical violence. Although rape is not a sex crime or a crime of passion, it is difficult to predict whether it would increase or decrease, although the former seems more likely if physical violence in general rises. In those classes and cultures in which males are more highly valued than females there might be an even greater disproportion of males, resulting in interclass and interracial tension. An imbalance in the number of males and females could give rise to a kind of supply-and-demand situation. As the number of women decreased, their value might increase, leading to an eventual evening out of the gender ratio or to a sudden increase in the number of females conceived by artificial insemination. Some scientists and sociologists believe that a sudden increase in the number of males born would soon correct itself because society would seek to emulate the balance of nature. A correction would be quickly sought because societal problems would be evident. In the 1970 National Fertility Study, Westhoff and Rindfuss[8] found that 63% of childless women wanted their first child to be a boy, and Fidell found the same was true of 85% of the female undergraduates at California State University at Northbridge. Because of the influence of the women's movement, however, it is likely that the number of women desiring firstborn males will decrease. Nonetheless, since firstborn children regardless of their gender tend to have characteristics that are considered more masculine than feminine (for example, assertiveness, aggressiveness, and independence), a preponderance of firstborn males might change the character of society in ways that are not predictable.

> If firstborn children really do reap a disproportionate share of the good things in life—or if people become convinced they do—then a campaign could arise to increase the proportion of firstborn girls. Cults dedicated to the increase of a single sex might appear, and political factions might pressure sex-control policies that seemed to complement their other aims. If an imbalance in the sex ratio became too threatening, governments would surely enforce new ratios, perhaps by means of premiums and fines on the model now imposed in India. Politicians might also decide to manipulate ratios for "positive" reasons. A nation bent on making war, for instance, could breed millions of male warriors.[9]

Gender control might be a way of slowing too-rapid population growth. As the ratio of males to females grew more imbalanced, the number of women as potential childbearers would decrease (and it could be predicted that many women would refuse to bear children in light of the imbalance), and men would realize that the species would be in serious jeopardy if more women were not permitted to be born. This would not only decrease the total population but would tend to balance the gender ratio, and natural selection could ensue.

While such an imbalance existed, however (and it might take several generations or even a century to correct), women would be at a great social, cultural, and economic disadvantage. Rape would probably increase, as would kidnap for ransom, and women would suffer all the indignities generally heaped on minority groups—employment discrimination and a general societal contempt. Men would surely have a great many advantages, but the quality of life would diminish for them too. If, as seems likely, women would be reduced to slavery at worst or a sort of refined concubinage at best, men would be denied the joys of relating to women as equals and as full persons. Purchasing a wife or winning her in a contest would be a Pyrrhic victory at best and would so diminish the joy involved that the nature of marriage itself would change.

ARTIFICIAL INSEMINATION

Artificial insemination is the process of injecting a syringe filled with viable and motile spermatozoa into the uterus or cervix of a woman who has been unable to conceive. There are two types of artificial insemination: homologous, or artificial insemination by the husband (AIH), and heterologous, or artificial insemination by a donor (AID). AIH is more common by far and is used if no known cause for the infertility exists or if the woman's vaginal or cervical secretions are somehow inhospitable to her husband's semen. It can also be used if the husband's sperm are viable and motile but low in number. In this case several samples of his semen are collected, usually several days apart, kept frozen, and then mixed together to produce the required concentration of sperm. AID is used when the husband is found to be totally aspermatogenic or if evidence shows that he is the carrier of a genetic disease. A suitable donor is located or frozen sperm from a sperm bank is used, but in neither case are the identities of the donor and recipient made known to each other. An effort is usually made, however, to match some of the physical characteristics of the donor to the recipient mother or couple. AID is also used when a single woman wishes to become pregnant.

Artificial insemination is now considered to be a routine part of the treatment for infertility, although for the couple it is usually their last hope to have a child and is far from routine for them. Many couples see artificial insemination as the final effort to conceive before they consider adoption, which may involve a wait of 5 to 10 years.

One of the major sources of sperm for AID is that which is frozen and stored in sperm banks. There are about 18 or so of these banks in the United States with a total of at least 100,000 sperm samples for sale, resulting in approximately 20,000 AID births each year.[10] This is a remarkable number, especially in view of the drastic decrease in healthy infants available for adoption within the past two decades. The Tyler Medical Clinic in Los Angeles is one of the largest sperm banks and fertility clinics in the country. It performs 15 donor inseminations a day (at a charge, in 1980, of $66 per insemination, which is not covered by health insurance), resulting in 200 pregnancies a year.[11] Most sperm banks are commercial enterprises, and although they will not sell sperm to anyone who walks through the door, they do operate on a profit basis and therefore may not have the most stringent control measures.

Most discussion of AID focuses almost entirely on the infertile woman or couple, but the sperm donor is an essential ingredient in the process. Most medical centers and major infertility clinics have a pool of regular donors who are almost always medical or other students. The donors and their sperm are subjected to fairly rigorous examination. They must have a sperm count far above average (100 million per mililiter as compared with the usual 50 to 60 million) to withstand the freeze-store-thaw process in which the sperm are subjected to liquid nitrogen at $-196°$ C. If they pass the sperm count test, donors are given a thorough physical examination, including tests for many genetic diseases. They must provide a detailed medical history, and most clinics will not accept donors that do not "look right." In addition to the objective tests, there is a great deal of subjectivity in the donor selection process. For example, the persons selecting donors are likely to be biased in terms of physical appearance. Everyone has preferences about those he finds to be physically appealing, and it seems natural for donors to be selected, at least in part, on the basis of how they appeal to the selector. There are also liable to be ethnic and sociocultural biases in the selection process. And because the process is so expensive and time consuming, the donors contribute sperm on a routine basis (usually about once or twice a week) for several years. However, every private physician who practices AID does not necessarily go through this screening process.

Annas[12] describes two major problems that could lead to future ethical dilemmas now that artificial insemination has become so popular and success-ful: donor selection and record keeping. Donors who contribute sperm on a one-to-one basis through a private physician may not be as carefully screened as those who donate through large commercial or medical center sperm banks. In fact, Annas uses the phrase "sperm vendor" to refer to those men who sell their ejaculate to private physicians as if it were an ordinary commercial commodity.

> While this distinction may seem trivial, it has legal consequences. For example, it makes no sense to designate the form signed by the vendor as a "consent form" since he is not a patient and is not really consenting to anything. It is a contract in which the vendor is agreeing to do certain things for pay. Moreover, continued use of the term "donor" gives the impression that the sperm vendor is doing some service for the good of humanity and deserves some special protection, rather than simply performing a service for pay.[13]

Annas points out that private physicians are actually making eugenic deci-sions for their clients when they purchase the sperm of certain individuals—individuals much like themselves (80% of the time physicians purchase sperm from medical students). "Physicians may believe that society needs more indi-viduals with the attributes of physicians, but it is unlikely that society as a whole does."[14] Moreover, many physicians do not bother with any but the most superficial genetic screening, and many do not even take a family history. Annas also points out that these physicians are acting as genetic counselors when they may not be qualified for that role. The second problem area Annas mentions, that of record keeping, will be discussed in a section to follow.

Artificial insemination is becoming a practical and desirable alternative for single women who wish to avoid the social, emotional, and possible legal problems of having sexual intercourse with a man who may be a relative stranger. There are, however, problems in addition to the ones usually associated with single motherhood. For instance, there is the dilemma of what to tell the child. Even though children have a prima facie right to the truth about their conception, and mothers are obligated to tell their children the truth, there are circumstances in which the truth might cause more harm than good, for example, when young children will be subjected to the taunts and ridicule of their peers or when a mother and child live in a very conservative community and might suffer social ostracism if the truth were known. Many single women find it difficult to obtain artificial insemination from private physicians and clinics, although Tyler does inseminate single women. Another alternative, and one that is especially practical for lesbians who face even greater problems than heterosexual women, is for women to manage their own artificial insemination. For example, a California woman[15] purchased a sample of sperm each month (for $38 in 1980) from a commercial sperm bank, which packed it in dry ice for her to carry to the Feminists Woman's Health Center in Los Angeles where staff physicians performed the insemination. This procedure is repeated in many places around the country.

Religious views

Religious questions about artificial insemination center around two major issues, masturbation and the debate between natural and artificial methods of procreation. The Catholic Church is opposed to masturbation under any circumstances; therefore AID is prohibited, and AIH is approved only if the husband's semen is obtained by aspirating it directly from the testes by inserting a needle into the testis itself. This is a procedure to which most men are not willing to subject themselves, and most Catholic couples who wish AID will ignore the Church's prohibition against masturbation for the same reason that many Catholic laypersons disregard other of the Church's reproductive sanctions— because it is widely believed that these matters of reproductive privacy should not fall within the realm of official Church dogma. This matter is discussed in some detail in the chapters on contraception and abortion.

The Church opposes AID for reasons other than the ban on masturbation. It is considered adulterous by nature and harmful to the sanctity of the family; it is contrary to natural law because the husband has not copulated with his wife; and it would be an injustice to the child resulting from AID, who would be considered illegitimate because AID is an act of adultery.

Many moral theologians have argued against the Catholic view. The first reason, concerning the unnatural manipulation of what should be a natural process, may be countered by the idea that human beings with more control over their natural lives can rise to a loftier moral plane where they are free to devote themselves to activities that will improve the quality of their lives. In other instances the Church looks with favor on interferences with other life processes (for example, pharmacologic intervention in various diseases) that allow people to transcend a base concern for survival.

> Should men attempt to suppress their reasoning faculty and the emancipating fruits of it because there are risks entailed? To transcend natural restrictions, to seek ends by means devised through choice rather than by physical determinism, is a human and spiritual victory. With many of us it is a matter of reasoned conviction that our march toward freedom and control is an irreversible trend. Man's moral and spiritual need is to exercise his moral faculties, including those of self-control as well as control over external circumstances. His task is not to suppress and deny his intellectual faculties.[16]

Many fear and consequently wish to prohibit any technologic advance. Some believe that possible future knowledge or technology could not be controlled and might be used to do evil. This argument has been around a long time and has never held much moral weight; one can imagine that ethical debates raged over the first use of fire. Knowledge and the use to which it is put can be controlled and in some cases probably should be, but to prevent a childless couple from conceiving because of the fear of some remote scientific evil does not seem in the best interest of intellectual integrity.

The second reason the Church prohibits AID, that it is unnatural because the husband has not copulated with his wife and because the donor is required to masturbate, may be countered in two ways. The couple has copulated, probably more frequently and more diligently with the intent of procreating (in the Church's view, the primary reason for copulation) than those who are not thinking about fertility or who are hoping that pregnancy will not result. A couple who has had and will most likely continue to have natural intercourse for the express purpose of conception would seem to come closer to fulfilling the Church's requirements than a couple who has intercourse without the desire to have children. The fact that their copulation does not result in conception is an accident of nature and punishing the couple by denying them AID would seem an injustice that is incongruent with the tenets of the Church.

Protestants are divided about AID. In general, conservatives view the marriage bond in terms of what is seen as God's desire for monogamy; copulation should take place within marriage or it should not take place at all. AID might be seen as adulterous in this view. But Protestant theologians have not made definitive statements about the moral correctness or permissibility of AID, which thus has not been decreed adultery. However, nowhere in the Bible is there a specific injunction in favor of monogamous marriage; there is only a prohibition against adultery, which provides leeway in the interpretation of the definition of AID as adultery.

Protestants, like Reform and Conservative Jews, as a rule debate which traditional Biblical commands (both positive and negative) should be obeyed in modern life and in light of modern technology. Those who tend to relax their observance of strict injunctions maintain that moral sensitivity and human relationships are more important than certain rules and the institutions created by those rules. Many also argue that no commandment can be proved a clear expression of God's will and that therefore no conduct specifically must be performed or prohibited. Theologians are awash in a sea of ambiguities about what is good and moral in view of the difference between historic situations and new ones, current technologic developments, and anticipated future changes. Religious liberals can point to almost any moral issue in health care and show how technology or knowledge transcends or at least circumvents traditional religious values.

Sperm and zygote banks

Sperm banks are cold storage vaults where sperm are kept frozen in liquid nitrogen. The process is quite successful on a relatively short-term basis, and when the semen sample is thawed, about two thirds of the spermatozoa are viable and motile. Ovum banking (the term *bank* or *banking* here will also include the freezing process) is not yet done, although research is currently going on to overcome the technical difficulties.

However, animal zygotes are now being frozen. In this process an oocyte is removed from the female by laparoscopy (a needle is inserted through the abdominal wall into the ovary), fertilized in vitro, and then frozen in liquid helium from $-196°$ to $-296°$ C. At some time in the future the frozen zygote would be implanted into a uterus, either the one from which the oocyte was originally removed or another. The problems of experimenting on zygote freezing, storage, and reimplantation in humans are so enormous and the actuality so far in the future that it will not be discussed further here.

In addition to storing the sperm used to inseminate infertile women, there are other reasons for the existence of sperm banks. One that is growing in popularity is the desire of men who are about to undergo vasectomy to store sperm in the event they wish to father more children. Some women are asking their husbands to store sperm in case they die and the women wish to impregnate themselves with their husbands' sperm, although this is not common and has some emotionally unhealthy overtones. Men who believe, for a variety of reasons, that they wish to have their genetic characteristics outlive them and are not content with the number of children they have already sired, can donate to a sperm bank.

Since the success rate of stored and frozen sperm has been so high, one could believe this to be an almost perfect reproductive technology. But there are problems. For example, sperm that has been frozen for 6 months or longer cannot be used successfully in artificial insemination because pregnancy almost never occurs. Therefore the record-keeping procedure of a sperm bank must be minutely accurate because, although pregnancy almost never occurs after long-term freezing, there is a slight chance that it will, and one must assume that the chance of defect would increase with aged sperm. Although there is little research to show that there is a higher incidence of congenital malformations in artificial insemination using frozen sperm rather than fresh, there is always the danger of damage during the freeze-store-thaw process; thus there is always the risk of a deformed fetus. If such damage does occur, should the resulting child be entitled to compensation for the damage, and if so, how can it be proved that the defect was caused by damaged sperm and not by unknown and unknowable factors? Since so few conceptions have occurred with frozen sperm when compared with the total number of natural conceptions that have ever occurred, it seems reasonable to suggest that women who subject themselves to AID with frozen sperm be considered human research subjects (and entitled to all the protections and compensations therefrom) rather than recipients of a health service.

Although it seems farfetched and perhaps even bizarre, there could be questions about the rights of ownership of sperm and zygotes. Does a sperm donor relinquish ownership after he has been paid (or even if he has not) and handed it to the sperm bank or physician? If not, is he then legally permitted to claim part ownership of the child that results? The legal aspects of artificial insemination will be discussed in the following section, but almost all case law and legal precedent pertains to the child, not to the sperm itself. It seems as unlikely, and as legally indefensible, that a man could lay claim to donated sperm as one could claim ownership of donated blood, but the issues involved in reproductive technology are so complex that one cannot dismiss the likelihood of future claims.

Legal and social views

Currie-Cohen et al.[17] surveyed 379 practitioners of AID and found that while 93% kept permanent records on recipients, only 37% kept permanent records of the children born of those inseminations and only 30% kept records on the donors. Annas attempts to explain this apparently contradictory phenomenon as follows:

> The fear of record-keeping seems to be based primarily on the idea, common in the legal literature, that if identifiable, the donor might be sued for parental obligations (for example, child support, inheritance, and so on) by one of his "biological children" sired by the AID process, and that this suit might be successful. The underlying rationale is that unless anonymity is assured, there would be no donors.[18]

Annas responds to this fear by making the following four key points:
1. Accurate records should be kept to see how a particular donor's sperm "works." For example, if a defective child is born, the sperm should be destroyed. Most physicians, according to the Currie-Cohen study, have no policy on the number of times they use a donor's sperm; therefore the chances of producing a defective child increase significantly.
2. No meaningful research on the characteristics and success of donors can ever be done if records are not kept.
3. AID children should have information about their family history; this can be available to them as adults only if records containing appropriate and accurate information are kept at the time of their conception.
4. Although it may or may not be in the best interests of AID children to know who their fathers are, it is surely not in their best interest to make certain that they can never find out. If donors have so strong a desire to protect themselves from ever being revealed as fathers of AID children, it is perhaps best that they not donate in the first place.

The Currie-Cohen study also showed that 32% of all physicians mixed the sperm of several donors for a single insemination. This could have severe untoward genetic and legal consequences for the children, and this information should surely be available to them.

Fifteen state legislatures have laws regarding AID, and the only thing they have in common is that the resulting child is considered legitimate—the child of both the mother and her husband. Many states have laws that protect the identity of the donor in much the same way as the identity of a natural mother is kept from adoptive parents and the adopted child. However, the number of adopted and AID children who are seeking the identity of natural parents is increasing, and many are questioning the wisdom of so much secrecy and confidentiality surrounding the circumstances of their conception and birth.

Although AID is common, it is by no means without risk, particularly to the children born of this new technology. For this reason Annas proposes that the following five points be considered in the development of public policy regarding AID:
1. AID should be removed from the practice of medicine and placed in the hands of genetic counselors and other nonmedical personnel.
2. Uniform national standards and criteria for donor selection should be established.
3. Permanent records on all donors, recipients, pregnancies, and births should be kept.
4. The number of pregnancies per donor should be limited, and each insemination should contain the sperm of only one donor.

5. There should be research on the psychologic development of AID
   children.

Of the 15 states that have laws concerning artificial insemination, five
require that the woman's husband consent in writing to AID (presumably if he
refused to consent and she went ahead with the procedure anyway, he would
not be held responsible for the ensuing child). Aside from legitimacy and
consent statutes, there are no laws governing artificial insemination, and this
lack of regulation has led to some of the questionable practices described
previously. Neither are there legal limits on sperm donation:

> single donors might father several babies, two of whom, who would be
> half siblings, might one day meet and marry—the so-called "intermarriage
> risk". And, finally, there are no guidelines about who should be inseminated.
> Can women with low I.Q.s or homosexual women or single women be
> denied donor insemination? In the first case of its kind, the American Civil
> Liberties Union has filed suit against the Mott Clinic at Wayne State Uni-
> versity because the clinic will not allow single women to apply for anony-
> mous donor inseminations. To deal with most of these legal issues, an ad
> hoc committee of the American Fertility Society is now trying to establish
> guidelines.[19]

If the legal issues of artificial insemination are in a welter of confusion, so are
the social ones, although there are not so many considerations of "naturalness"
here as there are in in vitro fertilization, which will be discussed later. The
major social and ethical issue is whether or not human beings have the right to
interfere in the natural process of reproduction. One's view on this matter will
depend to a great extent on one's view of natural law and the right that human
beings have to interfere (or intercede) in any natural biologic process. (The
reader is referred to Chapter 1 on ethical theory, especially the matter of consistency in solving ethical problems, when human intervention is permissible
and when it is not.)

One problem that particularly seems to worry those who are generally
opposed to technologic intervention in human reproduction is when and
where it will all end. Will we perhaps eventually end up with totally artificial
babies? That hardly seems likely, but this depends on one's interpretation of the
meaning of *artificial*; that is, if technology still requires a human ovum and
sperm to make a human, then the end product will surely not be artificial,
although the means to that end might be. If human sperm and ova are not
necessary, we may indeed end up with artificial life. But if we can now cope
with mechanical robots putting cars together on assembly lines, perhaps we
will in the distant future be able to cope with biologic robots as playmates and

professional colleagues. The only problem will likely be in distinguishing them from the real.

IN VITRO FERTILIZATION

In vitro fertilization (IVF) is the next step down the road of reproductive technology and represents a significant scientific achievement, one that excites and/or frightens almost everyone. Although several successful live births have occurred using the IVF technique, it still must be considered experimental (*in vitro* means "in glass," from which derives the term *test-tube baby*, even though a test tube is not part of the equipment used, nor is there a baby in that equipment).

The procedure consists of removing several oocytes from a woman's body by laparoscopy. A needle is passed through the laparoscope into her ovary, and the oocytes are aspirated and placed in a glass petri dish that has been filled with a nourishing culture medium. Some researchers and fertility clinics pretreat the woman with pituitary hormones, both to standardize her menstrual cycle and to ensure that several ova will mature at once. The husband's semen has been obtained by masturbation, and the spermatozoa are isolated from the semen by centrifugal force. They are then washed and placed in the culture medium with the ova, where fertilization takes place. This matter-of-fact description hardly does justice to the difficulty of achieving fertilization and the hundred years of research before the first baby was born of IVF. Even now, after the technique has been done successfully many times, for each completed fertilization there are thousands of unsuccessful attempts.

After fertilization occurs, the procedure becomes risky. Placement of the blastocyst (the fertilized ovum after mitosis has begun but while the cells are still undifferentiated) in the uterus must be done at the precise time at which the endometrium is appropriately developed, and it is at this point where the greatest risk of injury lies. Although the endocrine balances of the menstrual cycle are still not fully understood, it is believed that artificial removal of ova can be analogous to natural ovulation in that the endometrium will still undergo the same changes as if the ovum had been released naturally. The blastocyst is aspirated from the petri dish into a syringe, which is then inserted into the woman's uterus via her vagina and cervix. The blastocyst is released into the uterus, where it is hoped that it will attach itself to the endometrium, and the pregnancy will proceed naturally. Although amniocentesis can be done in midtrimester to detect certain birth defects, until birth occurs there is no way of being absolutely certain that serious damage has not taken place. The first successful IVF was the birth of Louise Brown in England in 1978 as a result of work done by Edwards and Steptoe.

Experimental and therapeutic procedures

It seems almost too obvious to say that IVF is used therapeutically to relieve infertility, but there seems no other reason why a woman would subject herself to this procedure, which entails considerable risk (some to herself but most to the embryo/fetus) if she and her husband were not desperate to bear a child and all other efforts had failed.

However, much of the work done in IVF is termed *laboratory IVF research*, and the blastocysts created thereby are not intended for eventual insertion into a human woman. Mastroianni[20] lists several ways in which IVF research can be used as follows:

1. The effectiveness of antifertility agents could be tested in vitro without subjecting human subjects to an untried drug. The agents might be used to deliberately destroy blastocysts or to prevent the penetration of ova by spermatozoa.

2. "The in vitro system could be used to evaluate the fertilizability of ova of patients with infertility and to assess the structural and biochemical normality of the conceptus in patients who have had repeated spontaneous abortion."[21]

3. The effect of teratogens and other noxious agents on the conceptus could be tested.

4. IVF can be used to study the progress of genetic disease and possibly to develop methods to predict or to prevent them.

5. General knowledge of cell growth and differentiation could be increased.

IVF is used both therapeutically and experimentally, and because the therapeutic use is still mainly in the experimental stage, it is difficult to draw a line between what is permissible for human therapeutic IVF and what is not. Although the major ethical issues will be summarized in the following section, they cannot be ignored here when attempting to distinguish between therapeutic and experimental uses. One example of the blurring of distinctions is the fate of the blastocyst. In therapeutic use the blastocyst is nurtured carefully to place it intact in the woman's uterus. However, if it were to be damaged inadvertently (and that fact were known before it was transferred), it would be destroyed, even though the original purpose was the opposite. On the other hand, in purely experimental IVF the blastocyst is destined for destruction even though in some experiments the researchers might try to keep it alive and developing for as long as possible. Although we will examine the problem in greater detail later, one of the major distinguishing factors may indeed be the intent of the researchers in regard to the blastocyst.

Undoubtedly there is considerable risk to the blastocyst (and some minimal risk to the woman) in IVF, but it is difficult, if not impossible, to assess precisely what those risks are. Although definitive answers will not be forthcoming for many years, it is becoming clear that certain questions about IVF research must be asked.[22]

1. Will the fertilization process in vitro and the transfer of the blastocyst to the woman's uterus significantly increase the likelihood of birth defects?
2. If so, will natural screening and spontaneous abortion work in the same way they do in natural reproduction?
3. Will a greater number of induced abortions take place as a result of defects being detected by amniocentesis?
4. Will there be long-term negative psychologic consequences for a child of successful IVF?
5. What will be the physical and psychologic risks to the woman?
6. Will there be an increasing callousness or coldness toward all embryos as a result of so much deliberate destruction of blastocysts in the laboratory?

As a result of a pressing need to address these and other questions, in March 1979, the Ethics Advisory Board of the National Commission for the Protection of Human Subjects (now defunct), after a series of debates and public hearings, established a set of guidelines to be used when doing IVF research on humans. A summary of those guidelines follows:

1. The research must comply with all provisions of the Department of Health and Human Services (DHHS) guidelines for biomedical and behavioral research on human subjects.
2. The research must be designed primarily to establish safety and efficacy of embryo (blastocyst) transfer and only when this knowledge cannot be gained in any other way.
3. All human gametes to be used in IVF research are to be obtained only from those persons who have been informed of the purpose of the research.
4. No embryo (blastocyst) will be sustained in vitro beyond the point normally associated with implantation (14 days after fertilization).
5. If research begins to show that IVF entails a higher risk of deformed offspring than that associated with natural reproduction, all interested parties and the general public will be informed of this fact.
6. IVF will be done only on lawfully married couples.

The transition from IVF research to the provision of therapeutic services has been accomplished, among other places, at a clinic at Norfolk (Virginia) General Hospital. Since the physicians and researchers at the Norfolk Clinic had to have their original proposal minutely scrutinized by the institutional review board (IRB) of the Eastern Virginia Medical School on the basis of the National Commission guidelines just mentioned, it would be appropriate here to describe the procedure used at the Norfolk Clinic.

The screening of couples who wish to undergo IVF is an integral part of the process, and it engendered considerable debate during the clinic's planning stage. Initially it was thought that only the woman's infertility problem should be considered, since it is she who must go through the actual physical procedures, but because infertility affects the couple as a unit and because the husband may have a medical condition exacerbating the problem, he too is considered in the screening process. The couple must meet the following selection criteria:

1. The couple must be married and childless and must be without any medically known way to achieve pregnancy. They must also demonstrate a stable marriage to the satisfaction of the attending physician.
2. Both husband and wife must be generally healthy and pass a physical examination.
3. The woman must have a normal uterus and normal endocrine and menstrual function.
4. The wife must be between 25 and 35 years of age.
5. The couple must be able to pay for the treatment, which in 1980 cost about $4000 and is not covered by insurance.
6. The husband must not have a sperm count below 20 million per milliliter (normal is 50 to 60 million).

The procedure followed at the Norfolk Clinic is the same as that described previously except that the woman is not given pituitary hormones; therefore only one oocyte is removed and fertilized. The policy of the Norfolk Clinic is never to comment publicly on the progress of work done or success achieved, although at least one IVF pregnancy has been successfully carried to term. This is done to assure the couple's confidentiality and privacy, but it is therefore impossible to assess the clinic's success. The couple may, however, make such information public if they choose, but it is understandable that many would wish to remain silent.

Ethical issues

Ethical issues in human IVF focus on two major questions, which in turn give rise to many ethical dilemmas. The two basic questions are as follows: (1) Do human beings have the right to interfere so drastically in natural reproduction, and (2) is it permissible to deliberately destroy blastocysts before transfer to the woman's uterus if they are found to be defective? Moreover, is it permissible to create these blastocysts for purely experimental purposes when the intent is to destroy rather than to transfer them? To answer the first question involves the issue of what is indeed natural and what the purposes are for interfering in natural reproductive processes. To this end, the reader is referred to the chapter on genetic engineering that considers questions of human intervention in reproduction. The second question is essentially a matter of abortion ethics; that is, is a blastocyst, a collection of undifferentiated cells, human? If so, then one might be opposed to destroying it; if not, then the question of destroying it is not ethically applicable. The guidelines of the Ethics Advisory Board, mentioned previously, specifically state that blastocysts may be destroyed (admittedly not everyone agrees with this conclusion, and there was some serious opposition, notably from the Catholic Church), but they also state that a blastocyst may not be kept for experimental purposes beyond 14 days after fertilization. This is a somewhat arbitrary decision, and one could reasonably conjecture that it is a compromise position.

With these two basic questions in mind, I shall summarize what Walters has delineated as the major ethical issues and questions in human IVF.[23]

1. What is the basic need for IVF research? Are there a sufficient number of women who (a) wish desperately to bear children and (b) have no other medical recourse? In other words, is it cost-effective?
2. Is the desire to bear a child of one's own really a medical need, and how can it be compared with other health care needs?
3. Has IVF been adequately studied biochemically and in animals before subjecting human subjects to such research?
4. Are the benefits worth the risks; that is, how big a risk should society be willing to take that more defective children will be born just so a few infertile women can bear children? What are acceptable levels of risk?
5. Is the couple's ability to give informed consent diminished by their desperation to have a child, and will this desperation lead them to take risks they either should not take or will regret later?
6. Who is liable for compensation if injury occurs during either therapeutic or experimental IVF? Who is responsible if a defective child is born?
7. What are appropriate institutional frameworks for doing IVF; that is, who should be responsible for setting standards, and how can criteria for objectivity be established?
8. How should selection criteria be established and on what basis? How can medical, social, and personal criteria be separated, or should they be evaluated together?
9. Are there certain types of knowledge that can be gained only from human IVF and not from research on other mammalian species?
10. Should research be done on blastocysts/embryos that have been allowed to develop past the point at which implantation normally occurs?

Kass asks some difficult questions about the right of scientists to do IVF, and in this regard he is almost directly opposed to the views of Joseph Fletcher. Kass believes that the ultimate moral question about IVF is as follows: "Does the parents' desire for a child (or the obstetrician's desire to help them) entitle them to have it by methods that deliberately impose upon that child an unknown and untested risk of deformity or malformation?"[24] Although the risks are still very much unknown, Kass states that they exist; moreover, the fact that scientists and researchers do not know what the risks are is in itself an unacceptable risk. Kass' major objection to IVF is the matter of informed consent, that is, that the fetus cannot consent to a procedure that is bound to affect it in serious and permanent ways—even if it is lucky enough to escape malformation.

> The problem of risks and mishaps that accompany the experimental phase of this new technology provides a powerful moral objection sufficient to rebut the . . . implantation experiments. This moral objection should be widely shared, for it rests upon that minimal principle of medical practice, do no harm. In these prospective experiments upon the unconceived and the unborn, it is not enough not to know of any grave defects; one needs to know that there will be no such defects—or at least no more than there are without the procedure. The general presumption of ignorance is caution. When the subject-at-risk cannot give consent, the presumption should be abstention.[25]

Kass is quick to point out that although all medical and scientific progress is indeed risky, there is a vast difference between accepting, with full knowledge of what is entailed, a risk for oneself and deliberately submitting an embryo or conceptus to what still remains a hazardous experiment, particularly when there is no possible therapeutic benefit to that embryo. The procedure of IVF is therapeutic only for the parents in that it treats their desire for a child.

Moreover, Kass does not view infertility as a disease in the usual medical sense; he refers to it as more of a social disease that is found ordinarily in only one partner but that takes the interaction of both partners to treat. Infertility may be a symptom of a disease, but it surely is not a disease in itself, nor is it life-threatening, crippling, or damaging to the body in any way. Kass then makes one other telling point:

> Just as infertility is not a disease, so providing a child by artificial means to a woman with blocked oviducts is not treatment (as surgical reconstruction of her oviducts would be). She remains as infertile as before. What is being "treated" is her desire—a perfectly normal and unobjectionable desire—to bear a child. There is no clear medical therapeutic purpose that requires or demands the use of new and untested technologies for initiating human life and that might possibly justify the unconsented-to use of a human subject for the benefit of others and at risk to himself.[26]

In addition to exposing an embryo/fetus to unknown and possibly serious risk is the issue of the motivation for doing so. It is acknowledged that the desire of some people to have children naturally is extremely strong; it may even be acknowledged that this is so in most people because indeed, where would the species be if most of its members had a half-hearted instinct for procreation? However, it is also true that the vast majority of human beings are fertile, as the current population explosion attests. Therefore it matters not at all to the survival of the species if a few of its females are infertile. In fact many population experts and demographers would consider this a blessing. And if, in addition, infertility is not a medical disease for which a cure should be sought, why is it important to devote scarce research funds and the time and talents of scientists toward artificially creating the ability to bear a child in a handful of women who, as Kass says, have a perfectly normal desire to do so? The only answer it seems is to satisfy that desire, to fulfill a personal need, and to achieve whatever measure of happiness that bearing a child will provide. Considering the likelihood of risk to that child, considering all the life-threatening diseases that remain incurable partly because of the lack of research funds, and considering all the tangible suffering in the world that could be assuaged, it seems unjustifiable to devote resources to IVF. This is a luxury that scientists and infertile women ought to enjoy only if it is not done at the expense of others.

EMBRYO TRANSFER

Embryo transfer is a technology that has not yet been accomplished in humans, although because it has been used in cattle breeding for more than a decade; it seems only a matter of time before it is possible in humans. The question is, however, whether it should be. Embryo transfer is the removal of a blastocyst immediately after fertilization from the uterus of one female and its insertion into another uterus. It is sometimes referred to as "prenatal adoption." This is not the same as surrogate motherhood, which will be discussed later, because the woman who is the recipient of the transfer bears and keeps the child. It is hers in every sense but the genetic.

The procedure is quite complex and in humans will require the cooperation of the two women for far longer than the actual removal-transfer. First, over a period of several months before the transfer, the menstrual cycles of the two women must be hormonally synchronized so that when the donor ovulates and conceives, the recipient's uterus will be in the proper cyclical phase for the fertilized ovum. Second, when the menstrual cycles are in synchronization, the donor is inseminated with the sperm of the recipient's husband, and 4 days later the donor's uterus is flushed out via a catheter inserted through her cervix. It is hoped that the free-floating fertilized ovum will be flushed out, recovered from the fluid, and then inserted in the recipient's uterus. The delicacy with which this procedure must be done, the precision of timing, and the danger of damage to the fertilized ovum make it a highly precarious and risky venture. It is also expensive for the recipient—about as much as the cost of a new car, according to Randolph Seed, M.D., and his brother Richard W. Seed, Ph.D., who have been conducting embryo transfer research in Chicago.[27] The Seed brothers pay the donor $50 for each flush of her uterus, with a $200 bonus if a fertilized ovum is recovered.

The obvious benefit of this technology is that women who either have no fallopian tubes or whose tubes are permanently occluded may become pregnant, although in vitro fertilization would work as well in this circumstance. Embryo transfer would, however, be the treatment of choice if the woman has an absence of ova but otherwise has a normal endocrine cycle. Considering the rise in prevalence of gonorrhea over the past several years, which frequently leaves fallopian tubes damaged, there may indeed be a great number of requests for embryo transfer when it is possible in humans.

The procedure carries with it all the risks of IVF plus some additional ones when the ovum is flushed from the donor's uterus. There is also another risk to be considered. Infertile couples, particularly women who have tried for years to conceive, tend to view themselves as failures, not only in the reproductive aspect of their lives but in other spheres as well. When they finally see an infertility specialist, they are in such a state of depression and desperation that they will agree to any procedure, no matter how risky. They are often willing to take chances with the health and well-being of the future child to prove to themselves that they can indeed bear one. It is highly arguable that women in such a state of desperation are capable of giving voluntary informed consent.

PRENATAL DIAGNOSIS

Prenatal diagnosis is one of the newest and most dramatic forms of reproductive technology and is carried out by both invasive (amniocentesis and a variety of blood tests) and noninvasive (ultrasonography, radiography, and the like) techniques. It can diagnose about 200 fetal diseases, conditions, defects, and anomalies, but there is also an unknown number of such conditions that it cannot detect. Prenatal diagnosis is by no means foolproof, and it perhaps raises more ethical questions than it answers.

One way to describe the history and methods of prenatal diagnosis is to use a paradigm, in this case screening for maternal serum alpha-fetoprotein (MSAFP), which is an indicator of neural tube defects such as spina bifida, meningo-myelocele, and anencephaly. A neural tube defect (NTD) is a malformation that results from an abnormal closure of the neural tube in early embryonic development. There are a wide range of conditions, some fatal and all handicapping with varying degrees of severity. All forms of NTD are considered serious defects and have life-long effects. Approximately 1 in every 500 newborns in the United States has an NTD,[28] although because NTD often results in spontaneous abortion, it is impossible to know the total number of embryos and fetuses affected. Prenatal diagnosis is made definitively by measuring the alpha-fetoprotein level in amniotic fluid, although anencephaly can be diagnosed by ultrasonography. Such diagnosis is made during the second trimester. The total screening process consists of measuring the alpha-fetoprotein in the woman's blood and then doing an amniocentesis if the MSAFP level is shown to be at a certain point. If the fetus is found to have an NTD, the woman must make a decision whether or not to abort.

Because screening is expensive and entails a certain degree of risk, Haddow lists some of the critical points to be considered when making a decision to either establish a screening program or to suggest that individual women undergo screening[29]:

1. The problem exists of whether to make MSAFP screening mandatory, although Haddow believes this is unlikely.
2. Women need to be informed about the nature of all the blood tests they undergo during pregnancy and precisely what defects and diseases are being looked for.
3. Approximately 10% to 20% of all NTDs will remain undetected, even with the most rigorous screening; this presents a problem of whether or not to invest research funds in developing even more sophisticated detection techniques.
4. Amniocentesis will be performed on approximately 1% to 2% of all pregnant women (for this specific reason), and there is always a slight risk of fetal damage or death as a result.
5. About 2 of every 1000 pregnant women will have to decide whether to abort as a result of known NTD.
6. Access to screening is uneven because of program shortcomings, such as lack of publicity, and because of resistance from certain physicians and other health professionals.

There are also other issues that may be directly or indirectly linked to the establishment of screening programs. For example, the attitude of health professionals toward persons with NTD can have a profound influence on not only whether a woman undergoes screening but also whether she elects to abort a fetus identified as having NTD. Moreover, many physicians do not know about the screening programs, or if they do, they have negative attitudes for one reason or another. These attitudes can have serious adverse consequences for the pregnant woman.

A study performed in Maryland before the MSAFP pilot project began indicated that many physicians were not familiar with the fundamentals of the screening process. Based on experience in Maine, education of physicians regarding MSAFP screening must be viewed as a continuing process. The physician becomes much more receptive to information when first confronted with a patient having a positive MSAFP test. Because a wide variety of physicians, including both specialists such as obstetricians and generalists such as family practitioners and osteopaths, provide prenatal care, education must be individualized to suit the needs of a given office. Attention should be devoted to giving adequate information to the office nurse, whose role is critical.[30]

Ethical issues

The ethical issues to be discussed here involve all types of prenatal diagnosis, MSAFP, as well as tests for other diseases and defects. In the discussion to follow we shall assume that various screening and diagnostic procedures can and have detected fetuses with serious defects or diseases, that is, that the procedures work. I shall define *serious* when applied to a congenital or genetic defect to mean that either (1) it is incompatible with life, (2) it requires emergency treatment, or (3) it requires ongoing care and treatment. For example, anencephaly (absence of a cerebral cortex or even an entire brain) is serious because it is incompatible with life; a tracheoesophageal fistula ("tunnel" leading from trachea to esophagus) is serious because it requires immediate (but usually not ongoing) treatment; and meningomyelocele (absence of vertebrae [usually lumbar] and protrusion of spinal cord and meninges) is serious because it requires ongoing (usually life-long) treatment. This definition, of course, is not completely adequate because the seriousness of defects can be highly subjective and depends to a great extent on personal and sociocultural attitudes.

There are several major ethical issues in prenatal diagnosis, the first of which is the moral status of the fetus, that is, the moral obligations owed it, especially by the woman carrying it. The reader is referred to the chapter on abortion for a general discussion of moral responsibilities owed to fetuses, particularly in view of their developing potentiality as pregnancy progresses. One must then consider in what ways, if any, a seriously deformed fetus differs from a normal one in terms of individuals' responses to it. At first glance one could deny that there is a prima facie moral difference between a defective fetus and a normal one, but this might not necessarily be true in all cases. An anencephalic will be born alive only 20% to 25% of the time and even then will die shortly after birth, usually in an hour or so.[31] Because an anencephalic is, in essence, born dying, it is probably owed fewer moral obligations.

However, in most instances severely deformed and handicapped fetuses should be accorded the same moral status as normal ones, but it should be remembered that this does not necessarily mean they should be treated as persons. The area in which major differences occur is in individuals' reactions to it. If the defect is so severe that it causes mental retardation to a great extent, some may doubt the infant's personhood, and some may use a utilitarian approach to measure the suffering the deformed infant and its family will experience when compared with the happiness that would ordinarily accrue in the course of a lifetime. The question, however, that perhaps bothers most people is whether it is less bad to abort a deformed fetus than a healthy one. Is perfect health a prerequisite for continued fetal life?

Another ethical issue is the matter of resource allocation for prenatal diagnosis. There are two major questions, according to Walters[32]: (1) Who should have access to screening programs and prenatal diagnosis, and (2) what priority should be given to national screening programs and prenatal diagnosis in comparison with other health-care needs? Screening and diagnosis are expensive. For example, in 1980 it was estimated that an initial screening test for MSAFP cost $12, the secondary (repeat) blood test $27, $50 for an ultrasound scan, and $62 for amniocentesis (and $500 for a midtrimester abortion). Some women might be able to pay for the initial blood test or two but not for the more complex diagnostic procedures. Should they then be denied these procedures, or should public funds be committed to pay for them? Private insurance companies vary a great deal in their willingness to pay for prenatal diagnosis, and Medicaid is growing increasingly reluctant to do so. Surely justice would dictate that every woman who desires screening and diagnosis should have access not only to the initial blood tests but to the entire diagnostic process. "To put the matter bluntly, a woman who is told that her serum AFP value is elevated but who cannot afford genetic counseling, ultrasound, or amniocentesis is probably worse off than a woman who has not been screened at all."[33]

The matter of comparing prenatal diagnosis with other health-care needs when allocating funds is actually a matter of societal values. Do we value prevention over cure? Will we insist on abortion for a seriously deformed fetus if we pay for the diagnosis? Will we prevent a woman from aborting even when she knows she is carrying a seriously deformed fetus? Will we weigh the numbers of people who are affected directly and indirectly by birth defects as compared with cancer or cardiovascular disease? All these questions could be argued indefinitely, but society will have to make some allocation decisions in the immediate future, and there is no guarantee that those decisions will be ethically correct; it is entirely possible that political expediency will be the ultimate criterion.

Yet another issue is the matter of freedom and coercion. Should prenatal diagnosis be mandatory or voluntary? Although there is as yet no such mandatory program, there are those who believe that removal of voluntariness would prevent birth defects to some extent. However, more than screening itself would have to be mandatory; actions within the program would need to be mandated if fewer infants are to be born with birth defects. In other words, for a mandatory program to be truly effective, a pregnant woman must agree to either fetal surgery, if that were possible, or abortion. It is unlikely that this society would approve such a course of action in the foreseeable future.

It is not by any means clear who the ultimate beneficiaries of a prenatal diagnostic screening program would be, but the issue is closely tied to the goals of the program. If the goal is to prevent the birth of defective infants, then there would be several beneficiaries: parents, having avoided the physical, emotional, and economic burdens of caring for such a child; society, having benefited financially in both saving money and being able to allocate funds elsewhere; and the infant itself, because it can be argued that it is worse to live a life of intense suffering than not to live at all. If, however, the goal of the program is to simply inform parents that the fetus is defective, then the only beneficiaries are the parents who might be able to make some preparation for the birth of the child.

New technology creates new issues, and one of the newest, and some believe strangest, ethical/legal issue to arise out of prenatal diagnosis is the matter of "wrongful life." This somewhat ambiguous phrase generally has to do with a lawsuit filed in one of two ways. Either parents file suit against a physician for either withholding information about a defective fetus from the prospective parents or for neglecting to diagnose the presence of a defect when knowledge of that defect could have been obtained by means of technology in common use. Or children sue their parents for having given birth to them despite the knowledge that they would suffer from a serious disease or defect. The premise of the suit is that no life at all would have been preferable to a life of present and future suffering. These concepts and problems can be best illustrated by summarizing actual cases.

In *Park v. Chessin*[34] Hetty and Steven Park gave birth to a child with polycystic kidney disease. The child died 5 hours after birth, and the Parks asked their obstetrician what their chances were of having another child so affected. The physician responded (incorrectly) that the disease was not hereditary and the chances of another such child being born to the Parks was "practically nil." On the basis of this information they had another child— similarly affected with polycystic kidney disease—who lived for 2½ years. The Parks sued, and lower courts agreed,

> The parents and their children had standing to sue for both wrongful birth and money loss, but could not sue for psychiatric and emotional distress. The question before the Court of Appeals was not who would win the lawsuits if and when they were heard, but whether, *assuming everything the plaintiffs alleged was true*, the plaintiffs could recover damages.[35]

The Court of Appeals was faced with a basic question: should the parents of a defective child, whose birth would have been prevented had it not been for the negligence of the physician, be permitted to recover the costs of treating the child? The court found that because the child was born solely because of malpractice on the part of the physician and because the cost of caring for the child could be accurately assessed, damages for that cost should be awarded.

> The court, however, refused to permit recovery for emotional or psychiatric damages because permitting such an action would "inevitably lead to the drawing of arbitrary boundaries." One such consideration the court mentioned is balancing the emotional trauma with the parental "love that even an abnormality cannot fully dampen."[36]

This decision is much more limited than it could have been and that many believe it should have been. The parent's emotional suffering was entirely the result of the physician's gross malpractice, and although it is admittedly difficult to calculate an actual monetary sum for such suffering, it has been done in other malpractice suits.

The second concept, that of "wrongful life" is much more complex, and there has now been legal precedent both for and against awarding damages to a defective child. One of the most dramatic was the *Curlender* case.[37] Shauna Tamar Curlender was born with Tay-Sachs disease after a laboratory had specifically told her parents, as a result of genetic screening, that they were not carriers. Shauna was subject to severe suffering and had a life expectancy of only about 4 years.

> The child's lawsuit sought damages for emotional distress and the deprivation of 72.6 years of life. She sought an additional $3 million in punitive damages on the grounds that the defendants knew their testing procedures were likely to produce a substantial number of false negatives and yet proceeded to use them "in conscious disregard of the health, safety, and wellbeing of the plaintiff. . . ." Since the complaint did not allege the date of the plaintiff's birth, the court could not determine whether the parents relied upon the test to conceive a child or to forego amniocentesis; nor does the court seem to care.[38]

The court must first grapple with the concept and definition of "wrongful life" and decide *why* the child is suing—because she has actually been born or because the laboratory was negligent. Before it began deliberations, the court made the following observations about the handling of such cases by previous courts[39]:

1. There is a major difference between a healthy child who is unwanted and/or illegitimate and one who was wanted and born with a severe deformity or disease.
2. There is a trend in the law to recognize that children should be compensated for injuries that are serious, painful, and long-lasting when their injuries are the direct result of negligence by others.

3. Parents and children have continued to sue even though other people have lost such cases because the problem is so serious and because technology is increasingly available to prevent such genetic disasters.

Given these observations, the court recognized the right of the child to sue for the negligent acts of others. The court also saw that the metaphysical aspects of existing as compared with not existing are not the immediate problem and are probably not an appropriate matter for the court in the first place. The reality is the child's suffering and the negligence of the laboratory. Annas finds that there is no reason to doubt the parents' and child's suffering, the laboratory's negligence, and the fact that there are costs involved. What is a more imponderable issue is the permissibility of the child to sue the laboratory.

> He or she expected nothing, not even birth. He or she *never* had the possibility of being born healthy—only the chance to be aborted or not conceived at all. From one way of looking at it, the child *could not* be damaged by the testing laboratory's negligence, because without the negligence the child would not have existed at all. The argument is *not* that any life is better than none, no matter what the suffering, but rather that to be damaged one needs to be worse off after the negligent act complained of than before it. It cannot be said, in this sense, that the child is worse off existing than not existing if one assumes that nonexistence is a state in which there are no rights and no rightful expectations.[40]

This is a metaphysical approach that courts of the future (and it seems reasonable to assume that these kinds of suits will increase in number) may or may not be competent to tackle, and it may or may not be relevant to the legal issue.

SURROGATE MOTHERHOOD

Surrogate motherhood occurs when the sperm of the husband of a barren woman is inseminated into another woman who then carries the fetus to term and gives it to the barren woman and her husband. There is almost always a fee involved that can range from $5000 to $15,000 and perhaps even more. It is divided between the woman going through the pregnancy and the attorney who arranged the transaction.

Most physicians and clinics engaging in this form of reproductive technology require that the surrogate mother conform to certain criteria as follows: (1) she should already have children of her own but want no more; (2) she should be reasonably mentally and physically matched to the eventual parents; and (3) she will agree in writing to give up the child. Surrogate motherhood is increasing in popularity, and there appear to be three main reasons why women would want to carry and bear a child knowing they will give it away immediately:

altruism, the love of being pregnant, and economic need. These reasons are by no means discrete, and some surrogate mothers use all three to justify what many believe to be a rather unusual action.

The ethical issues in surrogate motherhood are the same as many of the legal questions, and the procedure is particularly likely to result in a lawsuit. The first issue is whether or not a legal adoption must take place as it would if the child were not biologically related to either parent. Second, if the surrogate mother chooses not to give up the child at birth, can she be legally forced to do so, and should the courts have this power? Third, should money change hands; that is, is the surrogate mother selling the child, or is she simply being reimbursed for the expenses incurred as a result of the pregnancy? Fourth, can the prospective parents prevent the surrogate from having an abortion if she changes her mind, or can they sue her for breach of contract if she does so?

Elizabeth Kane (not her real name), a married woman and mother of three children, bore a child for a couple and received $10,000 for her services. She said, "It's the father's child. I'm simply growing it for him."[41] The arrangement was made by a Kentucky attorney who claims to have done this more than 100 times before for an undisclosed, but presumably high, fee. Both Kane and her attorney have no moral qualms about the action and do not consider it "baby selling." Others do not agree.

Most states have laws against selling children either for money or for items of value. The laws were enacted to counteract the burgeoning business in blackmarket babies, but it is unclear if surrogate motherhood is adoption in the usual sense of the word. A Michigan court declared that a surrogate mother may not be paid, although she may provide the service free of charge to satisfy her own psychologic needs.[42] In early 1981 the Attorney General of the Commonwealth of Kentucky announced that contracts to bear a child were illegal and unenforceable in that state, and any consent for adoption would not be valid until the fifth day after the birth of the child. Exchange of fees for adoption is also illegal in Kentucky. Thus the attorney mentioned earlier has been enjoined from continuing his surrogate motherhood transactions. It seems likely that there will be appeals of both the Michigan and Kentucky rulings as well as legislative and/or judicial action in other states.

Surely the answer to all the relevant questions about surrogate motherhood should center on the best interests of the child, which admittedly are difficult to evaluate. These children may indeed be prone to a greater number of psychologic problems when they find out that not only were they given away at birth, but the mother who bore them never had any intention of keeping them. On the other hand, they must surely be greatly wanted by people who went through so much to arrange for their birth and "transfer." One of the problems of assessing the relative harms and benefits in surrogate motherhood is that there are so few data available, and what there is is anecdotal. No controlled studies have ever been done.

The only question about surrogate motherhood that has a clear legal answer, according to Annas,[43] is the one about to whom the child belongs. It is biologically the surrogate mother's and the sperm donor's, although it is "more" hers than his. That is, he would be required to prove beyond a reasonable doubt that he is the biologic father. This might be legally difficult if the surrogate mother is married because most states recognize a married couple as the legal parents of a child born within that marriage. Even if the surrogate mother is not married, she could almost certainly keep the child if she so chose. She might even sue the sperm donor for child support, and this would most likely result in a court fight—perhaps even a definitive decision.

SUMMARY

Human reproduction is now no longer simply a matter of engaging in sexual intercourse with pregnancy the inevitable outcome—if nothing is done to prevent that outcome. It is also more than simply a matter of bad luck or regrettable tragedy if pregnancy does not result. It is now possible, in increasing numbers of cases, to remedy barrenness in both the male and female with reproductive technology that is rapidly developing in sophistication. In addition to helping infertile couples bear a child, technology has moved in the direction of discovering information about the fetus, such as its gender and which of many genetic defects or diseases it may have. This ability, however, creates the problem of what to do about a fetus that is either the "wrong" gender or that has a serious defect or disease.

Artificial insemination is a reproductive technology that has been in common use for over a decade. It is most often done with the sperm of an infertile woman's husband, but it can also be done with that of an anonymous donor, and this leads to legal, social, and religious issues that have not been settled to everyone's satisfaction. The major ethical issue in both artificial insemination and in vitro fertilization (IVF), which is an even more advanced reproductive technology, is whether or not human beings should interfere in the natural process of human reproduction. IVF also poses considerable risk to the embryo, which has no way of giving informed consent to the procedure and thus may have legal redress if it is seriously damaged but not seriously enough to be aborted naturally.

In addition to questions of procedure if a fetus is found to be defective, prenatal diagnosis also raises the question of allocation, that is, who ought to receive the screening tests, which increase in complexity and expense as they increase in technologic sophistication. One could also question the wisdom of allocating research funds for reproductive technology when so many serious and painful diseases remain incurable.

Surrogate motherhood is a fairly new technology, and although it is not procedurally as difficult as some of the others discussed in this chapter, it raises some of the most difficult emotional, ethical, and legal questions. And though one might wish to do what is best for the child, the path to that correct action is not always clear.

Notes

1. Fletcher, J. C. Ethics and amniocentesis for fetal sex identification. *Hastings Center Report*, 1980, *10*(1), 15–17. Reprinted with permission of The Hastings Center.© Institute of Society, Ethics, and the Life Sciences, 360 Broadway, Hastings-on-Hudson, N.Y. 10706.
2. Kazazian, H. H., Jr. Prenatal diagnosis for sex choice: a medical view. *Hastings Center Report*, 1980, *10*(1), 17–18.
3. Fletcher, p. 17.
4. Largey, G. Sex selection. In W. T. Reich (Ed.), *Encyclopedia of bioethics*. New York: The Free Press, 1978. p. 1440.
5. Largey, p. 1440.
6. Largey, p. 1442.
7. Campbell, C. The manchild pill. *Psychology Today*, August, 1976, p. 86.
8. Westhoff, C. F., & Rindfuss, R. R. Sex preselection in the United States: some indications. *Science*, 1974, *184*(4127), 633–636.
9. Campbell, p. 90.
10. Fleming, A. T. New frontiers in conception. © 1980 by The New York Times Company. Reprinted by permission. *New York Times Magazine*, July 20, 1980, p. 14.
11. Fleming, p. 20.
12. Annas, G. J. Artificial insemination: beyond the best interests of the donor. *Hastings Center Report*, 1979, *9*(4), 14–15, 43. Reprinted with permission of The Hastings Center. © Institute of Society, Ethics, and the Life Sciences, 360 Broadway, Hastings-on-Hudson, N.Y. 10706.
13. Annas, p. 14.
14. Annas, p. 14.
15. Fleming, p. 23.
16. Fletcher, J. *Morals and medicine*. Princeton, N.J.: Princeton University Press, 1954. p. 117. Copyright 1954 by Princeton University Press.
17. Currie-Cohen, M., et al. Current practice of artificial insemination by donor in the United States. *New England Journal of Medicine*, 1979, *300*, 585.
18. Annas, p. 15.
19. Fleming, p. 22.
20. Mastroianni, L., Jr. In vitro fertilization. In *Encyclopedia of bioethics*, pp. 1449–1450.
21. Mastroianni, pp. 1449–1450.
22. Steinfels, M. O. In vitro fertilization: "ethically acceptable" research. *Hastings Center Report*, 1979, *9*(3), 5–8.

23. Walters, L. Human in vitro fertilization: a review of the ethical literature. *Hastings Center Report*, 1979, *9*(4), 23–43.
24. Kass, L. R. Babies by means of in vitro fertilization: unethical experiments on the unborn? *New England Journal of Medicine*, 1971, *285*, 1175. Reprinted, by permission of The New England Journal of Medicine.
25. Kass, p. 1176.
26. Kass, p. 1177.
27. Fleming, p. 24.
28. Holmes, L. B. The health problem: neural tube defects. *Maternal serum alpha-fetoprotein: issues in the prenatal screening and diagnosis of neural tube defects*. Proceedings of a conference. National Center for Health Care Technology, U.S. Department of Health and Human Services, Office of Health, Research, Statistics, and Technology, July 28–30, 1980, Washington, D.C.
29. Haddow, J. E. Workgroup paper: general issues in maternal serum alpha-fetoprotein screening. In *Maternal serum alpha-fetoprotein*.
30. Haddow, J. E., & Holtzman, N. A. Workgroup summary: general issues in the prenatal screening and diagnosis of neural tube defects. In *Maternal serum alpha-fetoprotein*. p. 39.
31. Walters, L. Ethical perspectives in maternal serum alpha-fetoprotein screening. *Maternal serum alpha-fetoprotein*, p. 65.
32. Walters (Ethical perspectives), p. 68.
33. Walters, p. 68.
34. *Park v. Chessin*, No. 560, N.Y. Ct. Appeals (Dec. 27, 1978).
35. Annas, G. J. Medical paternity and "wrongful life." *Hastings Center Report*, 1979, *9*(3), 15.
36. Annas, p. 16.
37. *Curlender v. Bio-Science Laboratories*, 165 Cal. Rptr. 477 (Ct. App. 2nd Dist. Div. 1 [1980]).
38. Annas, G. J. Righting the wrong of "Wrongful life." *Hastings Center Report*, 1981, *11*(1), 8. Reprinted with permission of The Hastings Center. © Institute of Society, Ethics, and the Life Sciences, 360 Broadway, Hastings-on-Hudson, N.Y. 10706.
39. Annas, pp. 8–9.
40. Annas, p. 9.
41. Annas, G. J. Contracts to bear a child: compassion or commercialism? *Hastings Center Report*, 1981, *11*(2), 23.
42. *Doe v. Kelley*, 6 FLR 3011, Mich. (1980).
43. Annas (Contracts), p. 24.

Bibliography

Annas, G. J. Artificial insemination: beyond the best interests of the donor. *Hastings Center Report*, 1979, *9*(4), 14–15, 43.

Annas, G. J. Contracts to bear a child: compassion or commercialism? *Hastings Center Report*, 1981, *11*(2), 23–24.

Annas, G. J. Medical paternity and "wrongful Life." *Hastings Center Report*, 1979, *9*(3), 15–17.

Annas, G. J. Righting the wrong of "Wrongful Life." *Hastings Center Report*, 1981, *11*(1), 8–9.

Brock, D. J. H. Serum screening: alpha-fetoprotein. In *Maternal serum alpha-fetoprotein: issues in the prenatal screening and diagnosis of neural tube defects.* Proceedings of a conference. National Center for Health Care Technology, United States Department of Health and Human Services, Office of Health Research, Statistics, and Technology. July 28–30, 1980. Washington, D.C.

Campbell, C. The manchild pill. *Psychology Today*, August, 1976, pp. 86–91.

DeKretzer, D., et al. Transfer of a human zygote. *Lancet*, 1973, *2*, 728–729.

Edwards, R. G. Fertilization of human eggs in vitro: morals, ethics and the law. *Quarterly Review of Biology*, 1974, *49*, 3–26.

Edwards, R. G., & Steptoe, P. C. Physiologic aspects of human embryo transfer. In *Progress in infertility* (2nd ed.). S. J. Behrman & R. W. Kistner, (Eds.), Boston: Little, Brown & Co., 1975. pp. 377–409.

Etzioni, A. Sex control, science, and society. *Science*, 1968, *161*, 1107–1112.

Fleming, A. T. New frontiers in conception. *New York Times Magazine*, July 20, 1980, pp. 14–52.

Fletcher, J. C. Ethics and amniocentesis for fetal sex identification. *Hastings Center Report*, 1980, *10*(1), 15–17.

Fletcher, J. C. Moral and ethical problems of pre-natal diagnosis. *Clinical Genetics*, 1975, *8*, 251–257.

Fletcher, J. *Morals and medicine*, Princeton, N.J.: Princeton University Press, 1954.

Frankel, M. S. Sperm and zygote banking. In W. T. Reich (Ed.), *Encyclopedia of bioethics.* New York: The Free Press, 1978.

Fromer, M. J. *Ethical issues in health care.* St. Louis: The C.V. Mosby Co., 1981.

Glass, B. Science: endless horizons or Golden Age? *Science*, 1971, *171*, 23–29.

Haddow, J. E. Workgroup paper: general issues in maternal serum alpha-fetoprotein screening. In *Maternal serum alpha-fetoprotein.*

Haddow, J. E., & Holtzman, N. A. Workgroup summary: general issues in the prenatal screening and diagnosis of neural tube defects. In *Maternal serum alpha-fetoprotein.*

Holmes, L. B. The health problem: neural tube defects. In *Maternal serum alpha-fetoprotein.*

Kass, L. R. Babies by means of in vitro fertilization: unethical experiments on the unborn? *New England Journal of Medicine*, 1971, *285*, 1174–1179.

Kazazian, H. H., Jr. Prenatal diagnosis for sex choice: a medical view. *Hastings Center Report*, 1980, *10*(1), 17–18.

Lappé, M. Ethics at the center of life: protecting vulnerable subjects. *Hastings Center Report*, 1978, *8*(5), 11–13.

Lappé, M., & Steinfels, P. Choosing the sex of our children. *Hastings Center Report*, 1974, *4*(1), 1–4.

Largey, G. Sex selection. In *Encyclopedia of bioethics.*

Lenzer, G. Gender ethics. *Hastings Center Report*, 1980, *10*(1), 18–19.

Marsh, F. H., & Self, D. J. In vitro fertilization: moving from theory to therapy. *Hastings Center Report*, 1980, *10*(3), 5–6.

Mastroianni, L., Jr. In vitro fertilization. In *Encyclopedia of bioethics.*

Powledge, T. Prenatal diagnosis: new techniques, new questions. *Hastings Center Report*, 1979, *9*(3), 16–17.

Ramsey, P. Manufacturing our offspring: weighing the risks. *Hastings Center Report*, 1978, *8*(5), 7–9.

Robertson, J. A. In vitro conception and harm to the unborn. *Hastings Center Report*, 1978, *8*(5), 13–14.

Steinfels, M. O. In vitro fertilization: "ethically acceptable" research. *Hastings Center Report*, 1979, *9*(3), 5–8.

Toulmin, S. in vitro fertilization: answering the ethical objections. *Hastings Center Report*, 1978, *8*(5), 9–11.

Veatch, R. M. *Case studies in medical ethics*. Cambridge, Mass.: Harvard University Press, 1977.

Walters, L. Ethical perspectives on maternal serum alpha-fetoprotein screening. In *Maternal serum alpha-fetoprotein*.

Walters, L. Human in vitro fertilization: a review of the ethical literature. *Hastings Center Report*, 1979, *9*(4), 23–43.

Westhoff, C. F., & Rindfuss, R. R. Sex preselection in the United States: some indications. *Science*, 1974, *184*(4127), 633–636.

CHAPTER 9

FETAL RESEARCH

At the end of 1974 the National Commission for the Protection of Human Subjects of Biomedical and Behavioral Research (hereinafter known as the National Commission) was founded to investigate ways in which human beings as research subjects could be protected during the course of research. The National Commission succeeded admirably in this task and eventually produced a set of guidelines so comprehensive and complex that many believed them to hamper unnecessarily the conduct of research. In early 1981 the guidelines were amended to allow researchers more freedom, although they still remain the best protection that human subjects have had since experimentation began in ancient Greece.

The National Commission was given several tasks as follows: to identify basic ethical principles that ought to govern research using human subjects; to clarify the requirements of informed consent; to pay particular attention to the special requirements of particularly vulnerable groups such as children, prisoners, and the institutionalized mentally infirm; and to investigate the use of psychosurgery and recommend policies for its regulation.[1]

The National Research Act, which established the National Commission, also mandated that the commissioners investigate the nature and extent of research involving living fetuses, and at the same time it banned all such nontherapeutic research before or after an induced abortion. However, it was tacitly understood that the moratorium would be lifted when the commissioners devised a set of acceptable guidelines. By counting fetuses as among the subjects to be considered with others involved in human experimentation and by banning nontherapeutic research (that which does not directly benefit the subject) on living fetuses, the framers of the National Research Act involved themselves directly in what Steinfels and others refer to as "fetal politics," a phrase that implies a series of ongoing arguments about not only whether or not a fetus is a human being but also how it should be treated and what legal protections it should have.

The Supreme Court decided *Roe v. Wade* only 1 year before the establishment of the National Commission, but it did nothing to settle the issues and questions that are collectively known as fetal politics. In fact, there was considerable political backlash in reaction to *Roe v. Wade*, and this backlash seems to be growing more intense. Fetuses were included in the National Commission's mandate partly because it was politically expedient to do so but even more because fetal research presents a genuine ethical dilemma. Fetuses cannot be considered full consenting human subjects in the usual sense of the phrase "human subject," but neither can they be considered in the same category as other humans who cannot give informed consent for a variety of reasons (children, prisoners, the mentally retarded, and the like). Thus, fetuses must be considered a special class of beings when considering them as research subjects. Whether or not one believes them to be full human beings in the ontologic and metaphysical sense (see the chapter on abortion for arguments both for and against this position), they surely are not human beings in the physiologic sense, although they have all the physical potential to become so. For the purpose of avoiding bias as much as possible in this chapter, the fetus will be referred to as a "being unlike any other known being or entity."

FETAL-MATERNAL RELATIONSHIP

As soon as she becomes aware that she is pregnant (oftentimes before the actual confirmation by pregnancy test), a woman enters into a relationship with the fetus that changes and develops until it undergoes a transformation to a relationship with an infant, that is, a person-to-person relationship. The relationship with the fetus, however, is unique. Some women claim that their fetus has a personality even while it lies in utero. This may be ascribed more to the physical activity of the fetus than to anything else, but a pregnant woman's belief in this personality is indicative of her growing relationship with and attachment to the fetus.

The nature of this relationship depends on many variables, for example, the circumstances surrounding the conception, the woman's relationship with the father, the degree to which the pregnancy is desired, the woman's physical health and the way she is "weathering" the pregnancy, and the way in which she perceives childbirth and childrearing and her past experiences with them. The occasion of quickening (the perception of fetal movements by the woman) marks a turning point in the fetal-maternal relationship. Before quickening the fact of pregnancy was easy to recognize only in an intellectual sense; after quickening the fetus' physical presence makes itself known and the pregnancy becomes a part of the woman's everyday reality. She begins to incorporate it into her life, and her sense of responsibility for the fetus develops in intensity—for most women.

This chain of events is usual but by no means universal. Those women who are planning to abort during the first trimester do not usually feel that the fetus is a being to be protected and nurtured, although one woman, as she waited for the time to pass between the confirmation of her pregnancy and the scheduled abortion, began to take vitamins, pay attention to her nutrition, and drink milk. She said, "I'm taking care of it until the abortion—just in case I change my mind."

Those women who are either ambivalent or angry about being pregnant are generally slower to develop an attachment to the fetus, and some never do and either abort in the second trimester or give birth under far less than optimal circumstances.

> The phenomenon of maternal attachment to the fetus is presumably vulnerable, and failure of attachment might be expected to correlate with increased morbidity for the unborn infant or the postnatal child. Data to support this hypothesis are very few, in part because of the difficulties in designing a prospective study.[2]

It is sometimes possible to detect maternal attitudes toward the fetus by observing certain behaviors, although again these observations are by no means universally accurate, and it would be a mistake to make moral judgments solely on the basis of these observations. However, a woman who smokes cigarettes (and who understands the adverse effect of cigarette smoking on the fetus) must be said to have a less positive relationship with her fetus than a woman who refrains from smoking throughout her pregnancy. A woman who disregards the nutritional content of her diet demonstrates less respect for and responsibility to the fetus than a woman who guarantees the adequacy of the fetus's development in part by eating recommended nutrients.

Within certain limits (such as fate, genetics, accident, and the like) the pregnant woman is responsible for the fate of the fetus, yet at the same time it is an entity, separate as a being but physically connected, that is growing and developing in ways she cannot control and does not see. Although the fetus is inside the woman and is part of her body, it is not part of her self nor is she dependent on it. This makes the relationship extremely complex and difficult to discuss. According to Mahoney,[3] the complexity of the maternal-fetal duality creates even thornier ethical dilemmas than would any ethical question posed by the existence of either the pregnant woman or the fetus, who may, in any case, have conflicting interests. One of these conflicting interests may well be the continuation of one life at the expense of the other.

As pregnancy proceeds, these problems and conflicts increase in complexity as the fetus seems increasingly individualistic and appears more personlike with each passing week. Although the goal of this chapter will be to concentrate on the ethical issues in fetal research, the emotional or psychologic overtones cannot be ignored. By the time quickening has occurred, the fetus definitely looks like a person, and by the last trimester it has the appearance of a cuddly baby, especially with regard to its curled-up posture and vulnerable mien. It is cute. Its very cuteness and vulnerability create a certain emotional squeamishness when fetal experiments are considered, even when intellectualization about the research is positive. It is difficult to lay aside this emotionalism without appearing coldly calculating, yet an effort must be made to do so to correctly assess the right-making and wrong-making qualities of fetal research.

TYPES OF RESEARCH

Although there are ethical issues inherent in conducting research on dead fetuses, this chapter will concentrate on living ones for two major reasons: the ethical issues are more complex and more ultimately important, and the National Commission, which is responsible for the definitive work and most of the literature in the area, concerned itself only with living fetuses. I shall use the National Commission's definition of fetus as "a living human conceptus (1) *in utero* from the time of implantation to the time of delivery or abortion and (2) outside the uterus from a point eight days after fertilization to the point at which the organism is viable."[4] A living fetus is further defined as possessing at least one of the standard life signs such as heartbeat, spontaneous respiration, movement, or pulsation of the umbilical cord. Viable, according to the National Commission, means that the fetus is sufficiently mature to be able to live when the connection to the pregnant woman is severed, assuming standard neonatal care. (The reader is referred to the chapter on abortion for a more complete discussion of viability.) Therapeutic research is defined as the use of modes of treatment that are not yet established as standard but that are intended to directly benefit the subject (whether they are indeed beneficial is a secondary issue and one that causes ethical conflict). Nontherapeutic research is the use of procedures that also are not standard and that have the intent of adding to general scientific knowledge rather than directly benefitting the subject on whom they are being tested.

There are several ways in which to categorize fetal research as follows: that done either in utero or outside the uterus; that involving either induced or spontaneous abortion or premature delivery; research using either previable or viable fetuses; the differences, already mentioned, between therapeutic and nontherapeutic research; and research involving various degrees of risk to the fetus, either minimal, moderate, or serious. In theory there are 48 types of fetal research, but it is more practical to speak only of those that either have already been done or that are pragmatically feasible.

Research is most frequently done at the following four stages of fetal life: (1) when the fetus is in utero and will remain there for at least 1 week, (2) when the fetus is in utero but delivery by induced or spontaneous abortion is anticipated within a few hours or days, (3) during an abortion but while the maternal-feto-placenta unit is still intact, and (4) following the completion of an abortion when the fetus has been separated from the woman.[5] Research on live fetuses is done for a variety of reasons; for example, to diagnose fetal diseases or defects; to accomplish intrauterine therapy that corrects a defect; to study fetal behavior; to do fetal-maternal nutrition studies and to examine the mechanics and physiology of placental transfer; to study fetal physiology and metabolism; to study abortion techniques; to study oxygenation in various tissues and methods for prolonging fetal life; and to study techniques for facilitating delivery.

Most people will agree that the ultimate knowledge gained from these types of research will be beneficial and that the goal and intent of all of them is to improve the health of the fetus and ultimately that of the person for the rest of his life. Most of the ethical problems do not arise from the fact that the research is being done or from the intent of the researchers; instead they spring from the idea that fetuses may be unjustifiably harmed, that they cannot consent to the procedure, and that the pregnant woman may not be fully informed about the nature of the research.

Walters, in a report to the National Commission, chronicled the types of live-fetus research that had been reported in the literature for the previous 15 years. A summary of that chronicle follows[6]:

1. The fetus in utero more than 1 week before delivery or abortion—prenatal *diagnosis* by amniocentesis, ultrasonography, fetoscopy, and fetal blood sampling; intrauterine *therapy* with transfusions for Rh incompatibility, surgery for defects, and treatment for adrenogenital syndrome, fetal lung immaturity, and anemia; studies of *fetal behavior* in response to sound and light; studies of placental transfer in regard to drugs administered to the pregnant woman, including several rubella vaccine studies.

2. The fetus in utero a few hours or days before delivery or abortion—prenatal *diagnosis* by fetoscopy; *nutrition* studies, particularly maternal fasting for several days before abortion; studies of placental transfer of substances such as radioisotopes, ethyl alcohol, steroids, and other *drugs*; studies of *abortion techniques* that concentrate on maternal comfort and safety and the mechanism by which the fetus dies in saline-induced abortion; studies of techniques to *facilitate delivery*.

3. The fetus during the abortion procedure while the maternal-feto-placental unit is intact—*placental transfer* studies to detect whether substances travel from the fetal to the maternal side of the placenta; studies of fetal physiology or metabolism with such substances as arginine, sulfur, and I-glucagon.
4. The fetus outside the uterus following separation from the pregnant woman (the fetus is then called an abortus)—studies of fetal *physiology* or metabolism in which blood circulation can be used to detect the circulation and absorption of various substances throughout the fetus; the *removal or harvesting of fetal tissue*, which is the final step of fetal metabolism studies (the liver and brain are used most frequently); studies of *oxygenation* and prolongation of life by such methods as submersion in an oxygen-rich nutrient and attachment to an artificial placenta.

Therapeutic and nontherapeutic research

In fetal research, as well as that done on fully grown human subjects, one of the major controversies is the conflict between therapeutic and nontherapeutic research. At first glance, it might seem that the more beneficial the research is to the fetus under investigation, the more justifiable the research. This may indeed be true if the fetus is intended to be cured, treated, or simply not allowed to die. If, however, the fetus will die anyway as in the case of an induced or spontaneous abortion, in which the fetus is clearly previable, then it might seem unjustifiable not to use that fetus for research. If the fetus is doomed to death, there may be an obligation to use it to study conditions that might be beneficial to pregnant women and at the same time harmful to fetuses. For example, many drugs cannot be given to pregnant women because their effect on the fetus is not known. Nontherapeutic research on fetuses that are doomed to die would surely result in information about the fetal effect of such a drug. If future fetuses can thus be saved from harm, are not researchers obligated to do what they can to prevent such harm?

The development of a rubella vaccine is an example of this kind of research.[7] Exposure to German measles causes serious abnormalities in up to 40% of all fetuses. Before the development of the vaccine, no one knew how to prevent this tragedy. There were several courses of action open to researchers when they began to experiment with a vaccine that could prevent the pregnant woman from contracting the disease, but no one knew what effect the vaccine would have on the fetus. The only way to determine the answer was to do preabortion studies, that is, to give the vaccine to women who intended to abort and then examine the fetus. An alternative would have been to give the vaccine to pregnant women who wanted their children and then do a retrospective study of those children. This would have deliberately subjected the fetus to the risk of serious damage or death even though the vaccine might have provided adequate protection after the pregnant woman had been exposed to the disease. A third alternative would have been not to give the vaccine after the woman had been exposed to rubella, thereby leaving the situation to chance. The best choice of the three seemed to be to use the fetus that was destined for destruction, thereby giving a meaning to the fetal death and perhaps diluting the woman's negative perception of the abortion. This turned out to have been the best course of action, but it need not have been so.

There is a wide range of bacterial and viral agents, as well as environmental ones, that cause fetal defects, especially in the first trimester. The only way to counteract these effects is by fetal research, most of it nontherapeutic.

> We find ourselves, therefore, in a peculiar position. The total destruction of one or two *normal* fetuses to protect against the possible birth of one *abnormal* fetus, under current law in the United States, is not legally objectionable. We allow and sometimes encourage just such a practice in the case of a male fetus at risk for hemophilia. Here, abortion of the *normal* male, virtually indistinguishable from its affected brother, is sanctioned to ensure that half the time, a hemophiliac fetus is eliminated. Yet to do research that might save both infants on a fetus that is about to be destroyed is, if we accept the current status quo, morally objectionable. We will, in addition, have to permit the birth of many seriously crippled children when exposure to the virus or presence of genetic disease has not been detected, or the parent is morally opposed to abortion.[8]

The position of being legally permitted to abort an unlimited number of healthy fetuses while being prohibited from doing research on a limited number (limited by the consent of the pregnant woman and other factors) of live fetuses is as ridiculous as it is inconsistent. Those fetuses that are destined for certain destruction should not be wasted if their use can contribute to the improved health of future fetuses. Although the moratorium on live fetal research has now been lifted, there are indications that it may be reinstituted.

The real choice is not between experimentation on fetuses and no experimentation at all; it is between therapeutic and nontherapeutic research. The first position is not tenable in a highly technologic society that insists on moving ever forward in the quest for scientific knowledge. Research *will* be done; the only question is who or what should be the subjects of that research.

In utero and ex utero

Fetal research done solely in utero consists of various manipulations of the fetus, usually surgical, to correct deformities, exchange fetal blood via transfusion for Rh incompatibility, and the like. This is almost always accomplished by making a surgical incision in the pregnant woman's abdomen and then into the uterus, although a few experiments can be done by amnioscopy, a procedure in which a long hollow tube is inserted into the uterus through a very small abdominal incision. Fiberoptic bundles are then passed through the tube to visualize the fetus. Experiments done solely ex utero are those done after induced or spontaneous abortion and were described in the preceding section. Ex utero experiments can be done on either living or dead fetuses.

Most fetal research, however, is a combination of that done both inside and outside the uterus, typically in the manner already described when abortion or delivery will occur soon. This is the only way to test the effect of pharmacologic, biologic, and environmental substances on the fetus, that is, to subject the fetus to the substance and then physically and microscopically examine the effect. This, however, is the most ethically problematic type of research because it is done with the intent, or at least the very strong possibility, of harming the fetus in question, although it may prove highly beneficial to future fetuses.

The issue of consent is of major importance here. Obviously the fetus can consent to nothing; therefore two immediate questions arise: (1) Can another person (the pregnant woman or the researcher) consent for the fetus, that is, is fetal consent implied if the woman consents and (2) must the woman who is to undergo induced abortion give consent for fetal research, or does she, by intending to destroy the fetus, give up all rights to and responsibility for it?

The resolution of the first question rests partly on one's perception of the moral status of the fetus, that is, whether or not it is a person. Even if it is a person, it still cannot give its own consent as infants and some persons cannot; therefore the question of proxy consent arises. Proxy consent will be discussed in more detail in the chapter on infants as persons and the mentally retarded. Suffice it to say here that proxy consent applies to fetal research in theory only. None of the literature reports that proxy consent is actually obtained from the parent or guardian of the fetus. It should be noted that the consent of the pregnant woman to use the fetus for research is not precisely the same as proxy consent, although the differences are admittedly obscure.

However, the problem of the pregnant woman giving consent is a real one. One of the general functions of consent is to protect the research subject from as much harm as possible, but that is not precisely the case here. In electing abortion, the pregnant woman not only agrees to harm the fetus, she also intends it to some degree. Certainly she intends its death. On the other hand, there may be sensibilities and sensitivities about the fetus that are not easily dismissed simply because the woman does not wish to be pregnant. The grief of experiencing an abortion may be compounded if the woman were to find out later that the fetus was used as a research subject. Even if she were never to find out, the question of consent still exists. If the fetus is not exactly the woman's property, neither is it anyone else's, and she has a greater interest in deciding whether or not to consent to its use in research than does anyone else. In denying the woman the opportunity to consent to fetal research, it should be noted that a rather punitive attitude is displayed, almost as if the woman were to be doubly punished for having an abortion.

ETHICAL ISSUES

The ethics of fetal research are complicated by the fact that the endeavor is really several endeavors, involving subjects on a continuum of development and in various stages of probable viability. Walters[9] has identified the four most common ethical positions about fetal research before, during, and after induced abortion as follows:

1. Nontherapeutic fetal research should not be done under any circumstances.
2. Nontherapeutic fetal research should be done only to the extent that it is also permitted on those fetuses that will be carried to term or that is also permitted on children, that is, where the risk to the fetus is acceptably low.
3. Greater latitude should be allowed for nontherapeutic fetal research than would be permissible on fetuses that will be carried to term, although certain procedures should not be permitted even here.
4. Any type of nontherapeutic fetal research is permissible.

Walters attempts to defend the second position by appealing to McCormick's widely quoted argument in defending the permissibility of doing nontherapeutic research on children.[10] In his argument McCormick states that there are certain societal goods and benefits that are universally desirable, one of which is health. To secure this benefit, biomedical research, some of which entails risk, must take place, and it is a universal obligation to subject oneself to low-risk experiments. He thus concludes that because a child *ought* to consent to participation in such research, parents may give proxy consent for their participation; indeed they *should* do so because children would consent if they could.

Even though this argument can be logically attacked from several directions, Walters applies it to consenting to fetuses being used as subjects even though he acknowledges that the issue is somewhat more complex. In general, a parent who gives proxy consent for nontherapeutic research on a child has the best interests of that child at heart and can ordinarily be counted on not to subject the child to research that will be unduly risky, although admittedly the range of permissibility here is very wide and open to considerable debate. When fetal research is the issue, no such protective instincts exist because the pregnant woman does not intend the fetus to have a future. There are also different perceptions of risk, and it might be reasonable to assume that a pregnant woman would be willing to subject a doomed fetus to greater risk than would a mother her child. However, Walters does not find this an insurmountable problem.

> I suggest that it is possible to skirt these difficult problems as well as to be ethically consistent if one adopts the general rule: Nontherapeutic research procedures which are permissible in the case of fetuses which will be carried to term are also permissible in the case of (a) live fetuses which will be aborted and (b) live fetuses which have been aborted.[11]

Walters claims that he has found no factual proof demonstrating conclusively that there is a substantial measure of continuity between previable fetal life, viable fetal life, and infant life. Although he admits that the continuity thesis has some merit, the arguments against it are stronger.

First, he questions whether abortion and fetal experiments are either part of the same argument or are even analogous to each other; that is, he maintains that abortion is far worse than any fetal experiment and that the permissibility of abortion does not necessarily imply the permissibility of fetal research. He does not, however, say how most fetal experimentation can take place without abortion.

> The woman alleges a right to be rid of an immediate, serious threat to her previous pattern of life. This right is now guaranteed by the law for the stages of pregnancy prior to fetal viability. In the case of fetal research, however, there is, so far as I can see, no similar clear and immediate conflict between the previable fetus and society at large or any other social group. Thus, it would seem that the proponent of highly-invasive fetal research must build an entirely new case for such research rather than being able to piggyback his or her case on the fact of presumably-lethal abortion procedures.[12]

Walters' second point against the continuity argument is that there are undesirable consequences of fetal research, for example, the possibly dehumanizing social effects of performing highly risky invasive procedures on living fetuses that were destined to survive to become persons. Walters believes that a precedent might be set for performing such procedures on other classes of individuals whose personhood is questioned by some substantial segment of society, for example, the elderly senile, the comatose, and neonates.

Wasserstrom,[13] also in a report to the National Commission, summarized the arguments both for and against permitting experiments on nonviable living human fetuses ex utero. He divides the negative arguments into two groups, those taken from the utilitarian approach, that is, those having deleterious consequences, and those taken from the deontologic approach, that is, those being intrinsically wrong. He looks first at the utilitarian view.

1. If fetal research becomes widespread and well publicized, society in general will develop a desensitization toward or lessened respect for fetal life. The consequence could widen to a decreased respect for all human life.
2. All those persons who, for one reason or another, cannot look after themselves (the mentally retarded, the elderly, and the like) will command decreased respect from society.
3. "Individuals will become less sensitive than they ought to be to the claims of those persons whose deaths are reasonably thought to be certain and imminent, e.g., persons in the last stages of terminal illness."[14]
4. There will be a decreased sensitivity to the right of persons who are not willing to be subjects of experimentation.

All these arguments are based on what Walters referred to as the continuity argument; that is, the consequences of doing fetal research do not depend on the kind of entity that people perceive the fetus to be. Rather they depend on people's perception of human life in general, not of human persons in particular.

> Of course, the more one thinks the fetus is like other persons in most significant respects, the more one is also apt to think that individuals generally may confuse the case of the fetus with the case of those other entities whose claims to morally more sensitive treatment are nonetheless distinguishable.[15]

Wasserstrom also delineates other consequentialist arguments as follows:
5. If research on living nonviable fetuses becomes permissible, it will also become valuable, and the demand for fetuses will increase. This will result in subtle (or not so subtle) societal incentives for women to have abortions and to have them in such a way that the fetuses can be used for research.
6. Not only would abortion increase, it would do so disproportionately; that is, women of lower socioeconomic status would be more likely to succumb to the pressures and incentives to abort.
7. Significant numbers of people could react with severe and extreme revulsion to the idea of fetal research, much as people react strongly to cannibalism and to desecration of graves. The strength of this reaction, even if it affected only a minority of the population, would "substantially impair social peace and harmony."

Wasserstrom's deontologic arguments against fetal research are as follows:
1. The analogy can be made that if it is permissible to experiment on a living aborted fetus, then it is permissible to experiment on a living person who will die very soon (within a matter of hours or a day). Since the latter is clearly wrong, the former is also wrong.
2. The analogy can be extended to all living persons who have lost con-

sciousness and are not expected to regain it before death, regardless of how far in the future that death is expected to be.

3. Although viability is a continuum, there is clearly a range of time in which it can be expected that previable fetuses will not be able to survive no matter how much technology is applied to their care. However, this is by no means universal, and of all the previable fetuses delivered, a tiny minority will survive against all odds. Given that this is true and given that it is impossible to predict which of these ostensible previable fetuses will survive, it is wrong to experiment on any of them because to do the research would surely cause the demise of all of them, including those that would have lived.

4. If it is wrong to deliberately stop the heartbeat or respiration of a living fetus by direct action, then it is equally wrong to take steps that would hasten the cessation of heartbeat or respiration, no matter how indirect the method.

5. Even if the end results of fetal research are good in that the health of future fetuses will be improved, the means to that good end are wrong in that living fetuses are harmed. Therefore fetal research cannot be justified. Wasserstrom, however, admits to some problematic assumptions in this argument:

> To begin with, the argument assumes rather than explains the immorality of this kind of experimentation on non-viable fetuses. Unless independent grounds are offered to establish the impropriety of such experiments, the argument is at best hypothetical: if such grounds exist, they cannot be overridden by the worth of the end that is sought. In addition, the argument assumes both the possibility of separating clearly means from ends and the wrongness of using bad means to achieve a good end.[16]

6. All experiments that cause the fetus more pain than it would ordinarily experience are bad and cannot be justified. It does not seem to matter to Wasserstrom that we do not know for certain if fetuses can indeed experience pain; the possibility that they can is sufficient to justify this argument.

Wasserstrom's arguments in favor of fetal research are fewer in number and not stated in as compelling a way as his arguments against it.

1. Things of great usefulness in terms of the preservation and improvement of human lives will result from fetal research and can be learned only from fetal research.

2. The legitimacy of the research takes precedence over whatever harm might come to the fetus because not only have social utility and need been sufficiently established, the proof that some nonviable fetuses might indeed live has not been sufficiently established.

3. Fetuses are entities different from human beings, even those human beings who are permanently unconscious or totally outside their own control; this fact makes it permissible to experiment on fetuses when it would not be permissible on these classes of human beings. Nonviability in the fetus is not precisely analogous to irreversible coma in the person.

4. If there is no rational reason to prohibit fetal research, then a societal decision to prohibit it encourages irrational decisions in other biomedical contexts, and this is not a wise thing to do. Scientific investigation in general should not be restricted unless there are logical and compelling reasons to do so.

Other philosophers have established other views on fetal research. The most liberal permissive position is taken by Joseph Fletcher.[17] He maintains that it is impossible to injure, harm, or assault a fetus because these terms apply only to living persons who are independent biologic individuals. This may be true in a strictly legalistic sense, but it is no more true in an ethical sense than it would be to say that it is permissible to whip a dog because the dog cannot take the person who beat it to court. Fletcher further maintains that it is erroneous to think of fetal research as having a brutalizing effect because there was no such effect in evidence between the time fetal research began and the time the moratorium was called. This may or may not be true, but even if it is, there is no reason to believe that the absence of a brutalizing effect will continue; societal decisions often engender a delayed reaction, and there is no way of knowing whether or not the cumulative effect will be as benign as Fletcher predicts.

Fletcher further states that those who hold the minority view (that is, opposition to fetal research of any kind) would probably prefer a compromise position, hoping to have large classes of fetal research banned if they could not put a halt to all of it. But he believes that the minority view should be subordinated to the majority one, particularly when formulating public policy, because those who are opposed to fetal research need not consent to it for themselves and they should leave others alone to move ahead with medical and scientific knowledge. Although Fletcher does believe that the consent of the pregnant woman should be obtained, he sees no other permissible restrictions to fetal research. He tends to sweep aside arguments against and objections to fetal research without proving that they have no ethical or social merit. He attacks them as "doctrinaire and regulatory" rather than arguing against them by means of reason. In so doing he weakens his own case for the permissibility of fetal research.

Seymour Siegel takes the opposite approach and argues for a ban on all fetal research. He does this by affirming what he believes to be certain basic principles.[18]

1. The primary and most general principle is the "bias for life" that directs all persons in the healing arts to sustain life wherever it exists. All means or procedures that terminate life or hasten its end are unethical. "Another implication of this 'bias' is that any individual life which claims our efforts and attention, and which is before us at this moment, has prece-

dence over life that may come afterwards."[19] In other words, no present fetus may be harmed or sacrificed for the ultimate benefit of future fetuses, regardless of what the pregnant woman determines should be its fate.

2. The future can never be predicted accurately; therefore hoped-for bene-fits of fetal research may not come to pass. Moreover, some of the experiments must necessarily involve the pregnant woman, and there is no way of knowing whether or not her general health or reproductive capacities will be adversely affected by present experiments.

3. Although a fetus is not the same as a human being, and feticide is not the same as homicide because there is a physical, ontologic, and metaphysi-cal difference, this does not mean "that from an ethical standpoint there is no difference between a fetus and a tooth or a fingernail of the mother —to be disposed of as the mother wishes."[20] The special status that the fetus enjoys because it is a unique part of the pregnant woman's body gives it special rights and privileges. It is therefore wrong to harm the fetus unless it poses a specific threat to the pregnant woman. Even then, although she may under narrowly defined circumstances rid herself of the fetus, she may not subject it to further harm by causing it to be a research subject.

4. Because the fetus has rights, it must be guarded and protected from harm; therefore only therapeutic research is permissible or that which will help the pregnant woman successfully complete the pregnancy.

5. The dividing line between the life and death of a fetus is crucial and can determine permissibility of fetal research. Viability, which is only an indicator of the potentiality for survival, has nothing to do with this distinction. Actual life or death is the only appropriate indicator.

In view of these principles, Siegel would find it permissible to experiment only on those fetuses that will not only not be harmed but also will have an enhanced chance at a healthy life as a result of the research. Since no guarantee exists that these criteria will be met, the range of permissibility is indeed narrow.

Between these two extreme views is a moderate one in which fetal research would be allowed with certain restrictions. This position holds that the fetus does not have primary rights, but neither can its interests be ignored. However, other considerations take precedence. The pregnant woman has an interest in the disposal of the fetus, and both the pregnant woman and society in general can be expected to face a certain amount of emotional pain at the knowledge of casual fetal experimentation. Medical researchers should not be permitted to handle live or dead fetuses in a brutal or even casual manner, nor should they be permitted to exhibit an arrogant attitude toward the fetus or toward the woman from whom it issued. It is difficult to know how many researchers do indeed exhibit a casual attitude toward fetuses used in research or what observable effect these attitudes will have on the future of research.

The cases both for and against fetal research have already been enumerated, and points may be "pulled" from each side to arrive at a moderate consensus. Knowing which points to use creates the dilemma. Obviously there must be a balance struck between risks and benefits, and there must be an establishment of institutional safeguards and protocols that protect the safety and dignity of the fetus. In both therapeutic and nontherapeutic research the risks must be low enough and the benefits sufficiently important to justify the research, but this is difficult to assess. In addition, there must be no alternate way to achieve the desired results. The consent of the pregnant woman should be mandatory for both therapeutic and nontherapeutic research, although it is arguable whether the consent of the father is also necessary and if it matters whether or not she is married to him. Consent is important for the reasons already discussed and because if the fetus survives the experiment, there may be a problem of to whom it "belongs." If the abortion was spontaneous, the pregnant woman (now a mother) has a living child rather than the expected stillborn one. If the abortion was induced, does the infant revert back to the woman who aborted it, or by deliberately aborting, has she deliberately renounced all claim to it? This question, although fascinating in all its ramifications, cannot concern us here, but its existence does underscore the importance of obtaining consent.

Moral status of the fetus

The argument about whether or not the fetus is metaphysically a full human being will have to be left to theologians and philosophers, although the reader is referred to the chapter on abortion for some of the methods of debate used in this argument. It can be logically argued, however, that the fetus is not a full human being in the physical sense because it is not capable, at least for the first two thirds of its development, of surviving in the world as other human beings do. Toward the end of pregnancy that premise becomes shaky, and many fetuses born before term become human beings simply because they are forced to. In this way a nonswimmer might try valiantly to become an instant swimmer when his sailboat capsizes. If he manages to stay afloat, it is by dint of his struggling to do so, not by his swimming prowess. The swimmer is the same physical person before and after his struggle, and the fetus is the same physical being after it is born as it was beforehand; the only difference is the way in which it seeks to survive.

Although the fetus is not yet a human being, it is potentially not anything else. Thus the original decision to classify it as a unique entity is still valid when we discuss its unique position as a subject of research. In a paper for the National Commission about the status of the fetus, Wasserstrom[21] delineates four different views that are commonly held about the moral status of the fetus as follows:

1. The fetus is in most, if not all, morally relevant respects like a fully developed adult human being. This position tends to be supported by the concept of ensoulment (the soul enters the body at the moment of conception) and by the similarities between a fetus and a newborn infant. That is, a newborn infant is like an adult in that full moral obligations are owed it, and there are no significant morally relevant differences between a fetus and a newborn. Therefore a fetus is like an adult in its moral status. Furthermore, there is no specifically discernible point during fetal development when its moral status changes; therefore the fetus must be the same throughout its development, that is, the same as it is after birth.

2. The fetus is in most, if not all, morally relevant respects like a piece of tissue or a discrete human organ, for example, a bunch of hair or a kidney. This view focuses on the ways in which fetuses are different from adults in regard to the ability to think, to conceptualize, to communicate, and the like. The fetus is no more aware of its own existence than a bunch of hair or a kidney and is therefore no more a full human being than those pieces of tissue.

3. The fetus is in most, if not all, morally relevant respects like an animal such as a dog or monkey. In this view the fetus is clearly not a person, nor is it merely a collection of cells or a piece of tissue. It is surely an entity that is deserving of some respect but not that accorded to full human beings. It is wrong to inflict needless cruelty on animals because they do suffer, but it is proper to regard them as creatures that can be controlled, altered, and used by humans for the purpose of improving human life (for example, in animal experimentation and domestic breeding of farm animals). Fetuses are in this class of entity.

4. The fetus is in a distinctive, relatively unique moral category in which the status is close to but not identical with that of a typical adult. In this view the fetus is both different from and higher than animals, and although it is not fully human, its status is closest to (but not the same as) a newborn infant. This view also rests heavily on potentiality, that is, that the fetus is not yet fully human, but it soon will be and thus is deserving of special consideration.

With these four views in mind, let us look at the morality of fetal research based on the status of the fetus as the only criterion for permissibility. Social utility, the consent of the pregnant woman, and contributions to the store of medical and scientific knowledge will not be taken into consideration here. It should also be noted that we are discussing research on nonviable fetuses ex utero; little, if any, nontherapeutic research is done on viable fetuses. Although we are discussing only the moral status of the fetus here, one has to obtain the fetus to use it for experiments. That requires abortion, and Wasserstrom is unable to separate the fact of the necessary abortion from the fact of the fetal research. Because this point is shared with many others, it is worth noting here.

> It is evident, I think, that on this view abortion is a morally worrisome act because it involves the destruction of an entity that possesses the potential to produce and be things of the highest value. However, if an abortion has been performed and if the fetus is still nonviable, then experimentation on the fetus in no way affects the fetus's ability, or lack thereof, ever to realize any of its existing potential. On this view, especially, abortion, not experimentation upon the non-viable fetus, is the fundamental morally problematic activity.[22]

Based only on the status of the fetus, it would almost always seem unethical to use it as a research subject in the same way that it is unethical to use animals as research subjects (except in very narrowly defined and specific circumstances) because fetuses and animals have intrinsic value and worth; that is, they are valuable in and of themselves. Although we might not understand the meaning and purpose of their existence, we must acknowledge that there is a purpose, and it surely is not only to serve as a tool to implement the need or desire of human beings to increase their store of knowledge. If we can assume that the fetus is caused pain during the research process (and we must assume this is so until there is incontrovertible proof to the contrary), and if we ignore for the moment the social and scientific utility of fetal research, several conclusions can be drawn as follows:

1. The infliction of pain is prima facie wrong; therefore nontherapeutic research on beings that experience pain is impermissible.
2. Fetuses (and animals) have a natural right not to be harmed, and this right can be overridden, according to Regan,[23] only if (a) there is good reason to believe that overriding the right by itself will prevent vastly greater harm to other innocent individuals, (b) there is good reason to believe that allowing an individual to be harmed is a necessary link in a chain of events that collectively will prevent vastly greater harm to other individuals and is the only realistic way to prevent that harm, and (c) there is good reason to believe that one can reasonably hope to prevent vastly greater harm to other innocent individuals.

In view of these points, nontherapeutic fetal research would be allowable in only narrow and very circumscribed circumstances.

Legal status of the fetus

The fetus has no legal right to life in the first two trimesters, but it does have such a right in the last trimester. One of the most interesting aspects of the legal status of the fetus is that although it is protected by law to some degree against the external manipulations of others, it has no legal protection from the pregnant woman carrying it. For example, there are no laws requiring that a pregnant woman do certain things or refrain from doing other things during the course of the pregnancy, such as eating a balanced diet, receiving prenatal care, and refraining from smoking. In contrast, if the mother of a newborn infant was not feeding it, or if the diet it was receiving was found to be so unacceptable that the infant ran a serious risk of harm because of it, the mother could be charged with child abuse or neglect. However, if a pregnant woman consumes a diet that is so lacking in nutrients that the fetus is surely at great risk, she cannot be legally compelled to eat better. Thus the fetus has no legal protection from her harm. By the same token, a woman who repeatedly brought a child into a coal mine or an asbestos factory would surely be required to remove the child from such an environment or the state would take steps to remove the child from her. However, a pregnant woman who clouds the fetal environment with cigarette smoke, drugs, and alcohol is legally free to do so. It is ironic that the fetus has no legal protection from the person with the power to do the greatest harm and who ought to be the person with the greatest interest in protecting it.

Veatch[24] presents an interesting case in which a fetus was conceived for the sole purpose of destroying it to provide a kidney to be transplanted to its father. The situation is important in and of itself, but it also has enormous future implications.

The case involved a 28-year-old engineer who had been on kidney dialysis for 3 years and was becoming desperate because of the restrictions it placed on his life-style. He had been adopted as an infant and thus could find no genetically compatible donor. He had a rare tissue type that made the possibility of receiving a cadaver kidney unlikely. His mental and physical state continued to deteriorate, and he threatened to kill himself if he had to remain on dialysis indefinitely. His wife presented a novel solution to the transplant surgeon. She would become pregnant, have an abortion after 5 or 6 months, and have the fetus's kidneys transplanted into her husband. The surgeon knew that this was technically feasible and that the graft probably would not be rejected. He did not, however, know if it was ethically correct to transplant kidneys of a deliberately conceived and aborted fetus.

The case is accompanied by the reactions of Mary Anne Warren, a philosopher at San Francisco State University, Donald Maguire, a theologian at Marquette University, and Carol Levine, Managing Editor of the *Hastings Center Report*, where the case first appeared.

Warren viewed the dilemma in terms of the moral status of a 5- or 6-month-old fetus, that is, whether it should be considered a full human being with a right to life. In this situation the issue of abortion has nothing to do with the rights of the woman carrying an unwanted pregnancy but is a question of the moral correctness of killing a fetus at this age. If the fetus is considered a full human being, then the proposal is tantamount to murder, especially since the abortion would be done in such a way as to preserve the life of the fetus until its kidneys could be removed. If the fetus has no significant right to life, there is no reason why the wife cannot put into effect the plan to save her husband. Warren does not view a fetus as a full person and therefore sees no serious moral objection to killing it.

Maguire proposes an alternative to abortion. Because the fetus also inherits genetic characteristics of the mother, it may not be an appropriate donor; thus it should be allowed to be born and then it can be determined whether its tissue is genetically suitable. If the match is suitable and if the infant has two healthy kidneys, one could be transplanted to the father. Maguire believes that the transplant would occur more successfully if the kidney were more mature, and the fact that no abortion took place would make the transplant more ethically permissible. Terminating the life of a fetus is not the same as using an infant as a donor, but either way the fetus or the live infant would be used as a means to an end. Maguire confesses he is uneasy with either solution. He says the proposed abortion is not moral, but he also states that we cannot assume that the infant would give permission to donate if it had the mental capacity to do so. He points out that the autonomy of the infant should be protected until it can make its own decision, though this would not help the father who would probably be dead by then.

Levine objects to the planned action as an unwarranted manipulation of the procreative act as well as an abortion. Deliberately conceiving and aborting a fetus for an organ would not only be an affront to the dignity of the fetus as a potential human being but would also permit the wife to use herself as a means to an end. Levine does not see this situation as an issue of an altruistic sacrifice of one life to save another. The husband is not dying in a medical sense but is threatening to kill himself, although he may see being on dialysis indefinitely as a kind of death. Levine makes the point that even if a fetal kidney transplant could be successfully accomplished, it would probably not last for more than a few years. What then? Would the husband return to dialysis or would the wife need to become pregnant again? Even in the unlikely event that the procedure could be accomplished successfully twice in a row, a permanent solution would not have been achieved. Levine also considers the wife. Is her offer to use herself as an organ incubator entirely voluntary, or is she being coerced by her husbands threats of suicide? Levine believes that the abortion should not be considered and that the husband should receive psychiatric help in dealing with his feelings about continued dialysis. Marriage counseling is also indicated.

These three opinions, as considered and as rational as they are, do not take into account any possible legal rights of the fetus because those rights do not indeed exist.

PUBLIC POLICY

Policy making implies establishing a priority of societal values, and it must take factors other than ethics into consideration. This is particularly difficult to accomplish successfully in a highly pluralistic society such as our own. Public policy must take into account a variety of belief systems, but at the same time it must contain a high degree of internal consistency to make it both workable and relatively invulnerable to attack. The policy must be understandable to the public, which means that it cannot be on so abstract a level that it can be neither understood nor translated into regulations for action. This is no mean feat and is generally not accomplished to a satisfactory extent in the United States today.

In recommending that nontherapeutic fetal research should be done only to the extent that such research is permitted on fetuses that will be carried to term or on children, Walters argues that this position as public policy has the following several advantages:[25]

1. It is both formal and flexible in that it does not prohibit any specific research procedure but instead establishes a general test that all research protocols must pass.
2. It is a moderate position on the spectrum of opinion regarding fetal research.
3. It is continuous with other federal policies in regard to experimentation on the fetus in utero, and it protects the woman's right both to give consent and to change her mind after consent has been given.
4. There is no need to define viability, since the same guidelines apply to both previable and viable fetuses.
5. It takes into account the sensibilities of the large number of persons who object to highly invasive research on living aborted fetuses.
6. It would permit valuable types of research to continue such as that involving living tissue from dead fetuses and studies involving prenatal diagnosis, intrauterine therapy, fetal physiology, and placental transfer.

Walters is surely correct in stating that this is a moderate, or compromise, position that is generally a desirable course of action when formulating public policy in areas including but not limited to biomedical matters. Policy is concerned with the common good, but this may or may not be in the best interests of sizable minority portions of the populace. The problem when establishing public policy is to devise a plan of regulatory action that will meet with the approval of the majority while not causing so much affront to the dissenting minority that a serious backlash develops.

A case in point is the matter of cigarette smoking. In the 1970s the Department of Health and Human Services instituted a vigorous campaign, by means of heavy publicization, to discourage cigarette smoking among Americans. The campaign eventually began to have the desired effect, and cigarette smoking in the United States decreased somewhat. However, the tobacco growing and cigarette manufacturing industries stepped up their lobbying efforts directed at Congress and the administration in the late 1970s and early 1980s. Cigarette consumption increased and continues to do so. The growers and manufacturers believed the policy to be detrimental to their interests and sought to change it. The government's ethically correct position opposed that of private interests.

However, government is not always on the right side in an ethical debate, and sometimes the rights of significant numbers of individuals are abrogated in the search for the best compromise position. Even when the "will of the people" has been done, everyone's rights are not necessarily guaranteed. It is frequently impossible to devise a policy that will be at the same time fair to everyone and ethically correct.

> The common good of all persons cannot be unrelated to what is judged to be promotive or destructive to the individual, in other words judged to be moral or immoral. Morality and public policy are distinct because it is only when individual acts have ascertainable public consequences on the maintenance and stability of society that they are the proper concern of society, fit subjects for public policy.[26]

McCormick makes two additional points about the relationship between morality and public policy. First, actions that policy seeks to control ought to be determined not only by their morality but also by their feasibility. Feasibility implies that a policy is not only possible but that it is also practicable and adaptable to the social and cultural mores of the people who will be affected by it. If the policy is unenforceable or if it seems unlikely to be obeyed by significant numbers, then although it is theoretically possible to institute, it is not feasible to do so. "The answer to the feasibility tests depends on the temperature of a society at any given moment in its history."[27] McCormick believes that the feasibility test in regard to fetal research is particularly difficult because there is so much doubt and controversy about its morality.

Second, policy might sometimes go beyond morality; that is, some kinds of research may be morally justified for various reasons, but the danger of abuse or the degree of risk to the subjects might be so great that a policy ban should be instituted. There are forms of research in which the risk of potential abuse is so great that whatever knowledge might be gained from the performance of the research would not be worth the price paid by the subjects. This reasoning has been used before in biomedical research, for example, in psychosurgery and the sterilization of the mentally retarded.

In his report to the National Commission, McCormick, suggested that two additional concepts be kept in mind when developing public policy on fetal research: moral pluralism and cultural pragmatism. Moral pluralism creates difficulties in policy making, especially as fetal research is so closely allied with abortion, one of this country's most hotly debated moral dilemmas. McCormick believes the Commission is in a no-win situation.

> If it allows fetal experimentation without sufficient grounding and controls, it will alienate and galvanize those identified with right-to-life positions. If it disallows fetal experiments without sound and consistent reasoning, it will alienate and galvanize the "liberal" and research communities. If it tries to walk a middle path with a utilitarian sliding scale of costs and benefits, most ethicists in the country will be up in arms.[28]

The only way out of this predicament, according to McCormick, is by proxy consent, although one could easily question the motives and intentions of a pregnant woman who gives proxy consent for experimentation on a fetus she is about to abort. A woman in this position, who wants desperately to be rid of a fetus, is also in a vulnerable position in regard to coercion.

McCormick sees American culture as highly pragmatic in that technology is esteemed; moral judgments tend to be overshadowed by pragmatic cost-benefit analysis; youth, beauty, pleasure, and health are much valued and tend to be pursued with a vigor that is disproportionate to their ultimate worth; and maladaptations such as senility, retardation, illness, and defectiveness are treated destructively instead of being accepted and integrated into the general society. In view of these observations, McCormick interprets the general cultural mentality as one that values efficiency over morality, and he suggests that the Commission institute a policy that would protect the individual interest rather than allow more freedom for experimental research. In this way the proposed policy would be conceived of more as a balancing influence rather than one that reinforces undesirable cultural pragmatism.

The National Commission, before it made its final recommendations, noted some observations about the ethical history of fetal research, about the nature of the debate engaged in by the commissioners themselves, and about the application of ethical principles to the dilemmas at hand. First, the Commission noted that although fetal research has contributed substantially to the store of medical and scientific knowledge and has improved the general health and well-being of humankind, there have been serious abuses. Second, there is some information, vital to health and well-being, that can be obtained only by fetal research. Third, until the Commission can develop ethical principles, any policy proposal must be considered interim or temporary. Until such principles pertaining specifically to fetal research can be devised, the Commission proposes that the following general ethical principles be applied to the endeavor of fetal research:

1. Both scientific inquiry and the protection of individual integrity are endeavors to be valued. They are usually compatible pursuits, but when conflict arises, an effort must be made to resolve it by means of public deliberation.
2. The integrity of the individual is preeminent. Therefore the Commission must delineate the boundaries between respect for the fetus and the freedom of scientific inquiry.
3. General principles of research on human subjects should also guide fetal research, although there are necessary exceptions because of the nature of the difference in subjects. Those principles that apply to fetal subjects as well as to full human beings include, but are not limited to, avoiding or minimizing harm, avoiding injustice by not making racial or class distinctions when recruiting research subjects, and respecting the integrity of subjects by requiring informed consent (or proxy consent as the case may be).
4. Fetal research should have been preceded by research on animals or that done in vitro using bioassay and other techniques that do not require human fetuses. (It should be noted here that many ethicists such as Singer, Regan, and others have strong reservations about using animals as research subjects except in extremely limited and narrowly defined circumstances. One of the several ways in which they make their point is that animals have an equal or even greater right not to be unnecessarily harmed than do human fetuses. Although this view is a minority one, its proponents are increasing in number, and it deserves serious consideration.)
5. A variety of considerations should be carefully studied before approval is granted to a proposal that uses fetuses as subjects. Among these considerations are the value of therapeutic as opposed to nontherapeutic research; differences between directing the research toward the pregnant woman and toward the fetus; and the gestational age of the fetus.

The most important point to make in regard to public policy is that it is indeed public; that is, it must benefit all persons, or surely the overwhelming majority, while at the same time it must protect individual rights. This is a most delicate balance to achieve, and although the recommendations that the National Commission ultimately established come close to achieving that goal, they will not satisfy everyone and eventually will need to be revised.

SUMMARY: NATIONAL COMMISSION RECOMMENDATIONS

1. Therapeutic research directed toward the fetus may be conducted or supported by DHEW (now the Department of Health and Human Services [DHHS]) provided the research conforms to appropriate medical standards, has received the informed consent of the pregnant woman (the father need not consent and may not dissent), and has been approved by the existing institutional review procedures where the research will take place.

2. Therapeutic research directed toward the pregnant woman may be conducted or supported as in number 1, provided that the research has been evaluated for its possible impact on the fetus, that the fetus will be placed at the minimum amount of risk compatible with the health needs of the pregnant woman, and that she has given her fully informed consent.

3. Nontherapeutic research directed toward the pregnant woman may be conducted or supported as in number 1, provided the research has been evaluated for possible impact on the fetus, will impose minimal or no risk to the fetus, and has the fully informed consent of the woman, including possible impact on the fetus. It is further provided that such nontherapeutic research may be conducted only if the father has not objected, whether or not abortion is an issue.

4. Nontherapeutic research directed toward a fetus in utero (other than that conducted in anticipation of, or during, an abortion) may be conducted or supported as in number 1, provided that the purpose of such research is the development of important biomedical knowledge that cannot be obtained by any other means, that animal investigation and studies on nonpregnant humans have preceded such research, that minimal or no risk to the fetus be anticipated, that the pregnant woman has given her fully informed consent, and that the father has not objected.

5. Nontherapeutic research directed toward the fetus in anticipation of abortion may be conducted or supported as in number 1, provided such research is carried out within the guidelines established for all other nontherapeutic research on the fetus in utero. Research presenting special problems will be submitted to a national ethical review body.

6. Nontherapeutic research directed toward the fetus during the abortion procedure and nontherapeutic research directed toward the nonviable fetus ex utero may be conducted or supported as in number 1, provided the purpose of such research is the development of important biomedical knowledge that cannot be obtained by alternative means, that investigation on animals and nonpregnant humans has preceded it, that the pregnant woman has consented and the father has not objected, that the fetus is less than 20 weeks gestational age, that the abortion procedure itself is not changed in the interests of the research, and that no intrusion is made into the fetus that alters the duration of its life.

7. Nontherapeutic research directed toward the possibly viable fetus may be conducted or supported as in number 1, provided that the purpose of the research is the development of important biomedical knowledge that cannot be gained by alternative means, that investigation on animals and nonpregnant humans has preceded it, that no additional risk to the fetus is incurred, and that informed consent of the pregnant woman and the father has been given and neither has objected.

8. The institutional review procedures that must accompany or precede any human experimentation will remain in force. These procedures are mandated and required by DHHS.

9. Research on the dead fetus and fetal tissue may be conducted as long as it is consistent with local law, the Uniform Anatomical Gift Act, and commonly held convictions about respect for the dead.

10. The design and conduct of a nontherapeutic research protocol should not determine recommendations by a physician regarding the advisability, timing, or method of abortion.

11. Decisions made by a personal physician concerning the health care of a pregnant woman or fetus should not be compromised for research purposes, nor should the personal physician be involved in research protocol decisions. Review panels should be established to assure the independent nature of the medical judgments and to mediate conflicts of interest.

12. No individual should be required to perform or assist in research activities that would be contrary to his religious beliefs or moral convictions. (This provision is already made in the National Research Act [PL 93-348]; the National Commission merely seeks to reinforce it.)

13. No monetary or other inducements should be offered to procure an abortion for research purposes.

14. Research to be conducted outside the United States should comply with these standards.

15. The moratorium on fetal research that was currently in effect should be lifted immediately, allowing fetal research to proceed.

Notes

1. Steinfels, P. The National Commission and fetal research. *Hastings Center Report*, 1975, *5*(3), 11.
2. Mahoney, M. J. Fetal-maternal relationship. In W. T. Reich (Ed.), *Encyclopedia of bioethics*. New York: The Free Press, 1978. p. 486.
3. Mahoney, p. 487.
4. Walters, L. Ethical and public-policy issues in fetal research. In *Research on the fetus: appendix*. National Commission for the Protection of Human Subjects of Biomedical and Behavioral Research. Washington, D.C.: U.S. Department of Health, Education and Welfare, 1975.
5. Walters.
6. Walters.
7. Gaylin, W. & Lappé, M. Fetal politics: the debate on experimenting with the unborn. *Atlantic Monthly*, May, 1975, pp. 66–71. Copyright by the authors.
8. Gaylin & Lappé, p. 68.
9. Walters.
10. McCormick, R. A. Proxy consent in the experimentation situation. *Perspectives in Biology and Medicine*, 1974, *18*(1), 2–20.
11. Walters.
12. Walters.
13. Wasserstrom, R. Ethical issues involved in experimentation on the non-viable human fetus. Report to the National Commission.
14. Wasserstrom.
15. Wasserstrom.
16. Wasserstrom.
17. Fletcher, J. Pragmatists and doctrinaires. Report to the National Commission.
18. Siegel, S. A bias for life. Report to the National Commission.
19. Siegel.
20. Siegel.
21. Wasserstrom, R. The Status of the fetus. Report to the National Commission.
22. Wasserstrom.
23. Regan, T. Animal rights, human wrongs. *Environmental Ethics*, 1980, *2*(2), 113.
24. Warren, M. A., Maguire, D., & Levine, C. Can the fetus be an organ farm? *Hastings Center Report*, 1978, *8*(5), 23–25.
25. Walters.
26. McCormick, R. A. Fetal research, morality, and public policy. Report to the National Commission.
27. McCormick.
28. McCormick.

Bibliography

Bok, S. Research: casual or planned? *Research on the fetus: appendix*. National Commission for the Protection of Human Subjects of Biomedical and Behavioral Research. Washington, D.C.: Department of Health, Education and Welfare, 1975.
Fletcher, J. Pragmatists and doctrinaires. Report to the National Commission.

Fromer, M. J. Ethical issues in animal experimentation (Unpublished paper). Washington, D.C., 1981.

Gaylin, W. & Lappé, M. Fetal politics: the debate on experimenting with the unborn. *Atlantic Monthly*, May, 1975, pp. 66–71. Copyright by the authors.

Hellegers, A. Fetal research. In W. T. Reich (Ed.), *Encyclopedia of bioethics*. New York: The Free Press, 1978.

Jacobovitz, I. *Jewish medical ethics*. New York: Bloch Publishing Co., Inc., 1959.

Klaus, M. H., & Kennell, J. H. Mothers separated from their newborn infants. *Pediatric Clinics of North America*, 1970, *17*, 1015–1037.

Mahoney, M. J. Fetal-maternal relationship. In *Encyclopedia of bioethics*.

McCormick, R. A. Fetal research, morality, and public policy. Report to the National Commission.

McCormick, R. A. Proxy consent in the experimentation situation. *Perspectives in Biology and Medicine*, 1974, *18*(1), 2–20.

Morison, R. S., & Twiss, S. B. The human fetus as useful research material. *Hastings Center Report*, 1973, *3*(2), 8–10.

Ramsey, P. *The ethics of fetal research*. New Haven, Conn.: Yale University Press, 1975.

Regan, T. Animal rights, human wrongs. *Environmental Ethics*, 1980, *2*(2), 99–120.

Siegel, S. A bias for life. Report to the National Commission.

Steinfels, P. The national commission and fetal research. *Hastings Center Report*, 1975, *5*(3), 11–12.

Toulmin, S. Exploring the moderate consensus. Report to the National Commission.

Veatch, R. M. *Case studies in medical ethics*. Cambridge, Mass.: Harvard University Press, 1977.

Walters, L. Ethical and public-policy issues in fetal research. Report to the National Commission.

Warren, M. A., Maguire, D., & Levine, C. Can the fetus be an organ farm? *Hastings Center Report*, 1978, *8*(5), 23–25.

Wasserstrom, R. Ethical issues involved in experimentation on the non-viable human fetus. Report to the National Commission.

Wasserstrom, R. The status of the fetus. Report to the National Commission.

CHAPTER 10

INFANTS AS HUMAN BEINGS

STATUS OF THE INFANT

One might wonder why a chapter is titled "Infants as Human Beings." It is tempting to ask what there is to say about infants as persons aside from acknowledging that they indeed are persons. But that is precisely the problem: are they? Are they full human beings in the same way that you and I are—rational, responsible, and aware of ourselves as existing in relation to ourselves and to others? Infants, especially newborns, are not the same as fully developed adults except insofar as they are legally considered persons. Thus the moral conflicts arising over the care of infants spring from their ontologic status, that is, the degree to which they are owed full moral rights and obligations as persons. Moreover, if the degree differs from that which is owed to adults, where and in what way do the differences occur?

Engelhardt, in making a case against considering a human fetus a person, discusses the importance of the concept of continuity of development, what Aristotle described as distinctions in the identification of discrete stages in human ontogeny; that is, when does animal life become personal human life? Because there is now so much more sophisticated knowledge about biologic development, it is more difficult for us than it was for Aristotle to make these distinctions.

> Human life is an unbroken continuum which not only extends from one person to another but to the very origin or terrestial life. Along this continuum, there are significant qualitative differences, but they are tied to quantitative

increments which grade one into the other. That is, the qualitative differences are spread over a spectrum so that there is a progression of one into the other: no particular increment of quantitative changes is crucial. Yet, there are differences. Adult intact mature humans have a significance, and they command one's moral acknowledgment in a fashion quite different from ova and sperm. When does a human individual develop, then, to a stage at which one can recognize it as a person to whom one has obligations? This is the problem of identifying where quantitative changes become of qualitative significance, of categorizing a qualitative change along a spectrum manifesting only gradual quantitative progression.[1]

According to Engelhardt, the dilemma seems not to be whether or not moral obligations at all are owed to persons at various points on the developmental continuum, but rather how the nature of the obligations change, both qualitatively and quantitatively. No one would argue that one is obligated to feed, clothe, and provide for the physical needs of infants. We may even go further and agree that we are obligated to nurture them and protect them from harm and to provide them with the kind of environment that will assure their maximum development. But here we start to run into trouble: how far do we have to go in providing that environment? Yes, we must spend a few dollars each week on food and formula, but must we spend a half million dollars on several months of hospitalization to care for an infant with multiple severe birth defects? Yes, we must dress an infant warmly in winter and change its diapers regularly, but must we spend a lifetime's fortune to place it in an institution for the profoundly retarded and/or handicapped? Or can we expect the state to do it in our stead? In addition to assessing the ontologic status of an infant, perhaps the dilemma also involves weighing values. That is, do we value adults more than infants, and do we value different infants differently, depending on a variety of circumstances and characteristics? Some see distinct differences among infants and some, Lederberg for example, do not count very young infants as full persons.

> An operationally useful point of divergence of the developing [human] organism would be at approximately the first year of life when the human infant continues his intellectual development, proceeds to the acquisition of language, and then participates in a meaningful cognitive interaction with his mother and with the rest of society. At this point only does he enter into the cultural tradition which has the special attribute of man by which he is set apart from the rest of the species.[2]

This position is problematic because of its lack of specificity. When during that first year does the infant change sufficiently to enter this meaningful cognitive interaction? And how meaningful are the babblings and cooings of a 1-year-old? They surely cannot be considered rational, and although the infant is using cognitive processes, they are rudimentary, and he is by no means a responsible member of the moral community. By the same token, how does a 6-month-old differ qualitatively from a 12-month-old? And what should society do about whatever differences exist; what ethical principles can be used to defend and justify whatever actions are taken?

Engelhardt points out the difficulty of accepting Lederberg's position.

> If a stringent definition of "human person" is accepted, one would have to allow not only abortion but infanticide as well. Unlike abortion, however, infanticide would involve the destruction of members of the species who had begun to play an explicit role within the social structure of the family and society, even though they had not yet assumed a full personal life.[3]

This, Engelhardt goes on to say, would so undermine the fabric of society that the status of the individual within that society would be irrevocably eroded. Acquisition of language is not an acceptable criterion for full personhood because many full persons do not have a fully developed ability to use language, most specifically human infants. In earliest infancy the tiny being, by its mere existence and by its characteristic behaviors, elicits a series of responses that are socially acknowledged in every human culture as the response of one human being to another regardless of the ontologic or intellectual development of either human being in the interaction. In other words, we acknowledge infants as full persons even though we do not relate to them in the same way we relate to adult persons and even though their capacity for language is not fully developed. Although, according to Engelhardt, the infant is not actually a person, its social role is unique.

> The infant, in being able to assume the role "child", is socialized in virtue of this role, and the social significance "person" is imputed to it. Although the infant is irrational and not yet actually a human person, it can play a relatively independent role in a social matrix which is rational. A relation of obligation is then granted because the infant can engage in crude interactions with others, and thus, play the role "child". A social structure not simply a biological structure is available, namely the "mother-child relationship".[4]

Thus the ontologic status of the infant draws its strength from the social structure rather than from moral obligations owed to one person by another. The socialization of the infant, because it occurs universally and because the existence of infants is ubiquitous and ongoing, eventually becomes a moral obligation and as such is accepted by almost everyone. It appears to be a commonly accepted maxim in Western society that we are morally obligated to do everything humanly possible to not only nurture and care for infants, but also to save their lives regardless of the quality of that present and future life.

However, there is sufficient debate over this seemingly acceptable maxim to make it worth investigating and discussing. In a sense, Engelhardt's view is a bipolar one. On one hand he makes a case for personhood not coming into full being until late infancy on the basis of personhood as rational and self-conscious. On the other hand, there is a social category of "child" that is separate from, but related to, the category of person in much the same way as the category of fetus relates to that of infant. Because this special category is social in nature and because the act of providing health care is a social endeavor, it is understandable that many providers of health care would see an inherent moral obligation to treat infants as full persons. The vast majority of health care providers believe this, probably because of the socialization into their respective professions.

Another way to define "person" is as an individual having a serious right to life. Tooley[5] and others hold the view that withholding life-saving procedures from infants is tantamount to depriving them of their right to life. It is interesting to note that the existence of these life-saving procedures is not only what caused the dilemmas in the first place, it is the major reason why modern philosophers have begun to rethink the status of the fetus and infant. However, according to Reich and Ost,[6] having a right to something generally implies that (1) one is capable of desiring that thing, and (2) merely having this desire places other individuals under a prima facie obligation to refrain from denying its fulfillment.

The essential problem with this premise lies in its concept of desire. Reich and Ost explain that when we desire something, we must first understand the concepts involved in desiring it, that is, that some proposition is true, for example, "I desire an apple because I like the taste of apples." But to want a proposition to be true, one must first understand the concepts involved in it. Therein lies one of the differences between normal adults and infants—the former can understand the concept of himself as a self-conscious subject of desires, whereas the latter cannot. One could then conclude that an infant is not a person because it cannot grasp this basic concept about rights.

> Once the infant has developed the necessary concepts, particularly the concept of himself as an enduring self-conscious subject of experience, however, he would possess such a right.[7]

Aside from the negative emotional reaction that many would have to this position, it is problematic from ethical and pragmatic views. First, using such a justification to deny treatment to a defective infant would be no more morally impermissible than actually killing a perfectly normal, healthy infant because the latter's right to life depends on the same criterion as the former, that is, the ability to conceptualize that right. If killing a normal infant is impermissible, which it surely is, then so too is it impermissible to deny treatment to a defective one using the right to life as a criterion. Second, even if infants do not have a serious right to life, they do have other rights such as not being subjected to deliberate harm, pain, or other cruelty. Refusing to provide treatment to an infant in need of it will likely cause serious pain and suffering and would therefore be impermissible. Third, there are some actions that are morally wrong even if no one's rights have been violated. For example, cheating on one's income tax is wrong even though no individual's rights have been violated. Fourth, waiting until the infant was fully able to conceptualize the idea of desire would mean waiting at least until midchildhood, an impractical resolution of the dilemma.

This definition of personhood in regard to infants is particularly narrow and not of much practical use when trying to solve the dilemma of which obligations are owed them.

There are broader definitions that encompass a wider set of criteria. For example, infants have undeniable value for what they are now, for what they represent to adult persons, and for what they will become. They have both intrinsic and extrinsic value, that is, what they are in and of themselves and what they provide to others because they are who they are. Because they elicit certain feelings such as love, joy, and the desire to protect and nurture, they are valuable and have the right to exist. Because infants have the kind of social status described by Engelhardt and because of their intrinsic value, regardless of the fact that they may not conform to a narrow definiton of personhood based on rights or rationality, strong justification has to be made to deny them treatment, regardless of their physical or mental condition. In other words, the burden of proof falls on the person who seeks to make such a decision. But by the same token, one of the criteria that might be used in justifying a decision to withhold treatment is the degree to which the infant in question has the potential to achieve full personhood. For example, an anencephalic might, by a remote chance, survive birth and the immediate postnatal period, thus necessitating a decision about whether or not to institute ongoing intensive care. The fact that the infant will never be able to achieve full personhood can be used as one criterion when making the decision to treat or not.

Yet another view would take the opposite position. "From the perspective of the infant (or the person that the infant might become), one might further argue that there can be, under some circumstances, an obligation *not* to treat the infant."[8] This argument would be based on the belief that some conditions of life (for example, those characterized by severe and continuous pain) would be worse than no life at all. In such cases continued life would hold so much negative value that perhaps the physicians' maxim to do no harm would require that the life in question not be sustained. This is an arguable point; in fact it is one of the points around which the dilemma of euthanasia revolves and has to do with the intrinsic value of existence to the person in question. The dilemma, of course, intensifies when that person is an infant and others must make guesses about the value the infant would place on continued existence if he were able to conceptualize the matter.

Tooley[9] proposes yet another way to define personhood in regard to infants. He first discusses the common claim that only beings with a mental life can be classed as persons. He points out that many nonhuman animals have mental lives, some of them quite highly developed (certainly some are more developed than infant humans), yet no one regards them as persons. Therefore having a mental life, while it is a necessary condition for being a person, is surely not a sufficient one. Tooley suggests the following criteria:

1. A person has mental states that vary with time and condition and that are unified by memory.
2. A person possesses both consciousness and the capacity for thought.
3. A person is not only conscious, but is also self-conscious, that is, aware of himself existing through time.
4. A person is aware of not only possessing certain states but is aware of being a potential agent, that is, of the possibility of doing and feeling things in the future.
5. A person possesses consciousness and is capable of both envisaging a future and of having desires about that future.
6. A person is capable of interacting socially and morally with other human beings with similar capacities.

The problem with listing these criteria, all of which are reasonable and plausible, is deciding which are correct and can be used as realistic criteria. Tooley says that appealing to intuition is generally unsatisfactory because intuition differs so drastically in such matters. More acceptable would be to appeal to general moral principles in seeking an answer to the dilemma of whether or not nontreatment of infants is ever permissible. But while it may be possible to formulate a coherent outlook based on principles that are widely applicable, they are not universally so, and again we run headlong into differing intuitions about which principles are applicable and which foundations of morality would form the bases of correct moral principles. This is a matter of such great controversy that many philosophers believe it is impossible to accomplish.[10]

Tooley acknowledges that there may be no solution to the problem of principles, but he posits one idea that may be helpful. Even if moral principles cannot be justified because they turn out not to have been true values, it may still be possible to justify them in a different way, that is, by showing that it would be rational for a society to persuade all its members to act on those principles, regardless of whether or not they were intrinsically true. The society would have to believe that it was in its best interest to act on them and to believe that what is in the best interest of a society is a function of the needs and desires of individual members of that society. That is, if a moral principle is to be justified in this manner, it would have to be related to the satisfaction of individual members of society. This is an extremely utilitarian approach, and if it is used to choose among the six possible criteria mentioned, it could best satisfy the sixth criterion, which rests on envisaging a future and having desires about that future. That is, if one destroys the possibility of meeting future needs and desires, an unjustifiable action would have been taken.

Another way of assessing the personhood of infants is to determine whether they have developed to the point where they have sufficient properties or characteristics to be considered persons. At first glance it might seem impossible to determine this, but Tooley believes it is possible, although in a negative sort of way. There are a finite number of human properties. Normal adults possess them all so that even if there can be no agreement about exactly what the properties are, it can be agreed that whatever they are, an individual must have them all to be considered a person. On the other hand, infants to be considered persons need only possess some of the properties, and it does not matter which ones. If, however, an individual infant possesses none of them, it cannot be considered a person. Thus it is not necessary that the properties be either named or agreed on in kind and quantity, only that they exist.

But is it ever reasonable to believe that an infant does not indeed possess any of the properties? This is the most difficult question to answer because it depends on one's interpretation of thought, memory, consciousness, self-consciousness, and all the other concepts that are the foundation for Tooley's broad definition of personhood. It may also depend on empirical research that is within the realm of possibility but that has not yet been done. For example, when an infant exhibits certain behaviors such as smiling, reaching for an object dangling over its crib, and poking its fingers into its navel, what is it doing? Various theories have been proposed, for example, the infant is exploring and learning about its world or is interacting socially and emotionally with others. However, no one really knows what processes are going on inside that infant's head. Until we do know, it would seem foolhardy to believe that infants do not have the mental status necessary for personhood.

According to Tooley,[11] studies of the newborn infant's brain indicate that it has not developed to the point where higher mental functions are possible, that the electroencephalogram of a newborn is neither of the same character nor intensity as that of a fully developed adult. There is also the evidence of direct anatomic studies that the brain of newborn humans is not fully developed. "The complex functional systems of conjointly working cortical zones, which are the basis of the higher mental functions, rather than maturing independently, do so only as a result of the child's interaction with its environment."[12]

When this rationale is used to state that an infant is not a person, which seems to occur to no small extent in the United States today, one is tempted to ask, "So what?" Infants do not yet have the capacity or ability of many things; they are utterly dependent creatures. But we do not say that an infant is not a person because it cannot provide its own nourishment, or "doesn't have sense enough to come in out of the rain," or can't find itself an apartment or job. We accept this dependent status and devote ourselves to helping it achieve certain goals. We can also accept its lack of ability to perform complex mental functions as being the nature of an infant. Using the physiologic differences between infants and adults to declare the former nonpersons is as nonsensical as calling a legless person a nonperson because he is not physiologically like others.

One sometimes sees in the literature the attempt to prove that infants are not persons by comparing their mental capacities to those of animals; that is, if some nonhuman animals have a higher mental capacity than infants, then infants cannot be persons. This argument is illogical because it rests on a false premise—that all persons have higher mental capabilities than all nonhuman animals. There are many animals that are much smarter than many people, and there may be entire species of animals that are better equipped mentally than some groups of people. This does not mean that persons are not persons and animals are not animals.

BIRTH DEFECTS

Although it is interesting to discuss the personhood of infants in general, ethicists and health care providers generally use the positive and negative arguments only when they are faced with an infant who has a severe birth defect resulting in serious life-long consequences. Hemphill and Freeman[13] have identified four categories of birth defects that almost always raise questions about the quality of the infant's life and about which actions (or nonactions) may be appropriate in view of the defect. They first define a static disease or condition as one that is already present and is unlikely to get worse. Progressive disease is that which will in all likelihood get worse and will surely shorten the infant's life span. The four categories of birth defects are as follows:

1. Static conditions associated with mental retardation. Although intelligence cannot be determined at birth, there are many types of mental retardation in which physical signs are immediately apparent such as phenylketonuria (PKU), bleeding into the brain, and Down's syndrome. Frequently there are other physical anomalies that accompany the retardation. One issue here is what should be done about the other, correctable anomalies in view of the retardation. To put it bluntly, is it worth expending considerable resources on an infant who will always be retarded? Other issues include the degree of certainty about the extent of the retardation, the comparison of a retarded child

with other physical anomalies with a retarded child who is otherwise healthy, and who should make the decisions about treatment. This last issue is a constant thread running through not only all dilemmas about infants with birth defects but all bioethical dilemmas.

2. Progressive conditions associated with mental retardation. There are conditions detectable at birth or shortly thereafter that are untreatable or that if treated will cause further impairment, such as Tay-Sachs disease in the former category and certain forms of spina bifida in the latter. The issues here are most complex and in many cases tragically paradoxic. One involves the effort expended to forestall the inevitable death or progression of retardation. That is, when the child becomes very ill, should ordinary measures to care for it be carried to the extreme of extraordinary ones? A second issue involves research.

> As technology advances, *new forms of therapy* will be directed at the disease process itself. When new therapy becomes available, one option would be to treat advanced cases first, so that, if the therapy is unsuccessful or harmful, the harm will be done to those children with the poorest diagnosis.[14]

However, this choice could create further problems because it might turn out that the therapy did not cure the disease, but only halted it for a time, thus preserving the lives of the most handicapped and ignoring those who might be more treatable.

Yet another issue is the timing of diagnosis and treatment; that is, if an illness is diagnosed at birth, or even before, should treatment be instituted immediately or at all, even though death will occur in early childhood? For example, should Tay-Sachs infants be treated symptomatically?

3. Static conditions with physical disability but normal intelligence. Examples of such conditions that are considered serious include spina bifida, congenital limb amputations, craniofacial anomalies, and various gastrointestinal and genitourinary anomalies. Other conditions that are common but less serious include cleft lip and palate, major facial birth marks (nevi), hypospadius (malformation and misplacement of the urethra), and ambiguous genitalia (but not true hermaphrodism). There are other conditions that may be very serious but that require little medical intervention because no treatment exists; these include congenital deafness and blindness, dwarfism, and giantism.

In these conditions the personhood of infants is not in question. The problem is whether or not to institute every possible treatment to lessen the degree of handicap and/or to help the infant adapt to the handicap as quickly and as well as possible. This decision does not always rest on the fact of personhood.

Hemphill and Freeman provide an example of the dilemmas that exist even when the infant in question is undeniably a person.[15] They describe an infant born with omphalocele (intestines exposed outside the abdomen). When the surgeon operates, he finds that most of the intestine has died and must be removed. After the repair only about 10 inches of intestine will remain, which is not enough to absorb adequate nutrition. The infant will have to be fed special nutrients intravenously for the rest of its life, but it is normal in all other respects. In all likelihood the child will have to be hospitalized all or most of the time, and there is a high risk of infection and other complications from the intravenous feeding. Its life will be sustained by artificial means even though it will be normal in other respects. As being fed intravenously is not a normal way to exist, as is living one's life in a hospital, can the life itself be considered normal? There is almost no possibility that the infant will grow into a self-sustaining person; it will always be dependent on others for nutrients. Thus should the infant's life be sustained at all? Or should the life be kept going until the infant has developed sufficiently to make its own decision? It is not appropriate in such cases as this to use the principles and justifications that are employed when debating adult euthanasia because there are distinct differences between the lives of infants and those of adults or even of older children. An infant has no conscious past, no knowledge of the future, and cannot participate in a decision about itself. This means that the entire weight of the responsibility rests on others.

4. Progressive conditions with physical disabilities but normal intelligence. Some examples of these conditions are cystic fibrosis, some types of congenital heart disease, sicke-cell anemia, and muscular dystrophy. Many progressive conditions eventually result in death, and the rest cause severe, even crippling, disability. As they grow these infants require increasingly complex and expensive treatment, and acute episodes of the disability or disease usually appear closer together. Should the child be treated episodically knowing that conditions will surely worsen, and if not, what should be done when the child becomes critically or terminally ill?

In addition to these issues, there are other complicating factors inherent in dealing with an infant with a serious birth defect. The first is that the outcome of any treatment is unpredictable. An infant with one birth defect is more likely to have another defect than is an otherwise normal child likely to have that second defect. For example, if an infant requires surgery for esophageal atresia (a condition in which the esophagus ends in a blind pouch instead of connecting with the stomach), the surgeon may find other anomalies of the gastrointestinal tract; therefore the outcome of the surgery is unpredictable.

Second, rapid advances in technology have made it possible to save the lives of infants who would have died even a decade ago. However, the ability to assess the quality of these infants' lives has not been as rapid as the technologic developments that create the dilemmas. Moreover, technology itself can create unforeseen side effects, such as problems with vision or hearing, increased chance of infection, and growth retardation.

Third, a great deal of the exotic therapy used in the treatment of these infants is experimental, although much of it is not part of controlled studies for formal protocols. The infants then become subjects of therapeutic research and must be protected as such. However, too much "protection" could result in too little or too conservative therapy. "Unless such experimentation is carried out in controlled fashion, each newborn receives randomized therapy based on the whim or prejudice of the physician, without the information about benefits that controlled studies could provide."[16] This situation then leads us back to the familiar question, Who decides?

Because there is such a wide variety of birth defects with an equally wide range of severity, the ethical problems involved in what, if anything, should be done about these affected infants are sometimes complicated by confusion. It is therefore worthwhile to use one serious defect as an example, to discuss the treatment options, the ramifications of each, and to explore the views of various philosophers and physicians who have written on the subject. I have chosen spina bifida with meningomyelocele because it is not uncommon (about 2 per 1000 live births), is extremely serious, requires long and complicated treatment, affects other body systems permanently, and has been the target of much research and new forms of treatment in the past decade.

Spina bifida with meningomyelocele (SBM) is one of the most serious birth defects that is still compatible with life. It is the result of faulty embryologic development where the spinal cord and vertebral column fail to close and there is a gap between vertebrae (spina bifida only). In most cases there is a sac protruding through this space that is filled with cerebral spinal fluid (CSF) and part of a defective spinal cord (meningomyelocele). The sac is usually covered by only the thinnest membrane; it is easily damaged and may leak CSF. Most occur in the lower lumbar region (small of the back), although some are higher or lower. As a consequence of the deformity the infant is paralyzed below the level of the lesion, has no bladder or bowel control, and may have dysfunctional kidneys. Circulation of CSF is impaired, often leading to hydrocephalus, which also is a frequent sequela of corrective surgery. Hydrocephalus can, but does not necessarily, lead to mental retardation, although infants born with SBM usually have normal or even superior intelligence. Parents who give birth to an infant with spina bifida have a higher than average chance of having another child so affected. Although it is difficult to estimate the cost of treatment for so severe and long-lasting a defect, a million dollars would seem a reasonably conservative estimate in today's economy.

There are various opinions about treatment of SBM and much research is being done, but a major treatment goal is to surgically close the defect to prevent the ever-present risk of infection and to control the loss of CSF. Surgery used to be performed immediately after birth, but it is believed that some delay to adequately evaluate the extent of damage will not significantly lower the infant's chances of achieving whatever repair is possible. Sometimes a surgical shunt is done to alleviate or prevent hydrocephalus, and leg deformities can be corrected by the use of casts. Later treatment includes devices to restore some degree of bladder and bowel control.

Even with extensive treatment, the prognosis for infants with SBM is not good. Only about half survive to middle childhood, and all are left with permanent disability ranging from intermittent incontinence to permanent paraplegia and/or mental retardation. Predictions of therapeutic outcome are notoriously inaccurate.

The effects of an SBM infant ripple out to include not only the infant and its immediate family but the community and the larger society as well. The diagnosis of SBM is made at or before birth, and a decision about what to do must be made shortly thereafter, although not necessarily within the first day or two. There is time to reflect on the three alternatives: to kill the infant, to allow it to die by withholding treatment and nourishment, or to actively treat it. This choice will be discussed in more detail later in the chapter, but for now let us assume that the decision has been made to treat the infant. Now there are more decisions to be made. Which treatment regimen will be best in the long run? Does one operate and perhaps risk further neurologic damage and hydro-cephalus, or does one refrain from performing neurologic surgery but try to protect the lesion with skin grafts and concentrate on minimizing other prob-lems and deformities? Neurosurgeons and neurologists are by no means in agreement on which course of action will be ultimately most beneficial, and much therapeutic research is currently being done.

> There is no necessary connection between early operation and survival. It is true that in a large series of cases treated with and without operation, the results favor surgery as far as mortality is concerned. Yet this is probably not a valid reflection of the effect of operation on survival-rates. Surgical patients are receiving active treatment from all points of view; infections are treated vigorously whether they are local infections, systemic infections, or ventriculitis, and the child will probably be getting better attention to the renal tract than those who are receiving no treatment at all. I do not think it has been proved, from a concurrent study of two large series of cases, that the mortality is less in those receiving early operation than in those who do not have early operation but in every other respect receive the same care and attention as the surgical series.
>
> The question at issue is whether there are advantages of early operation which outweigh any possible extra risks that such operation might have for the life of the child.[17]

Zachary goes on to say that the surgeon (and one would presume the family as well) should consider the maximum development of the child rather than making an effort to reduce all possible handicaps to a minimum. Keeping the long-term development of the child in mind might mean that fewer operations are performed and length of hospital stays are shortened in order to attend to the child's social and emotional development. Even with treatment there will be severe residual handicaps; it might be better in the long run to teach the child to live productively with the handicaps he does have than to try to correct them to the extent that his whole social and emotional world revolve around the health-care system.

The effect on the family of an infant with SBM is almost incalculable. Not only is there acute disappointment in not having a perfectly healthy baby, there is guilt and blaming of the spouse when a genetically defective infant is born. Thus the parents must cope with their own feelings in addition to having to make critical decisions about the infant—all when they are in an emotionally and judgmentally vulnerable position. Siblings must be told that there is something seriously wrong with the infant, and the family unit is likely to undergo one of the most serious crises in its history. Many marriages do not survive, especially if there was marital discord before the birth. Rejection of the child is a distinct possibility, especially when there has been a decision either not to operate or not to treat at all. Because the infant must remain in the hospital for so long, it is tempting to visit less and less frequently and to put off thinking about posthospital problems and decisions.

The financial burden is a major issue in itself. It is safe to say that almost no family has the resources to pay for the care required. Those with health insurance will find that the benefits terminate before treatment is complete, and those without insurance will find themselves almost financially helpless.

SBM and other serious birth defects are not merely private matters. The community is involved not only in an economic regard but in others as well. As treatment becomes more sophisticated and effective, these children will live longer, and community involvement will increase. There are many questions and issues.

1. Should hospitals establish special care units for infants with SBM, or should there be only a few special treatment centers in the country to which all such infants are sent as soon as they can be transported?

2. Should the financial burden of the care be assigned to the community in which the infant was born, or should state or federal funds be spent for this purpose? If public funds are not allocated, which private agencies should be responsible? What if no one takes on the financial obligation?

3. How shall these children be educated? The law now states that public schools must accept handicapped students, and reports indicate that this

is not working as well as might have been expected and hoped. Children with SBM have a great many physical needs throughout the day; is it fair to expect public school personnel to attend to them, and if not, what alternative arrangements should be made to educate these children?

4. What of their future lives? If they live to adulthood (and as research continues this will become a distinct possibility), they will need vocational training or higher education to prepare them for earning a living and generally getting along in society. Who will pay for it?

If vigorous treatment of an SBM infant is instituted, there will be certain residual handicaps, some quite severe. This creates an ethically interesting question: would the child, as it develops, have wished for things to be as they are, or would he have preferred to die in infancy? There is, of course, no possible way to predict the future in this regard and thus to answer the question, but physicians and philosophers do discuss this, and because they are in positions of power and influence, their views affect the lives of people who respect and trust them. Slater believes that the consequences of saving the lives of these infants are mostly negative in the long run.

> These children are now beginning to come into puberty and adolescence, when their sufferings will really begin. Only the most miserably impaired social life will be open to them; they will be equipped with normal sex drive but no normal sex function; all around them they will see the normal, the vigorous, and the healthy. Will they really be grateful to the fates, the all too human fates, but for whose intervention, they would have died before their miseries began?
>
> Perhaps the whole procedure is mistaken. If this is one of the necessary consequences of the sanctity-of-life ethic perhaps our formulation of the principle should be revised. The spina bifida baby is a mistake of nature not equipped to survive. Who suffers if he dies at birth? Certainly not the child, though if he is forced to survive he faces years of suffering. Do the parents suffer if he dies? Yes, in the disappointment of not having a baby when they had hoped for a normal little boy or girl; but in a few months they can try again. If the child survives, however, they have years of servitude, of tortured love, trying to make up to him for all his disadvantages. And society, the community? The death costs nothing; the life costs not only money, but the preemption of precious medical, nursing, social, and educational resources.[18]

This is an extremely utilitarian, even act-utilitarian, view that, although it was written a decade ago, seems current in view of today's popular cost-benefit analyses. It is also not an uncommon or unpopular view. Freeman[19] points out that many infants with SBM do die, and they do so slowly and with great suffering. They endure pain and hardship for no discernible purpose. He believes that if it is permissible not to treat these infants, or even to abort them in utero (SBM can be diagnosed during pregnancy; the reader is referred to the chapter on reproductive technology), then it is equally permissible to deliberately end their present suffering and to prevent increased future suffering by killing them.

> It is time that society and medicine stopped perpetuating the fiction that withholding treatment is ethically different from terminating life. It is time that society began to discuss mechanisms by which we can alleviate the pain and suffering for these individuals whom we cannot help.[20]

Cooke disagrees.[21] He claims that medicine in particular and society in general would change for the worse if "the physician joined too fully in the new discomfort-free society." Although Cooke is careful to state that he is not a "harbinger of the ethic of suffering," he disagrees with the permissibility of killing infants who have serious noncorrectable deformities. It is wrong to kill infants, healthy or deformed. It is, according to Cooke, pure and simple murder and is thus unjustifiable in any circumstances. Although he does not necessarily condone abortion, he makes a distinction between that and infanticide. "The difference in attitude toward the fetus and neonate does not exist because of the law, rather the law exists because of the attitude of the public."[22] Thus, he concludes, physicians (and presumably parents and others) must accept the suffering of the infant and must offer whatever corrective action is possible and available. Even when there is no possibility of cure, care is a necessary part of medicine, despite the fact that the physician himself must suffer as a result of his inability to do as much as he might wish. Death is not an acceptable means of dealing with the suffering of others.

Calculation of handicap

Handicapped or defective people are generally considered ill by the rest of society. Not ill in the usual sense of having the flu or cancer or suffering a heart attack, but ill in the sense of not being healthy or whole. On the other hand, many (if not most) defective or handicapped people see themselves as quite healthy; they simply operate with a particular physical disadvantage that others do not have. This difference in perception exists, and understanding its origin and ramifications would be useful in calculating degrees of handicap or even in assessing whether or not a particular infant should be treated.

Sedgwick[23] maintains that there is no such thing as illness in nature except that which is defined and labeled as such by humans. For example, a tree afflicted with parasites is not ill, nor is a tiger that has been bitten and scratched by another in a fight. They may be uncomfortable, or even dying, but the concept of being ill does not exist for them except as it is described about them by human beings. There are, of course, events and occurrences in nature, such as the existence of contagious viruses and bacteria, the fracture of bones, and the malignant multiplication of certain cells, but Sedgwick claims that simply because these things exist does not mean they are illness. He likens the fracture of an old man's leg to the snapping of a branch of an old tree. It happens in nature. It is by itself neither good nor bad, nor is it illness until it is judged as such by social systems.

Sedgwick acknowledges that some will disagree that only natural occurrences, not illnesses, exist in nature, but, he claims, if we examine the concept of illness in humankind, the same kind of value-laden concepts will be revealed. Some occurrences will be compared with others, and not all will be declared equally desirable. Concepts of illness among humans have been in existence for centuries and have changed as societal and cultural characteristics have changed. Although the meanings and origins of illness have been differently perceived, the human concept of illness has had some remarkable similarities throughout history. This is why, Sedgwick believes, primitive cultures have been able to take advantage of modern medical technology without too much trouble.

> Sickness and disease may be conceptualized, in different cultures, as originating within bodily states, or within perturbations of the spirit, or as a mixture of both. Yet there appear to be common features in the declaration or attribution of the sick state, regardless of the causal explanation that is invoked.[24]

An illness is considered deviancy in some way, a comparison with a state of affairs that is seen as more desirable. It is "better" to have two legs than one, better to be of average intelligence than mentally retarded, and better not to have cancer than to have it. If, however, there were no societally imposed value norms, then having one leg would not be worse than having two, it would only be different. Certain conditions that are considered illness in one culture are viewed as a normal or usual part of life in another. For example, parasite infestations of hookworm and others are so common in many North African people that those who are not parasite infested are considered deviant. The same is true in some South American Indian tribes with regard to a disease called dyschromic spirochetosis.[25] In our own culture certain ailments or conditions are part of everyday life. For example, most of us do not think of a tension headache or indigestion as illness per se. They are minor annoyances of modern life and are dealt with quickly and and with almost no thought. Other cultures, however, might view head pain as a serious deviation from normal or as an indication of the presence of spirtis or demons.

The point is that illness, like beauty, can be in the eye of the beholder, and if a society believes that a hunchback is ugly and misshapen, he will in all likelihood regard himself as such. Thus if a society or a powerful system within that society such as the health care-system regards infants born with SBM or other serious defects as so defective that they are possibly unworthy of continued life, they indeed may be so in that time and place. Those who hold this view are ethical relativists and would be strongly opposed by the absolutist who holds that all human life, regardless of how defective or how diseased, is of value. Therefore when one calculates the degree of handicap and makes an effort to determine how difficult a time a particular infant will have in living with certain defects or deformities, the general societal context should be taken into consideration; that is, how much "normalcy" is required to be considered within the bounds of normal health? Or conversely, how much deviancy from that norm is acceptable?

To treat or not to treat

The question of whether or not to treat infants with serious birth defects (and other infants as well) is in many instances too complex to answer. Most of the arguments revolve around the value or quality of life that is anticipated for that infant. However, sometimes decisions for treatment are taken out of parents' hands and given over to the courts. Beauchamp and Childress[26] describe such an instance.

A woman who was a practicing Jehovah's Witness had refused to sign a consent for blood transfusion before the delivery of her daughter. During birth an accident occurred that necessitated transfusions for the infant to prevent mental retardation and possible death. The parents refused permission for the transfusion and a hearing took place at the hospital to decide whether the parents' objections should be overridden. A Superior Court judge appointed a temporary guardian to sign the consent form, and the infant was given the transfusions. In this case the court decided that parents do not have a right to make a decision not to treat an infant, and it is presumed that had the physician concurred with the parents in this case (instead of disagreeing and seeking a court order) and not transfused the infant, this judge might have found him guilty of malpractice, manslaughter, or an even more serious charge.

There was another dramatic development in this case. During the hearing the infant's mother began to hemorrhage, and physicians said she needed an emergency hysterectomy to stop the bleeding. Her husband, also a Jehovah's Witness, gave permission for the surgery but not for a transfusion. The judge declined to override these decisions and the woman bled to death a few hours later.

If a decision is made to treat, the subsequent actions are fairly clear—engage in those activities and procedures that will cure or ameliorate the problem as quickly and as effectively as possible. However, if the decision is not to treat, several options for management follow, all of them problematic. The infant can be given routine nursing care and can receive nourishment but nothing else (in the case of certain gastrointestinal deformities, nourishment cannot be given by mouth, and the infant may be left to dehydrate and starve; death will usually occur in 1 to 3 weeks). The infant could also be given sedation and analgesics to ease its suffering (it should also be noted that the sedation will cause it to cry less, which is less upsetting for the professional staff in the nursery). It could be given intravenous fluids but no food, which simply prolongs death from starvation but is not as painful or distressing to the infant as not being given any fluids. The infant could be nourished indefinitely, either in the usual way or intravenously, depending on the nature of the defect, but not subjected to surgery or any other treatment for the birth defect. The last option is that the infant could be killed by an intravenous injection of potassium or some other appropriate substance to prevent prolonged suffering. Two major questions arise when deciding on the appropriate management of the untreated infant. One is whether distress and suffering experienced or anticipated before the infant dies justifies active euthanasia, and if so, under what circumstances. The second is whether the decision not to treat is morally equivalent to active euthanasia and whether any effort to maintain life is reasonable after the decision not to treat has been made. "If a patient dies, is it ethically relevant whether the physician wanted him to die or just didn't want him to have to live with his handicap?"[27]

It is unlikely that most of society or even most health professionals will ever agree about whether or not to treat infants with certain serious defects. A major reason is that it is difficult to justify a decision either way based on ethical principles, while the principles, interests, and rights most often used in the debate conflict with each other. For example, the two major principles that guide physicians and other health professionals are (1) to preserve life and overcome illness and disease and (2) to do no harm. They clash head-on in the decision to treat or not to treat a defective infant. For instance, in the process of saving the life of an infant with SBM and preserving whatever function is possible, the parents and physicians may be condemning that infant to a life of intolerable pain and misery. However, preventing that future misery would mean condemning the infant to death. Ordinarily, the principle of nonmaleficence, to do no harm, takes precedence over all others in medical practice, except for the principle of the sanctity of life. There may be no way to resolve the conflict between the two in such cases as we have been discussing.

The decision for or against treatment also involves a complex conflict of interest. Usually when a health-care decision must be made, the best course of action is for the person to be treated to make up his own mind after he has been informed of the facts by health personnel. He then makes a decision that he thinks will be in his best interest. By the same token, if an adult is not conscious or otherwise not competent, others make the decision for him with the person's best interest in mind. However, in the case of defective infants there are other interests to be considered. In addition to the family and the community at large, which were discussed earlier, the health professionals involved in the care of the infant have an interest in the ultimate decision. For example, if a decision is made not to treat, the nurses and physicians who work in the nursery will be profoundly affected.

One of the most dramatic cases of this kind (known as the Johns Hopkins case) is presented by Beauchamp and Childress.[28] A child with Down's syndrome was born to a nurse (the mother) and an attorney (the father), ages 34 and 35, respectively. The infant also suffered from a form of intestinal blockage known as duodenal atresia, which could be corrected with a relatively low-risk operation. Without the operation the infant could not be fed and would die. When the mother found out at birth that the child was a mongoloid, she indicated that she did not want to keep it. The next day when she was consulted by the pediatric surgeon and told of the necessity for the operation and the consequences of withholding consent, she maintained her position by saying, "It would be unfair to the other children of the household to raise them with a mongoloid." The physician tried to convince her to change her mind by pointing out that mongoloids are almost never profoundly retarded, can be trained to do simple jobs, and are famous for having loving natures and sunny dispositions. The parents remained adamant. In view of the parents' decision, the hospital staff did not seek a court order to perform the surgery, and the infant was put in a side room and allowed to starve to death. It took 15 days.

In this case, which has been widely discussed in the literature and about which a film was made,* the hospital staff surely had an interest in the fate of the infant. It has never been made clear why the physicians, nurses, hospital attorneys, and others stood by and let the infant suffer for so long nor why no attempt was made to obtain a court order to perform the surgery as it was in the case of the infant of the Jehovah's Witnesses. The event took place in 1970 when there was already a good deal of legal precedent in this regard. In the Hopkins case, the staff not only had an interest in the decision, it could be argued that they shared responsibility for the outcome.

INFANTICIDE

Infanticide is defined as the killing of an infant, and the common sensibility in Western society is that infanticide is tantamount to murder and is thus indefensible. However, if we define murder as the unjustified killing of an innocent person, then infanticide may be seen by some to be not always wrong

---

*The film, *Who Should Survive*, was made in 1971 by the Joseph P. Kennedy Jr. Foundation, Washington, D.C.

because in some few cases, such as the ones we have been discussing, the killing may be justified. This is not a popular view, but it is held, or at least seriously debated, by enough people to make it worth discussing here.

Let us assume that under most circumstances it is wrong to kill people, and the exceptions to this maxim are few in number and fall within a narrow range of permissibility. The one exception that most everyone agrees on is killing in self-defense, a concept that can be broadened somewhat to killing enemy combatants in war. Another less universally accepted exception is the execution of murderers and certain other criminals. The justification for killing in these two instances usually rests on the fact that the person killed is not innocent, at least not in regard to the reason why he is being killed. Although these two examples are endlessly debatable, they point out that there are arguments to justify killing people.

But what morally reasonable argument can be made for killing a deformed infant who without doubt must be classed as an innocent person? Tooley[29] believes that to be able to even attempt to answer the question one must distinguish between potential and nonpotential properties of persons. Potential properties are those that an individual will come to have if it is not interfered with in the normal course of events. Nonpotential properties are the characteristics an individual already possesses. It is mostly with the former that we will be concerned in the discussion of infanticide. The argument of potentiality against infanticide, according to Tooley, follows:

> It is wrong to kill persons. But it is also wrong, and seriously so, to destroy potential persons, that is, to destroy things that, in view of their biological or ontological nature . . . will become persons. Since normal human infants . . . are certainly potential persons, their destruction is seriously wrong.[30]

We can take this one step further and say that seriously defective infants are as much potentially persons as are normal ones, with the possible exception of those with no potential for mental ability. Because all definitions of personhood rest on a foundation of mental ability, this is the only criterion that should be used to establish personhood and even then the assessment of personhood based on mental status should not be made immediately except in very obvious cases such as anencephaly. That is, physical defects, no matter how profound or permanent, are irrelevant when assigning the status of personhood. The infanticide argument should not rest on the presence of physical defect.

Tooley poses two challenges to this potentiality argument. First, if it is wrong to destroy potential persons, then it must also be wrong to prevent an organism from realizing its potential. If it were not, then one could simply destroy an infant's brain, and then because it is no longer potentially a person, destroy the infant. Second, if there is a system of organized and interrelated occurrences that, if not interfered with, will eventually give rise to a person, then it would also be wrong to destroy or interfere with this system because it has the potentiality to create a person. If these arguments are carried to their extremes, it would be wrong to destroy a potential person, that is, a normal infant, only if it is seriously wrong to practice certain methods of contraception or to perform some risky brain operations on infants. Although the argument may be theoretically defensible, it is nonsensical. There is surely a quantitative and qualitative ethical difference between taking birth control pills and killing infants.

There is also a problem with regarding infants, no matter how deformed, as potential persons. Engelhardt and Tooley may indeed make perfectly logical points about the ontologic and mental status of infants as opposed to adults or even older children, but to become accustomed to thinking about actual infants, which exist and eat and cry and soil their diapers, as only potential persons is a serious mistake. Just as treating aborted fetuses routinely or casually can lead to a callous attitude about fetal research (the reader is referred to Chapter 9), so too can a callousness about infants develop when thinking of them as potential persons. The subject of infanticide is emotionally extremely difficult to deal with; thinking of infants as not real or actual persons can only desensitize those who debate the issue. This would be a highly undesirable state of affairs.

Before continuing the discussion of the rightness or wrongness of infanticide, a word should be said about the difference between active and passive euthanasia, between killing and letting die. Active euthanasia, the deliberate and conscious act of killing a person, is condoned less frequently and by fewer people than passive euthanasia, the act of letting someone die naturally by not engaging in "heroic" artificial means of sustaining life. The morality between the two is difficult to finely differentiate, and condoning one while condemning the other can create a more complex ethical dilemma than being categorically for or against all kinds of euthanasia.

The crucial issue may be one of cruelty. If one is opposed to a lethal injection for the surcease of suffering but is in favor of either not resuscitating a person who has died or deliberately leaving someone alone to die, one would be said to be in favor of pain, a position that could be seen as unnecessarily cruel. The issue of active and passive euthanasia often hinges on a time factor, as was well demonstrated in the Johns Hopkins case. The infant in question took 15 days to die of starvation and dehydration, during which time it surely suffered. That suffering could have been prevented by a lethal injection.

There may or may not be a moral difference between killing a person and letting that person die, depending on a variety of external circumstances. The following example illustrates this issue. Fred is swimming alone in a pond. He begins to drown and shouts for help. Larry, an excellent swimmer, sees a drowning man and immediately jumps into the pond and begins swimming toward Fred. As he draws near he recognizes Fred as the man who is having an affair with his wife. If Larry calmly and deliberately pushed Fred's head under the water, waited until he was dead, and then left, no one would deny that Larry killed him even though Fred was clearly in danger of dying on his own. But suppose Larry, after recognizing Fred, decides to swim back to shore leaving Fred to sink or swim on his own, though Larry knows he could have saved Fred. Fred then drowns. No one would deny that Larry let him die, but in the act of letting him die and in view of the fact that he had the power to save him, did Larry kill Fred? The motive and intent were the same, the end result was the same, but the means differed. Is there then a moral difference? Did letting Fred die when he could have saved him make Larry less guilty than he would have been if he had pushed Fred's head under the water?

The American Medical Association (AMA) condones the "cessation of the employment of extraordinary means to prolong the life of the body." In other words, the AMA approves passive but not active euthanasia, probably on the premise that killing a client is morally worse than letting him die and is therefore not to be permitted. Is killing always worse? Our feelings toward killing are almost always negative because we associate it with murder that involves an evil motive or a war that horrifies us with its brutality. Our associations with letting someone die are usually humanitarian. One learns to think of killing a person as worse than letting him die, but in the kinds of situations we have been discussing letting him die may be the same or worse than killing him. In a moral context, when a physician lets a person die when he could keep him alive, he is killing that person as surely as if he had injected the fatal dose.

In terms of decision making in euthanasia, a decision to do nothing is a decision and therefore an action, making passive euthanasia a positive action—or active euthanasia. In this light there is no moral difference between active and passive euthanasia, between killing and letting die, though the method differs.

Those who disagree with this view argue that the agent of death creates a moral difference in the responsibility for the death. If an infant suffers from duodenal atresia and is permitted to die, the birth defect is the cause of death, not the lethal injection by a physician. If Larry does nothing and lets Fred drown, the death is the result of accidental drowning, but if Larry pushes Fred's head under water, the death is the result of murder.

Another argument against morally equating killing and letting die concerns guilt. Society exacts a terrible price for the act of killing; the conscience of most people, unless they are amoral, exacts a worse price. One may feel less guilty having let someone die than after actually killing him. The physician's guilt is usually far less if he does nothing than if he acts to kill. This may reflect an internalization of society's standards.

Then what about the consequences of infanticide? There are surely legal ones, but there are ethical and social ones as well. First, there is a belief that the widespread practice of infanticide (the number of cases that would qualify a practice as widespread is, of course, open to discussion and is probably a function of one's views on the subject) would lead to a general decrease in the respect for human life and might cause other forms of sanctioned human killing to increase. This is the wedge or "slippery slope" argument; that is, if an action is permissible in certain circumstances, it will automatically become permissible in ever-widening sets of circumstances. For example, if infanticide of defectives is condoned, then society will be more willing to condone the killing of other groups of people who are sick or helpless, such as the mentally retarded, the comatose, or the senile elderly.

Second, acceptance of infanticide may weaken the parental bond and thus eventually all family ties. The suggestion is that parents will care less for their remaining children and treat them harshly, thus adversly affecting the children's development.

These two beliefs are seen fairly often in the bioethical literature, but there is no empirical evidence to prove them. The stronger argument, the one that rests on the edge of that slippery slope, states that if one is willing to violate the principle of the sanctity of life in one set of circumstances, then one would be equally willing to violate it in other circumstances. This implies that the person making the decision to violate a principle is unable to distinguish differences in intrinsic and extrinsic factors in sets of circumstances. Usually rational, thoughtful people do not behave this way. It is interesting to note that one of the arguments against euthanasia in the face of terminal illness is the wedge argument; that is, if it becomes acceptable to kill or let die persons dying of cancer, then respect for life in general will so diminish that other groups of people will also be killed. The first group mentioned is defective infants. This seems an irony.

The second consequence, that it would lead to parents treating their other children less well, does not seem realistic. There is a strong taboo against cruelty to children, and the decision to be cruel has little, if anything, to do with the decision not to treat a defective infant. According to Tooley, there is direct evidence from the observational experience of anthropologists that those societies practicing infanticide treat their remaining children with even greater loving kindness than does our own. If one wishes to argue that infanticide is morally wrong, it would be more appropriate to do it from a deontologic base than a utilitarian one, that is, that infanticide is intrinsically wrong, not that it has bad consequences.

Historic and anthropologic view

Active and passive infanticide have existed since the beginning of recorded history. Until very recently severely deformed infants were not expected to survive; therefore no active measures were taken to help them to do so. Their defects were ascribed to fate, evil spirits, or the devil, and that was all there was to it. Many societies practiced active infanticide and did not feel obligated to justify their actions to themselves and others. Some societies justified the practice in a more complex way. For example, Beauchamp and Childress[31] report that the Nuer tribe in Africa viewed defective infants as nonhuman "hippopotamuses" who were mistakenly born to human parents. They were put in the river, which was viewed as their natural habitat. These kinds of definitional flights of fancy are generally not allowed in our society, although after a good deal of reading about the ways in which the concept of personhood is defined, one could be excused for thinking that defining *person* to meet certain treatment criteria is not far from the Nuer practice of simply labeling a defective infant a hippopotamus. We are not, it might seem, as far removed from the expediency of the Nuers as we might like to believe.

Amundsen[32] discusses the history of the concept of the prolongation of doomed lives in medical practice. In the writings of Plutarch there is a saying of Pausanias, King of Sparta, from 408 to 394 BC, that the best physician is the one who does not cause his patients to linger on but buries them quickly.

> Although Pausanias was well known as an excoriator of physicians, his remark represents a quite commonly held attitude. The medical art's two functions were preserving life and restoring health. Preserving or restoring health was the emphasis, not prolonging life *per se*.[33]

Plato argued strongly for physicians not to prolong the life of patients who had no chance of regaining their health, and considering his special concern with eugenics as reflected in the *Republic*, we can assume that he favored infanticide of defectives. In Greek culture, in the fifth century BC and even later, there is strong evidence that health was a virtue and that the physical health of the community was more important than the personal worth of any individual.

> Health was an ideal, indeed the highest good, set above beauty, wealth, and inner nobility. Health was a goal in itself, for without health all else was without value. The statement in the *Hippocratic Corpus* that without health nothing avails, neither money, nor any other thing, expresses a strong popular, philosophic, and medical statement.[34]

In this context, infanticide was surely permissible, if not mandatory.

During early Greek and Roman times physicians were not licensed, nor were there any other formal controls over professional practice. A physician sold his services as a private entrepreneur and generally used his best judgment when making treatment decisions. Moreover, he could accept for treatment only those persons he wished to treat.

The Hippocratic Oath, which figures prominently in current debates about physicians' responsibilities, was almost certainly not written by Hippocrates himself, and there is even doubt about when it was written; it may not have been during Hippocrates' lifetime. Whenever it was written and by whomever, there is evidence, according to Amundsen, that physicians at the time did not pay it a great deal of attention, and it certainly was not a significant influence on the way they practiced medicine. Thus the admonition to do no harm and to preserve life, if they were part of the way the physician practiced, sprung more from the physician's own personal ethics and from the prevailing social ethic than from any formal oath or code. The Hippocratic Oath did not become a significant factor in medical practice until the first century AD.

The idea of the respect for life is not necessarily the same as the idea of the desirability of prolonging life, especially when such prolongation could be interpreted as harmful. So while the classical physician may not have actively terminated a life by aborting a fetus or killing a person, he surely would not act to sustain the life of a severely defective infant. The sanctions on his mode of practice were negative rather than positive; that is, he was obligated to refrain from taking certain actions rather than performing other acts.

> This negative tradition did indeed become stronger with the rise of Christianity: abortion, suicide, and euthanasia became sins. . . . Many early Christians and Church Fathers, however, insisted that God also either inflicts or permits disease and the practitioner of the secular healing arts thus works against divine purposes. Wide acceptance by Christians of the medical arts as conso-nant with the sacrificed life of faith took centuries. While abortion, suicide, and euthanasia became sins, the prolonging of life did not become either a virtue or a duty.[35]

Westermarck[36] describes many societies in which infanticide was widely practiced, not only as a means of getting rid of defective infants but also to rigidly determine family size, that is, as a means of conforming to societal expectations about population. This was common practice in many of the South Sea islands such as Melanesia and Polynesia, as well as in Australia by the Aborigines, where a woman could be punished for bearing too many children. Other cultures that are considered more highly developed also condoned or even mandated infanticide. The Arabs considered it a duty, and female infanti-cide was common in China. While killing healthy infants may have been regarded with only mild disapproval in many cultures, killing deformed infants was a social necessity and in some instances even required by law.

Explanations for this widespread practice are complex and varied. In some societies it was believed that devils and evil spirits lived in deformed persons; thus if the person was destroyed, the evil spirits would be also. Many societies that practiced infanticide did so without any moral conflict. It was perfectly natural and acceptable to either kill defective infants outright or to expose them to the elements.

However, because certain cultures believed (and some still do) that infanticide was a normal and natural part of life, it does not necessarily mean that it can be considered an ethical practice any more than slavery becomes an ethical practice simply because some societies practice it routinely. Those who believe that infanticide is ethically acceptable because the members of a particular society or culture believe it to be so are operating within a framework of ethical relativism.

The practice of infanticide as routine and casual had diminished in countries where Christianity was the dominant religion, although infanticide decreased much more slowly than did other practices that the Church considered wrong. In societies where infanticide was used to limit family size, the practice diminished even more slowly. Feeding one's family was a more pressing concern than adhering to theoretic Church tenets. The Church's arguments against infanticide, although somewhat philosophic in nature, are mainly theologic, that is, that persons are immortal, that unbaptized children will be in hellish torment forever, that life is a gift from God and remains always in divine stewardship, and that God created human life and thus always controls it.

There may indeed be cases where a logical argument can be put forth to justify infanticide, but it seems obvious that as a pluralistic society we cannot practice wholesale infanticide; we cannot simply let all seriously deformed infants die. Neither, many believe, can we absolutely forbid infanticide in some small number of cases. But where and how do we draw the line?

Who shall decide?

In 1975, Shaw et al.[37] surveyed members of the Surgical Section of the American Academy of Pediatrics. They sent questionnaires to pediatricians and pediatric surgeons in clinical practice as well as to those in hospital and academic administration concerning their attitudes and practices with respect to making difficult ethical choices. There were 457 responses to the survey, and some of the results are surprising. For example, the first question asked, "Do you believe that the life of each and every newborn infant should be saved if it is within our ability to do so?" Of the total number responding to the question, 18% said, "yes," and 82% said, "no." The overwhelming majority of these physicians did not feel morally obligated to save the life of every newborn infant.

Another question asked,

> Would you acquiesce in parents' decision to refuse consent for surgery in a
> newborn with intestinal atresia if the infant also had (a) Down's syndrome
> along with it, (b) Down's syndrome plus congenital heart disease, (c) anencephaly,
> (d) cloacal exstrophy, (e) meningomyelocele, (f) multiple limb or craniofacial
> malformation, (g) 13–15 trisomy, or (h) no other anomalies, i.e. normal aside
> from atresia?

Again, with the exception of the last choice (h), the pediatricians over-
whelmingly stated that they would concur with the parents' decision to refuse
surgery. Although there were some differences in the responses according to
the accompanying anomaly (ranging from a high of 100% "yes" in the face of
anencephaly to a low of 47.4% "yes" in limb or craniofacial anomaly), the
physicians' attitudes against surgery in such cases were evident.

Another response is worthy of note. The question was,

> If you accept parental withholding of lifesaving surgery, would you (a) stop all
> supportive treatment including all intravenous fluids and nasal gastric suction,
> (b) give oral feedings, (c) terminate the infant's life actively by an injection of
> drugs such as morphine or potassium, (d) insist that the parents take the baby
> out of the hospital if no treatment is to be allowed?

The response was 53% of the pediatricians would stop all supportive treatment;
24.6% would give oral feedings; 1.7% would actively kill the infant; and 8.2%
would insist that the infant be removed from the hospital.

In another question about what the physician would do if the parents were
undecided about the decision whether or not to treat, more physicians said
they would provide the parents with the necessary facts and let them decide
rather than take any other action (obtain a court order, make the decision
themselves, etc.). However, the physicians who would let the parents decide did
not represent a majority (45.1%) of those responding to the survey.

Shaw et al. drew the following four major conclusions from the survey:

1. Physicians are not morally obligated to save the life of every infant
   simply because they have the technology and skill to do so.
2. Parents and physicians (in that order) should take responsibility for
   deciding whether or not to treat deformed infants.
3. The decision should be made on the basis of medical predictions concerning the longevity and quality of life. Differences in the perception
   of the quality of life seem to spring mainly from the nature and severity
   of the defect.
4. Decisions to treat or not to treat are best made on a case-by-case basis,
   not as a result of predetermined policy.

It should be noted that these opinions are those of only pediatricians and pediatric surgeons, not all of whom are in clinical practice. They are, though, the most directly concerned with and experienced in these problems.

McCormick[38] presents a case that well illustrates the dilemmas we have been discussing. An infant son of Mr. and Mrs. Robert H. T. Houle died after emergency surgery at the Maine Medical Center. He was 15 days old and had been born horribly deformed. His entire left side was malformed; he had no left eye and practically no left ear. His left hand was deformed, and some of his vertebrae were not fused. He had a tracheoesophageal fistula and therefore could not be fed by mouth; air that should have gone into his lungs leaked into his stomach, and stomach fluids entered his lungs. The chance of there being other internal deformities was great, and as time passed the infant deteriorated. He contracted pneumonia, his reflexes became impaired, and severe brain damage was suspected because of poor circulation. The parents, who did not name the boy, refused to consent to surgical repair of the tracheoesophageal fistula (the anomaly that posed an immediate threat to life) because of the presence of the other deformities. Several physicians at the Maine Medical Center disagreed with the parents and sought a court order for the surgery from Maine Superior Court Judge David G. Roberts. He complied, citing the basic human right to life as justification to perform the surgery.

This case is not unlike the Johns Hopkins case described earlier and is similar to many (perhaps hundreds) that do not receive public attention and are not discussed in the medical press. McCormick believes that the essential dilemma in these cases is the definition of what is meant by "hopelessly ill" or other designations of that type. He says that this definitional problem creates so much ambiguity that decisions cannot be made.

Although McCormick admits that decisions in these cases can be achingly difficult, he does believe that certain guidelines can be established. He sees a guideline as

> not a slide rule that makes the decision. It is far less than that. But it is far more than the concrete decision of the parents and the physician, however seriously and conscientiously this is made. It is more like a light in a room, a light that allows the individual objects to be seen in the fullness of their context.[39]

One guideline could be the difference between active and passive euthanasia. Another might be the difference between ordinary and extraordinary means of treatment. McCormick defines the latter as those that would entail grave hardship for the person receiving the treatment, although he is not more specific than this. The second guideline is almost impossible to apply because the criteria for ordinariness change so rapidly and so drastically. High-technology care of the newborn, where the nursery looks more like the capsule of a space vehicle than a place where babies live, would have been so extraordinary as to have been astounding a decade ago. Today it is quite ordinary.

A middle course in decision making, according to McCormick, must rest somewhere between the premise that continued life is always precious and good and the one that death is always evil and to be prevented at all costs. There may indeed be a higher and more important good (a spiritual one, surely) than continued life or even death. However, it is impossible to know whether the means used to attain this higher good are worth the ultimate goal. Since human life is more than simply the maintenance of biologic functions, the means to achieve truly human life may not be worthwhile.

> One who must support his life with disproportionate effort focuses the time, attention, energy, and resources of himself and others not precisely on relationships, but on maintaining the condition of relationships. Such concentration easily becomes overconcentration and distorts one's view of and weakens one's pursuit of the very relational goals that define our growth and flourishing. The importance of relationships gets lost in the struggles for survival. The very Judeo-Christian meaning of life is seriously jeopardized when undue and unending effort must go into its maintenance.[40]

If the result of saving a deformed infant's life means a crushing economic hardship for the family (for example, perhaps other children will have to forego a higher education to pay for the defective's care); if it creates unending emotional stress and tension whereby the parents devote all or most of their energy to the infant; and if other children are emotionally and spiritually neglected, then perhaps the price of saving this one infant is not worth what it costs in the pain and suffering of others.

When addressing the question of who should decide these matters, Reich and Ost[41] list the following variety of considerations that should be taken into account: the values likely to be represented by an agent (the person making a decision), the qualifications for decision making, role expectations, the right to decide, and where the power of authority should reside. There are generally the following four groups that might be involved in the decision making process: parents, physicians, nurses, and committees.

There are reasons both for and against giving parents the right to make the ultimate decision to treat or not to treat a defective infant. Society generally invests parents with the legal and moral right to make all decisions for their children, and, unless they are proved incapable of decision making or are judged to be cruel or abusive, there is no reason to assume that parents do not have the best interests of the child at heart and in fact have a greater interest than anyone else in the fate of the child. Any decision will affect the parents to a greater extent than anyone else (except the infant). Since they will reap the greatest benefit or suffer the most harm, they should cast the deciding vote. On the other hand, parents are under more emotional stress and tension than all others involved in the decision. It is possible that these factors render them less able to make a rational decision than others who are not so emotionally involved, especially when there is no time for reflection. There is also the possibility that the parents will be motivated primarily by such factors as thoughts of the economic burden and the necessity of devoting more than the ordinary amount of time and energy to the care of the infant.

In terms of understanding the immediate and long-range medical consequences of a treatment decision, the physician is the best qualified, and this fact has led to the belief that the physician should be the one to make the decision, especially in view of his minimal emotional involvement. However, permitting the physician to have the final authority would surely foster paternalism in the physician-client relationship and give the physician an unwarranted amount of power in view of the fact that the infant does not belong to him, nor will he have the ultimate and enduring responsibility of caring for it. Physicians also cannot be depended on to make a decision based solely on medical criteria. Their own values, religious beliefs, and personal preferences will creep into the decision-making process, even if only on an unconscious level. This is not fair to the parents who may not know what is happening and who may have a different set of values and beliefs.

Reich and Ost believe that a mediating position can be struck in the conflict between parents and physicians. To do this, however, one should be particularly conscious of the kinds of judgments and roles that make up the decision. For example, the physician does have the necessary medical competence to predict treatment outcomes (insofar as predictions can be made at all). He also has the obligation to provide the parents with all available information in language they can understand. The physician can recommend (and can even try to obtain a court order if he strongly disagrees with the parents' decision) a particular course of action and can suggest various alternatives, but it is the parents to whom the decision belongs because they are the most directly and intimately affected by it.

Many people believe that nurses who work in neonatal intensive care units should take part in the decision-making process because they too are affected by the decision. It is likely, although there is no written evidence of this, that nurses do indeed make decisions to treat or withhold treatment in some nurseries and have probably acted on those decisions. However, it is not likely that they will be given a large official role.

There is a variety of kinds of committees that could participate in decision making, although in most hospitals they are not the final arbiters. A committee could review decisions already made, in particular the decision not to treat. Or it could act in a purely consultative role and as a legal proxy if the parents are incapable or incapacitated.

Although individual members may demonstrate emotionality, the advantages of committee participation are that the committee as a whole could probably be counted on to act in as unemotional a manner as possible. Because the members represent a variety of values and beliefs, the total committee is more likely to be objective than individual persons. There is a greater number of viewpoints that could be brought to bear on the decision than having it made by either the parents or the physician (or a combination of the two), and there may be, depending on the hospital and the composition of the committee, more ethical expertise available.

A committee's participation also has disadvantages. Sometimes the very objectivity that is possible creates a remoteness and impersonal detachment that would lessen the committee's value when it deals with these very human issues. There is no guarantee of consensus in any one decision, nor is it guaranteed that the committee will decide similarly in similar cases, thus leaving the committee open to accusations of capriciousness and outside influence.[42]

SUMMARY: THE QUALITY OF LIFE

While discussing the general ramifications of serious birth defects, this chapter has focused mainly on the question of infanticide. It is an unpleasant issue, even a horrible one, but it exists. Infanticide occurs and is probably more common than is reflected in the literature. To treat or not to treat defective infants is essentially a question of deciding their fate—helping them to live, to consign them to a life of possible pain and misery, or maybe to a life filled with as much joy and satisfaction as anyone else achieves. Or it is letting them die (or killing them outright, although active euthanasia is far less common than passive), saving them from a life of pain and misery or preventing them from experiencing joy and satisfaction. The difference in the way the infant's future is perceived is a matter of the definition of the quality of life, that amorphous phrase that one encounters so often in bioethics literature.

What is an acceptable quality of life, and how can we know what would be acceptable for others? Are there certain minimum standards that can be applied to everyone like some celestial regulatory agency saying that there can be only so many negative factors in one's life before the quality would be considered unacceptable? Or is it all a matter of personal preference subject to no objective standards?

In 1973 Duff and Campbell[43] published an article in the *New England Journal of Medicine* that could conservatively be described as a bombshell. They said that between January 1, 1970, and June 30, 1972, at the Yale-New Haven Hospital special care nursery 43 infants with severe birth defects died as a direct result of the discontinuation or withdrawal of treatment. The article was shocking, not because people in the medical profession had no idea that this kind of thing happened, but because Duff and Campbell were willing to admit to it in writing and expose their actions to public scrutiny and debate.

Although the rights and interests of the infants and families were discussed, as well as the feelings and attitudes of the physicians and nurses involved, the emphasis of the article was on quality of life. Many of the infants would have been institutionalized for life in places characterized as the most inhumane sort of repository, as one person said, "hardly more than dying bins." Duff and Campbell described the slow deterioration of infants with SBM and characterized it as a slow death even with vigorous treatment.

The 43 infants who died in the 2½-year period written about were by no means the only defectives born at Yale-New Haven. Parents who wanted full treatment for their infants were assured that everything possible would be done, and they were not talked into withholding or withdrawing treatment. No decision to withhold or withdraw treatment was made quickly or spontaneously. All the parents consulted physicians and other health personnel many times, and although Duff and Campbell supported their decision, parents were not encouraged to take one action or another. When the article was published more than a year after the time period mentioned, Duff and Campbell still had contact with most of the families.

> Thus far, these families appear to have experienced a normal mourning for their losses. Although some have exhibited doubt that the choices were correct, all appear to be as effective in their lives as they were before this experience. Some claim that their profoundly moving experience has provided a deeper meaning in life, and from this they believe they have become more effective people.[44]

But is there such a thing as a quality of life so impoverished that it is not worth the effort necessary to save it? Perhaps if the essence of human life is so overridden by the struggle for mere physical existence that most meaningful human contact is impossible, then the quality of that life is below standard. The problem, however, comes in defining what the essence of human life is. The characteristics could be defined, but once this has been done, one might well ask how many of these characteristics are necessary for an acceptable quality of life. For instance, most people would agree that the ability to communicate with others is one of these necessary conditions or characteristics. But how much can that ability be impaired before the quality of life is judged so poor that the life itself is not worth sustaining. And if a severely impaired ability might seem unacceptable to one person, or even many, this does not mean that it is universally unacceptable. This kind of evaluation can be applied to any human activity or characteristic. For example, one person might find the constant illness, infection, lack of excretory control, and paraplegia of SBM an unacceptable way to live, yet another, while surely preferring otherwise, will find enough satisfaction in life to create an acceptable life-style and even to achieve happiness.

Is quality of life perhaps a matter of personal preference like preferring to be an attorney rather than a molecular biologist? Or living in the city rather than in the country? This seems a fairly frivolous way to characterize it, but surely there are elements of preference. Is quality of life perhaps an ability to tolerate adversity, as in having a higher or lower pain threshold than other people? This perhaps is more on the mark, but it is so subjective that it seems impossible to use it as a definitive criterion for decision making. McCormick believes there may be a difference in the quality of life with respect to the time at which that quality diminished.

> Obviously there is a difference between having a terribly mutilitated body as a result of surgery, and having a terribly mutilitated body from birth. There is also a difference between a long, painful, oppressive convalescence resulting from surgery, and a life that is from birth one long, painful, oppressive convalescence. Similarly, there is a difference between being plunged into poverty by medical expenses and being poor without ever incurring such expenses. However, is there also not a similarity? Can not these conditions, whether caused by medical intervention or not, equally absorb attention and energies to the point where the "higher, more important good" is simply too difficult to attain? It would appear so. Indeed, is this not precisely why abject poverty (and the systems that support it) is such an enormous moral challenge to us? It simply dehumanizes.[45]

This is true; poverty and profound physical and mental disabilities dehumanize, and they surely are less than desirable when measuring quality of life. But we do not simply kill poor people to put them out of their misery, even those for whom there appears absolutely no hope to turn their lives around. This analogy is not precise because the cure for poverty is money and/or jobs, and there is no cure for the kinds of defects we have been discussing. But similar principles apply.

The solution to the problem of the quality of life is that there is no solution; it is impossible to know what the future will hold for these infants. In all likelihood it will be as bleak as can be imagined, but there is no way to know what the infant wants—now and if it could foresee the future. Decisions will continue to be made and actions taken on those decisions, but it is important to realize that with our present understanding of the nature of human existence, those decisions will be, for the most part, stabs in the dark.

NOTES

1. Engelhardt, H. T., Jr. The ontology of abortion. *Ethics*, 1974, *84*, 228. The University of Chicago Press.
2. Lederberg, J. A geneticist looks at contraception and abortion. *Annals of Internal Medicine*, 1967, *67*, 27.
3. Engelhardt, p. 230.
4. Engelhardt, p. 231.
5. Tooley, M. A defense of abortion and infanticide. Feinberg, J. (Ed.), *The problem of abortion*. Belmont, Calif.: Wadsworth Publishing Co., 1973. pp. 51-91.
6. Reich, W. T., & Ost, D. E. Ethical perspectives on the care of infants. In W. T. Reich (Ed.), *Encyclopedia of bioethics*. New York: The Free Press, 1978. p. 729.
7. Reich & Ost, p. 729.
8. Reich & Ost, p. 730.
9. Tooley, M. A. Infanticide: a philosophical perspective. In *Encyclopedia of bioethics*, p. 745.
10. Tooley, p. 745.
11. Tooley, p. 746.
12. Tooley, p. 746.
13. Hemphill, J. M., & Freeman, J. M. Infants: medical aspects and ethical dilemmas. In *Encyclopedia of bioethics*, pp. 718-720.
14. Hemphill & Freeman, p. 719.
15. Hemphill & Freeman, p. 719.
16. Hemphill & Freeman, p. 721.
17. Zachary, R. B. Ethical and social aspects of treatment of spina bifida. *The Lancet*, August 3, 1968, p. 274.
18. Slater, E. Health service or sickness service? *The British Medical Journal*, 1971, *4*, 734-735.
19. Freeman, J. M. Is there a right to die—quickly?. *Journal of Pediatrics*, 1972, *80*, 904-905. © The C.V. Mosby Co., St. Louis.
20. Freeman, p. 905.
21. Cooke, R. E. Whose suffering?. *Journal of Pediatrics*, 1972, *80*, 906-908. © The C.V. Mosby Co., St. Louis.
22. Cooke, p. 908.
23. Sedgwick, P. What is illness? In Sedgwick, P. (Ed.), *Psycho politics*. (First published in *Hastings Center Studies*, 1973, *1*(3).)
24. Sedgwick.
25. Sedgwick.
26. Beauchamp, T. L., & Childress, J. F. *Principles of biomedical ethics*. New York: Oxford University Press, 1979. pp. 260-261.
27. Hemphill & Freeman, p. 722.
28. Beauchamp & Childress, pp. 267-268.
29. Tooley, p. 743.
30. Tooley, p. 746.
31. Beauchamp & Childress, p. 121.

32. Amundsen, D. W. The physician's obligation to prolong life: a medical duty without classical roots. *Hastings Center Report*, 1978, *8*(4), 23–30. Reprinted with permission of The Hastings Center. © Institute of Society, Ethics, and the Life Sciences, 360 Broadway, Hastings-on-Hudson, N.Y. 10706.
33. Amundsen, p. 24.
34. Amundsen, p. 24.
35. Amundsen, p. 27.
36. Westermarck, E. A. The killing of parents, sick persons, children—feticide. In *The origin and development of the moral ideas* (Vol 1.). London: Macmillan, 1906–1908. Chap. 17.
37. Shaw, A., Randolph, J. G., & Manard, B. Ethical issues in pediatric surgery: a national survey of pediatricians and pediatric surgeons. *Pediatrics*, 1977, *60*, (suppl), 588–599.
38. McCormick, R. A. To save or let die: the dilemma of modern medicine. *Journal of the American Medical Association*, 1974, *229*(8), 172–176. Copyright 1974, American Medical Association.
39. McCormick, p. 172.
40. McCormick, p. 173.
41. Reich & Ost.
42. Reich & Ost, p. 739.
43. Duff, R. S., & Campbell, A. G. M. Moral and ethical dilemmas in the special-care nursery. *New England Journal of Medicine*, 1973, *289*(25), 890–894.
44. Duff & Campbell, p. 890.
45. McCormick, p. 175.

BIBLIOGRAPHY

Amundsen, D. W. The physician's obligation to prolong life: a medical duty without classical roots. *Hastings Center Report*, 1978, *8*(4), 23–30.

Beauchamp, T. L., & Childress, J. F. *Principles of biomedical ethics.* New York: Oxford University Press, 1979.

Boorse, C. On the distinction between disease and illness. *Philosophy and Public Affairs*, 1975, *5*(1), 49–68.

Cooke, R. E. Whose suffering? *Journal of Pediatrics*, 1972, *80*, 906–908. © The C.V. Mosby Co., St. Louis.

Duff, R. S., & Campbell, A. G. M. Moral and ethical dilemmas in the special-care nursery. *New England Journal of Medicine*, 1973, *289*(25), 890–894.

Engelhardt, H. T., Jr. The ontology of abortion. *Ethics*, 1974, *84*, 217–234.

Fletcher, G. P. Legal aspects of the decision not to prolong life. *Journal of the American Medical Association*, 1968, *203*(1), 119–122.

Freeman, J. M. Is there a right to die—quickly? *Journal of Pediatrics*, 1972, *80*, 904–905. © The C.V. Mosby Co., St. Louis.

Fromer, M. J. *Ethical issues in health care.* 1981. St. Louis: The C.V. Mosby Co.

Gorovitz, S. Spina bifida. *Teaching medical ethics: a report on one approach.* Moral Problems in Medicine Project, Department of Philosophy, Cleveland: Case-Western Reserve University, 1973. pp. 29–30.

Hemphill, J. M., & Freeman, J. M. Infants: medical aspects and ethical dilemmas. In W. T. Reich (Ed.), *Encyclopedia of bioethics*. New York: The Free Press, 1978.

Lederberg, J. A geneticist looks at contraception and abortion. *Annals of Internal Medicine*, 1967, *67*, 26–27.

McCormick, R. A. To save or let die: the dilemma of modern medicine. *Journal of the American Medical Association*, 1974, *229*(8), 172–176.

Reich, W. T., & Ost, D. E. Ethical perspectives on the care of infants. In *Encyclopedia of bioethics*.

Sedgwick, P. What is illness? In Sedgwick, P. (Ed.), *Psycho politics*. (First published in the *Hastings Center Studies*, 1973, *1*(3)).

Shaw, A., Randolph, J. G., & Manard, B. Ethical issues in pediatric surgery: a national survey of pediatricians and pediatric surgeons. *Pediatrics*, 1977, *60*(suppl), 588–599.

Slater, E. Health service or sickness service? *The British Medical Journal*, 1971, *4*, 734–735.

Tooley, M. A defense of abortion and infanticide. In Feinberg, Joel (Ed.), *The problem of abortion*. Belmont, Calif.: Wadsworth Publishing Co., 1973. pp. 51–91.

Tooley, M. Infanticide: a philosophical perspective. In *Encyclopedia of bioethics*.

Westermarck, E. A. The killing of parents, sick persons, children—feticide. In *The origin and development of the moral ideas* (Vol. 1). London: Macmillan, 1906–1908. (Chap. 17.)

Zachary, R. B. Ethical and social aspects of treatment of spina bifida. *The Lancet*, August 3, 1968, pp. 29–30.

INDEX

WITHDRAWN